Handbook of Sarcoidosis

Handbook of Sarcoidosis

Edited by **Karen McMahon**

FOSTER
A C A D E M I C S

New Jersey

Published by Foster Academics,
61 Van Reypen Street,
Jersey City, NJ 07306, USA
www.fosteracademics.com

Handbook of Sarcoidosis
Edited by Karen McMahon

International Standard Book Number: 978-1-63242-217-0 (Hardback)

Printed in the United States of America.

Contents

Preface

Over the recent decade, advancements and applications have progressed exponentially. This has led to the increased interest in this field and projects are being conducted to enhance knowledge. The main objective of this book is to present some of the critical challenges and provide insights into possible solutions. This book will answer the varied questions that arise in the field and also provide an increased scope for furthering studies.

This book discusses the severe chronic disease of Sarcoidosis. Even though Sir Jonathan Hutchinson explained sarcoid lesions more than a century ago but the cause of this granulomatous disease is still unrecognized. While many patients affected by this disease enter spontaneous remission, some patients relapse after intervention or get chronically affected which remains an unexplained characteristic of sarcoidosis. This book highlights advances and recent developments in the ongoing researches on sarcoidosis which contribute to our understanding of the complex nature of this disorder. It presents a variety of topics including a recent approach of etiology as an endogenous infection caused due to hypersensitivity to indigenous bacteria, new directions in therapy, new diagnostic approaches with FDG-PET and EBUS-TBNA, and latest immunopathogenesis and genetic factors. This book will assist the readers in their practice and researches of sarcoidosis.

I hope that this book, with its visionary approach, will be a valuable addition and will promote interest among readers. Each of the authors has provided their extraordinary competence in their specific fields by providing different perspectives as they come from diverse nations and regions. I thank them for their contributions.

Editor

Pathogenesis

Chapter 1

Propionibacterium acnes as a Cause of Sarcoidosis

Yoshinobu Eishi

Additional information is available at the end of the chapte

1. Introduction

Sarcoidosis is one of the best-known systemic granulomatous diseases. Despite intensive investigation, however, the etiology of sarcoidosis has remained unresolved for more than 100 years [1]. Sarcoidosis seems to result from the exposure of a genetically susceptible subject to an environmental agent, and microbial etiologies of sarcoidosis have long been considered based on the clinical similarities to infectious granulomatous diseases [2]. Several epidemiologic mechanisms may underlie the association of an infective agent or agents with the etiology of sarcoidosis, including spatial, seasonal, and occupational clustering [3]. The results of the ACCESS (A Case Control Etiologic Study of Sarcoidosis) study support an association between selected microbially-rich environments and sarcoidosis [4].

Mycobacterial and propionibacterial organisms are the most commonly implicated etiologic agents based on studies indicating the detection by polymerase chain reaction (PCR) of microbial DNA from these organisms in tissues from sarcoid patients around the world [5-7]. Different studies have produced considerably varying results, however, with microbial DNA detected in 0% to 80% of sarcoidosis tissues and in 0% to more than 30% of control tissues [8, 9]. The failure to detect microbial DNA from these organisms in samples from some sarcoid patients suggests other causes of sarcoidosis in those patients, whereas detection of the microbial DNA in some control samples suggests latent infection of the bacterium.

Immune responses against microbial antigens from these organisms, such as ESAT-6 and KatG peptides from *Mycobacterium tuberculosis* and a recombinant trigger-factor protein from *Propionibacterium acnes*, have been examined in sarcoid patients and control subjects [10, 11]. Immune responses are frequently detected in sarcoid patients as well as in some non-sarcoid patients and healthy subjects. Latent infection by these organisms complicates the interpretation of the results of these immunologic studies. Unless microbial antigens that cause a specific immune response found only in sarcoid patients can be used to stimulate an immune response, immunologic approaches will not be sufficient to unequivocally confirm that these organisms are causative.

Granuloma formation results from the persistence of a nondegradable product or a hypersensitivity response [12]. The two mechanisms overlap in most infectious diseases because microorganisms act as both foreign bodies and antigens to induce immunologic responses. Granulomas serve as protective mechanism to sequester and degrade the invading agent. The pathologic hallmark of sarcoidosis is an epithelioid cell granuloma, thus some etiologic agent of sarcoidosis must be present or have been present within the sarcoid granuloma. Histopathologic studies are therefore essential to demonstrate mycobacterial or propionibacterial organisms or antigens within sarcoid granulomas to demonstrate an etiologic link between sarcoidosis and these organisms.

P. acnes is so far the only microorganism isolated from sarcoid lesions by bacterial culture [13, 14]. P. acnes is an anaerobic, non-spore-forming, gram-positive rod bacterium indigenous to the skin and mucosal surfaces. A series of Japanese studies has provided accumulating evidence for a role of P. acnes in sarcoidosis. In this review, we propose mechanisms of granuloma formation in response to this indigenous bacterium in subjects with sarcoidosis based on our results obtained using histopathological and experimental approaches, and introduce a new concept of infectious disease in which endogenous infection is caused by indigenous bacteria.

2. Bacterial culture

The lung and its draining lymph nodes are the organs most commonly affected by sarcoidosis. As the lung constantly encounters airborne substances, including pathogens, many researchers have considered infection to trigger sarcoidosis and have thus tried to identify possible causative transmissible agents and their contribution to the mechanism of sarcoid granuloma formation [15, 16].

2.1. Bacterial culture from tissue samples affected by sarcoidosis

In the late 1970s, a large Japanese research project conducted by many clinicians and microbiologists with support by a grant from Japanese Ministry of Health was organized to seek the pathogens responsible for sarcoidosis. Extensive trials were performed to isolate microorganisms, including bacteria, viruses, and fungi, from tissue samples (especially biopsied lymph nodes) affected by sarcoidosis. Only P. acnes, and no other microorganism, was isolated from the large number of samples [13]. P. acnes was isolated in culture from biopsy samples of 31 (78%) of 40 lymph nodes from 40 patients with sarcoidosis [14], whereas this indigenous bacterium was also cultured from 20% of 141 control lymph nodes from patients with diseases other than sarcoidosis. The study was repeated twice to confirm that the initial samples had not been contaminated by cutaneous P. acnes during biopsy, and the results of both studies were the same.

2.2. Bacterial culture from tissue samples without sarcoidosis

Ishige *et al* cultured peripheral lung tissue and various lymph nodes obtained from patients with diseases other than sarcoidosis [17]. *P. acnes* was isolated from 24 of 43 lungs and 8 of 11 mediastinal lymph nodes, mostly in pure culture. *P. acnes* was isolated from 10 of 20 gastric and 3 of 12 intestinal lymph nodes; intestinal bacteria were also numerous. *P. acnes* was generally the only species isolated from these tissues. The number of *P. acnes* cells isolated was usually no more than 500 colony forming units (CFU)/g in the lungs and lymph nodes. Of 43 lungs from patients without sarcoidosis, only 4 (9%) had exceptionally high numbers of *P. acnes* cells. Random amplified polymorphic DNA analysis was used to compare the DNA of 45 isolates of *P. acnes* from these patients, 39 isolates from sarcoid lymph nodes, and 67 isolates from normal skin, conjunctiva, and intestine. The *P. acnes* strains in the lung and mediastinal lymph nodes differed genetically from those in the skin. Therefore, contamination from the skin during operative or culture procedures seems unlikely. These findings suggest that *P. acnes* normally resides in peripheral lung tissue and mediastinal lymph nodes.

2.3. Cell invasiveness of *P. acnes*

Studies of cell-invading *P. acnes* are essential for linking this indigenous bacterium to the cause of sarcoidosis because infectious granulomas are commonly caused by intracellular pathogens. Furukawa *et al* examined the cell invasiveness and serotype of *P. acnes* isolates from lymph nodes affected by sarcoidosis, together with isolates from non-sarcoid tissue obtained from the lymph nodes, lungs, prostate, skin, conjunctiva, and intestine [18]. The invasiveness of these *P. acnes* isolates into HEK293T cells was examined by cell-invasion assay according to the method described by Cue and Cleary [19] and intracellular localization of the invasive isolates was confirmed by electron microscopy (Figure 1). Cell invasiveness was found in 14 (40%) of 35 sarcoid isolates and 65 (51%) of 127 non-sarcoid isolates. The proportion of invasive isolates did not differ between isolates from sarcoid and non-sarcoid tissues. The whole-bacterium enzyme-linked immunosorbent assays with serotype-specific antibodies discriminated the serotype of all 162 isolates (112 strains of serotype I and 50 strains of serotype II). The proportion of the two serotypes did not differ between sarcoid and non-sarcoid tissues. Cell invasiveness was found in 79 (71%) of 112 serotype I isolates and in none of 50 serotype II isolates.

3. Polymerase chain reaction

Some investigators in Europe using PCR assays detected mycobacterial DNA in samples of affected tissue from patients with sarcoidosis [20-22], but others did not [23-25]. Quantification of the bacterial genomes detected in sarcoid lesions is essential for clarifying the etiologic correlation between lesions and bacteria detected therein because a tiny volume of bacteria or bacterial DNA can be detected even in conditions of latent infection or contamination with no etiologic correlation.

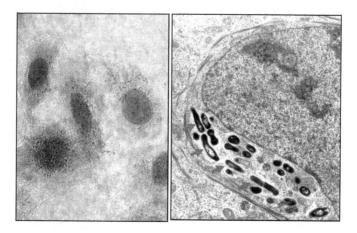

Figure 1. Invasiveness of *P. acnes* into epithelial cells. HEK293T cells infected with one of the serotype 1 *P. acnes* strains isolated from sarcoid lymph nodes were Giemsa-stained (left) and further examined by electron microscopy (right). The electron micrographs of the cells infected with an invasive isolate show intracellular localization of the bacterium (indicated by the red arrows).

3.1. Quantitative PCR for propionibacterial and mycobacterial DNA

Ishige *et al* used quantitative PCR to search for bacterial genomes of *P. acnes, P. granulosum,* and *M. tuberculosis* in histologic sections of lymph nodes from patients with sarcoidosis, tuberculosis, or gastric cancer [26]. They examined lymph node biopsy samples from 15 patients with sarcoidosis and 15 patients with tuberculosis lymphadenitis. As controls, they examined 15 lymph nodes without metastasis from 15 patients with gastric cancer undergoing surgery (Figure 2). Genomes of *M. tuberculosis* were found in samples from all 15 patients with tuberculosis, 3 patients with sarcoidosis, and 1 control sample. Genomes of *P. acnes* were found in 12 of 15 patients with sarcoidosis, 2 tuberculosis patients, and 3 controls. The difference in the estimated number of *P. acnes* genomes between individuals with and without sarcoidosis was similar to that in the number of *M. tuberculosis* between people with and without tuberculosis. Biopsy samples from the three patients with sarcoidosis but without *P. acnes* all contained many *P. granulosum* DNA. These findings suggest that propionibacteria resided in or proliferated ectopically in the sarcoid lesions, whether or not there was a connection with the disease. Propionibacteria are more likely than mycobacteria to cause sarcoidosis.

3.2. International collaborative study with quantitative real-time PCR

The international collaborative study evaluated the possible etiologic link between sarcoidosis and the suspected bacterial species [8]. Formalin-fixed and paraffin-embedded sections of biopsy samples of lymph nodes, 1 from each of 108 patients with sarcoidosis and 65 patients with tuberculosis, together with 86 control samples, were collected from 2 institutes in Japan and 3 institutes in Italy, Germany, and England (Figure 3). Genomes of *P. acnes, P. granulosum, M. tuberculosis, M. avium* subsp. *paratuberculosis,* and *Escherichia coli* (as the control) were estimated by quantitative real-time PCR. Either *P. acnes* or *P. granulosum* was found in all but

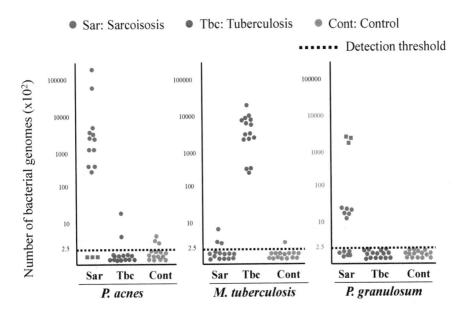

Figure 2. Quantitative PCR of bacterial DNA in lymph nodes from patients with sarcoidosis, tuberculosis, and gastric cancer. The horizontal dotted lines show the detection threshold and samples with results under this line were considered negative.

two of the sarcoid samples. *M. avium* subsp. *paratuberculosis* was not found in any sarcoid sample. *M. tuberculosis* was found in only 0% to 9% of the sarcoid samples, but in 65% to 100% of the tuberculosis samples. In sarcoid lymph nodes, the total numbers of genomes of *P. acnes* or *P. granulosum* far exceeded those of *M. tuberculosis*. *P. acnes* or *P. granulosum* was found in 0% to 60% of the tuberculosis and control samples, but the total numbers of genomes of *P. acnes* or *P. granulosum* in these samples were lower than those found in sarcoid samples. *Propionibacteria* spp. are more likely than *Mycobacteria* spp. to be involved in the etiology of sarcoidosis, not only in Japanese but also in European patients with sarcoidosis.

4. *In situ* hybridization

In situ localization of *P. acnes* genomes in sarcoid lymph nodes may help to elucidate an etiologic link between sarcoidosis and this indigenous bacterium. Formalin-fixed and paraffin-embedded biopsy samples of lymph nodes from nine patients with sarcoidosis, nine patients with tuberculosis, and nine patients with nonspecific lymphadenitis as controls were examined by quantitative real-time PCR (QPCR) for *P. acnes* and by *in situ* hybridization (ISH) using catalyzed reporter deposition (CARD) for signal amplification with digoxigenin-labeled oligonucleotide probes that complemented 16S rRNA of *P. acnes* [27]. The signals per 250 μm^2 of tissue sections from inside and outside sarcoidosis and tuberculosis granulomas and

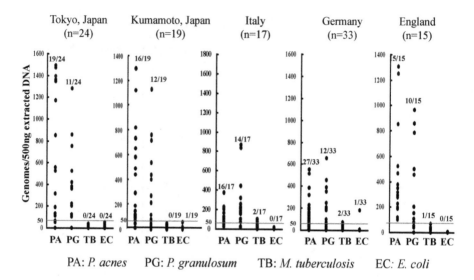

PA: *P. acnes*   PG: *P. granulosum*   TB: *M. tuberculosis*   EC: *E. coli*

Figure 3. Quantitative real-time PCR of bacterial DNA in lymph node samples from Japanese and European patients with sarcoidosis. The horizontal red lines show the detection threshold and samples with results under this line were considered negative.

from control lymph nodes were counted. The number of genomes determined by QPCR was examined for correlation with the mean signal count by ISH with CARD. In sarcoid samples, one or several signals were detected in the cytoplasm of some epithelioid cells in granulomas (Figure 4). The mean signal counts were higher in granulomatous areas than in other areas of sarcoid lymph nodes. The correlation between the QPCR and ISH with CARD results was significant ($r = 0.86$, $p < 0.001$). The accumulation of *P. acnes* genomes in and around sarcoid granulomas suggests that this indigenous bacterium is related to the cause of granulomatous inflammation in sarcoidosis.

5. Immunohistochemistry

Granulomatous reactions are basically a defense mechanism that the body uses to fight off poorly degradable antigens. Granulomas begin as a small collection of lymphocytes and macrophages surrounding poorly degradable antigens. The aggregating macrophages, called an early focus of granuloma, then change to epithelioid cells and become organized into a cluster of cells, called an immature granuloma. Further progression results in ball-like clusters of cells and fusion of macrophages into giant cells, called a mature granuloma. The questions that must be asked in searching for the cause of sarcoidosis, therefore, are: "What is the antigen that the granulomas are fighting?" and "How is the antigen localized within the sarcoid lesion?" To evaluate the pathogenic role of *P. acnes*, Negi *et al* screened for this indigenous bacterium in sarcoid and non-sarcoid tissues using immunohistochemical methods with novel *P. acnes*-specific monoclonal antibodies that react with cell-membrane-bound lipoteichoic acid

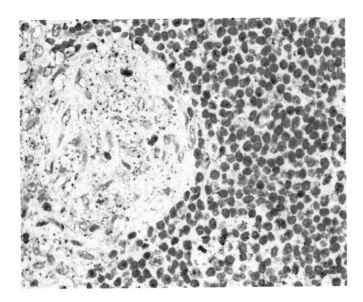

Figure 4. *In situ* hybridization using catalyzed reporter deposition for signal amplification with digoxigenin-labeled oligonucleotide probes that complemented 16S rRNA of *P. acnes*. Many signals were detected in the cytoplasm of sarcoid granuloma cells.

(PAB antibody) and ribosome-bound trigger factor protein (TIG antibody). They examined formalin-fixed and paraffin-embedded samples of lungs and lymph nodes from 196 patients with sarcoidosis, and corresponding control samples from 275 patients with non-sarcoidosis diseases. The samples were mostly from Japanese patients, with 64 lymph node samples from German patients [28].

5.1. Intracellular *P. acnes* detected within sarcoid granuloma

Immunohistochemistry with the PAB antibody revealed small round bodies within sarcoid granulomas in 20/27 (74%) video-assisted thoracic surgery lung samples, 24/50 (48%) transbronchial lung biopsy samples, 71/81 (88%) Japanese lymph node samples, and 34/38 (89%) German lymph node samples. The PAB antibody did not react with non-sarcoid granulomas in any of the 45 tuberculosis samples or the 34 samples with sarcoid reaction. The appearance of the small round bodies detected by the PAB antibody within sarcoid granulomas did not differ between lungs and lymph nodes. In sarcoid granulomas with many small round bodies, the cytoplasm of some granuloma cells was filled with small round bodies, consistent with the intracellular proliferation of the bacterium (Figure 5). In many sarcoid granulomas, a few small round bodies with occasional degraded or large-sized features were scattered among the granuloma cells. The amount of these small round bodies varied from each granuloma in identical sarcoid samples as well as from each sarcoid tissue sample (Figure 6). The appearance of the small round bodies detected by the PAB antibody within sarcoid granulomas did not differ between lungs and lymph nodes (Figure 7, 8).

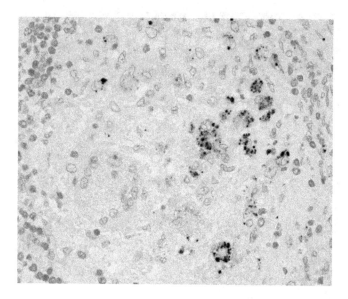

Figure 5. Immunohistochemistry with a *P. acnes*-specific monoclonal antibody (PAB antibody) that reacts with cell-membrane-bound lipoteichoic acid of the bacterium. Many small round bodies are shown within a non-caseating epithelioid cell granuloma of sarcoid lymph node.

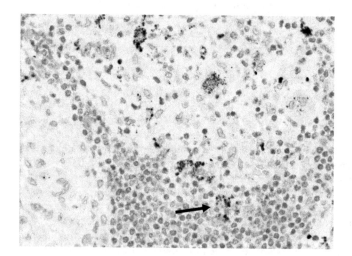

Figure 6. Many small round bodies detected by the PAB antibody are shown intermingled with many lymphocytes in one immature granuloma (right), but only a few are observed in the mature granuloma (left) of the sarcoid lymph node. Most of the *P. acnes* are present within the granuloma, but some are present outside of the granuloma (as indicated by the arrow)

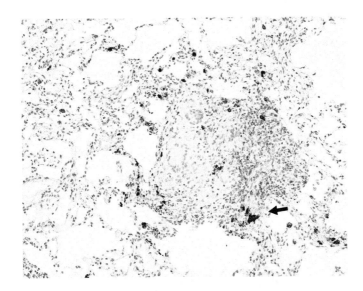

Figure 7. In the lung sarcoid granuloma lesion surrounded by prominent inflammatory cell infiltration, small round bodies are detected by the PAB antibody not only in the granuloma cells but also in some of the inflammatory cells. The arrow indicates the magnified region shown in Fig. 8.

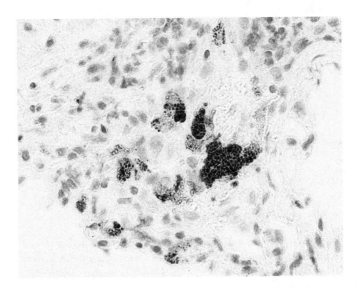

Figure 8. Higher magnification of the area indicated by the arrow in Figure 7. Some swollen macrophages of the immature granuloma are filled with many small round bodies detected by the PAB antibody.

5.2. Intracellular *P. acnes* in non-granulomatous areas

In non-granulomatous areas, small round bodies detected by the PAB antibody were found in alveolar macrophages of lungs and paracortical macrophages of lymph nodes from many sarcoid and some non-sarcoid patients. In the lymph nodes, paracortical macrophages with many small round bodies detected by the PAB antibody (Figure 9) were observed in 26 (22%) of 119 sarcoid samples and 18 (11%) of 165 non-sarcoid samples. The frequency was significantly higher in the sarcoid samples. Such small round bodies were observed in lymphatic endothelial cells in a few samples of sarcoid lymph nodes (Figure 10). In the lungs, alveolar macrophages with many small round bodies detected by the PAB antibody were found in 28 (36%) of 77 sarcoid samples and 18 (16%) of 110 non-sarcoid samples. The frequency was significantly higher in sarcoid samples. Such alveolar macrophages occasionally contained one or a few large spheroidal bodies detected by the PAB antibody that were acid-fast with Fite staining and also reacted with the TIG antibody.

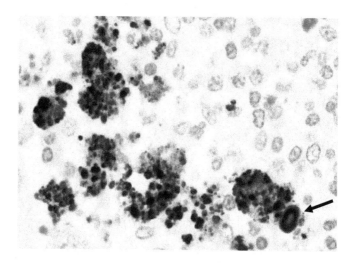

Figure 9. A cluster of some swollen macrophages filled with many small round bodies detected by the PAB antibody is occasionally found in paracortical areas of sarcoid lymph nodes. The arrow indicates a large-spheroidal body similar to Hamazaki-Wesenberg bodies.

5.3. Hamazaki-Wesenberg bodies

Hamazaki-Wesenberg (HW) bodies frequently appear in sarcoid lymph nodes although these bodies are not specific to sarcoidosis [29-31]. The large-spheroidal acid-fast bodies, HW bodies, which were found in 50% of sarcoid and 15% of non-sarcoid lymph node samples, reacted with both PAB and TIG antibodies. Electron microscopy revealed that these HW bodies had a single bacterial structure and lacked a cell wall with occasional protrusions from the body (Figure 11). Immunoelectron microscopy revealed that the immunoreactive products of the PAB

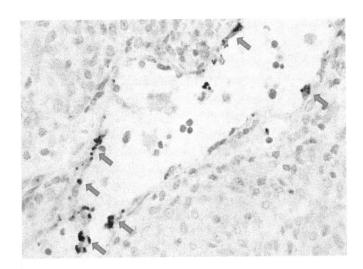

Figure 10. Some of the small round bodies detected by the PAB antibody (green arrows) were observed in lymphatic endothelial cells adjacent to sarcoid granulomas of the lymph node.

antibody and TIG antibody were differentially distributed in the outer and inner areas of the HW bodies, respectively (Figure 12). The localization of cell-membrane-bound lipoteichoic acid detected by the PAB antibody and ribosome-bound trigger factor detected by the TIG antibody suggests that HW might not be phagolysosomally-degraded products of *P. acnes*, but rather intact forms of intracellular bacteria because the original distribution pattern (plasma-lemmal and protoplasmic localization, respectively) of these bacterial components was preserved in terms of the morphologic structure of the bacterium. Furthermore, conventional electron microscopy revealed that these bodies lack a cell-wall structure and occasionally exhibit protrusions from the body that appear to be yeast-like proliferating features (not mitotic, but sprouting or branching), characteristic of cell-wall-deficient (L-form) bacteria (Figure 9). HW bodies may be cell-wall-deficient *P. acnes*.

5.4. Intracellular proliferation of *P. acnes*

Histopathologic analysis with the PAB antibody led us to formulate a hypothesis for the mechanism of granuloma formation in sarcoidosis (Figure 13). *P. acnes* causes latent infection and persists in macrophages. HW bodies are dormant and cell-wall-deficient *P. acnes*. This dormant form of *P. acnes* can be activated endogenously under certain environmental conditions and proliferate in cells at the sites of latent infection. Small round bodies proliferating in macrophages are infective forms of *P. acnes*. When these bodies spread out of macrophages, they infect other cells or organs via the lymph and blood streams. Sarcoid granulomas are formed as a host defense mechanism at the sites of activated bacteria proliferating intracellularly in patients with hypersensitive immune responses to *P. acnes* to prevent the spread of the infectious agent.

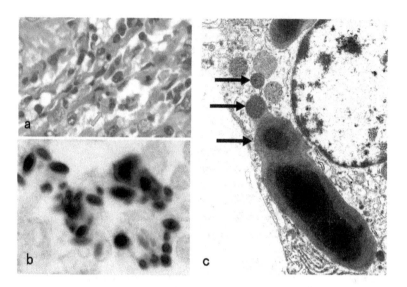

Figure 11. Hamazaki-Wesenberg (HW) bodies in sarcoid lymph nodes. HW bodies are large and spheroidal in shape with a yellow-brown color, as indicated by the green arrow, with hematoxylin and eosin staining (a). These bodies are strongly acid-fast with Fite staining (b). HW bodies with one-by-one protrusions (c), as indicated by black arrows, are rarely found in sinus macrophages of sarcoid lymph nodes.

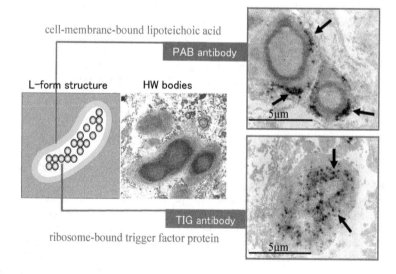

Figure 12. Immuno-electron-microscopic analysis with PAB and TIG antibodies suggests HW bodies may be cell-wall-deficient *P. acnes*.

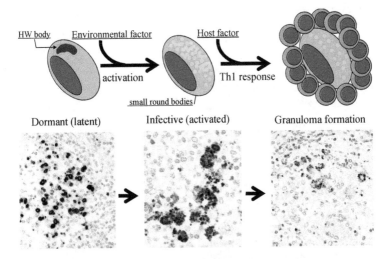

Dormant (latent)   Infective (activated)   Granuloma formation

Figure 13. Hypothesized mechanism of sarcoid granuloma formation caused by *P. acnes*. Intracellular proliferation of *P. acnes* in macrophages triggers granuloma formation in patients with hypersensitivity to this indigenous bacterium.

5.5. Histopathological diagnosis of sarcoidosis by the PAB antibody

The PAB antibody seems to be appropriate for detecting cell-wall-deficient *P. acnes* because an epitope of lipoteichoic acid detected by this antibody is more exposed in cell-wall-deficient forms than in conventional forms of the bacterium. The high frequency and specificity of *P. acnes* detected by the PAB antibody within sarcoid granulomas suggests an etiologic link between sarcoidosis and this indigenous bacterium. The PAB antibody may be useful for diagnosing sarcoidosis caused by *P. acnes*, when the reactivity is detected in idiopathic granulomas (Figures 14, 15). The TIG antibody seems to be appropriate for detecting latent forms of *P. acnes* because increased expression of the trigger-factor protein is found only in the HW bodies. The trigger-factor protein is a molecular chaperone, like some heat-shock proteins, and either overproduction or depletion of the trigger-factor protein causes filamentation indicative of cell division defects. Increased expression of the trigger-factor protein in HW bodies might be necessary to sustain the latent phase of intracellular persistent bacterium.

6. Host factor

Host factors may be more critical than agent factors in the etiology of sarcoidosis, as suggested by the Kveim test phenomenon [32], in which an intracutaneously injected suspension of sarcoid tissue causes sarcoid granulomas in patients with sarcoidosis but not in healthy people or patients with other diseases. The inflammatory response in sarcoidosis involves many activated T cells and macrophages [33], with a pattern of cytokine production in the lungs

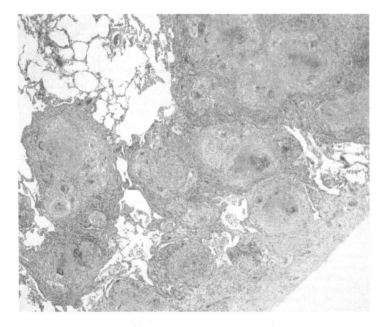

Figure 14. A lung sample with many epithelioid cell granulomas with central eosinophilic necrosis. This case required differential diagnosis from tuberculosis although the specimen contained no acid-fast bacilli and the clinical data of the patient suggested sarcoidosis.

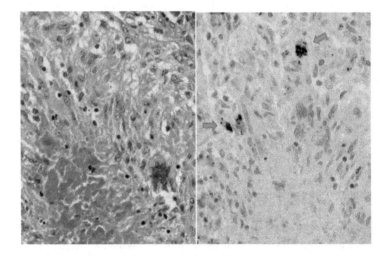

Figure 15. Immunohistochemistry with the PAB antibody for the specimen shown in Figure 14 revealed positive reaction products (green arrows) within granulomas accompanied by central eosinophilic necrosis.

consistent with a helper T-cell type 1 (Th1) immune response triggered by undefined antigen(s) [34]. If a propionibacterium caused a particular case of sarcoidosis, it is likely that an antigen arising from the bacterium gave rise to a Th1 immune response in the subject.

6.1. Hypersensitivity to *P. acnes* antigens

Ebe and colleagues searched for propionibacterial antigens that evoked cellular immune responses only in patients with sarcoidosis [11]. For this purpose, a λgt11 genomic DNA library of *P. acnes* was screened with sera from patients with sarcoidosis, because high levels of serum antibodies against the antigen usually accompany such an immune response. Of 180,000 plaques screened, 2 clones coded for an identical recombinant protein, RP35, recognized by sera. RP35, a recombinant protein of 256 amino acid residues with a calculated molecular mass of 28,133 Da, is a fragment (the C-terminal region) of the *P. acnes* trigger factor, which has 529 amino acid residues and a calculated molecular mass of 57,614 Da. The C-terminal sequence (Asp-463 to Lys-529) seems to be unique to *P. acnes*, with no similarity to sequences of other bacterial proteins deposited in the Swiss-Prot database. Conformational analysis of the Ser-491 to Lys-529 region at the C terminus revealed it to be highly antigenic. RP35 caused sarcoidosis-specific proliferation of peripheral blood mononuclear cells (PBMCs) from 9 (18%) of 50 patients with sarcoidosis (Figure 16). The same study established that serum levels of IgG and IgA antibodies to RP35 are high in patients with sarcoidosis and other lung diseases. In bronchoalveolar lavage (BAL) fluid, IgG and IgA antibody levels were high in 7 (18%) and 15 (39%), respectively, of 38 patients with sarcoidosis, and in 2 (3%) and 2 (3%), respectively, of 63 patients with other lung diseases. The results of the study suggested that this antigen from *P. acnes* is responsible for the formation or maintenance of granulomas in some patients with sarcoidosis.

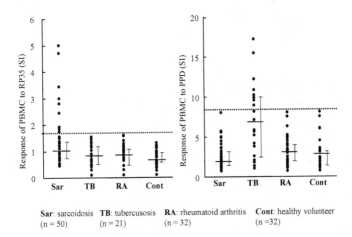

Sar: sarcoidosis TB: tubercusosis RA: rheumatoid arthritis Cont: healthy volunteer
(n = 50)   (n = 21)   (n = 32)   (n =32)

Figure 16. Response of peripheral blood mononuclear cells (PBMC) to recombinant trigger factor protein (RP35) from *P. acnes* and purified protein derivative (PPD) from *M. tuberculosis*. The horizontal bars show, from bottom to top, the 25th percentile, median, and 75th percentile, respectively. The dotted lines show the threshold, set at the mean + 3SD of the 32 control samples.

Recently, Furusawa *et al* [35] reported that interleukin-2 secretion from PBMCs after stimulation with viable *P. acnes* is higher in patients with sarcoidosis than in control subjects. Interleukin-2 and interleukin-12 mRNA expression of PBMCs after stimulation with *P. acnes* is also higher in patients with sarcoidosis than in control subjects. In contrast, interleukin-17 mRNA expression of PBMCs is lower in patients with sarcoidosis than in control subjects. The responses of the two groups to stimulation with *M. tuberculosis* antigens such as Bacille de Calmette et Guérin (BCG) or ESAT-6 recombinant protein were not significantly different. Sarcoidosis may arise from an imbalance of Th1/Th17 immune responses to viable *P. acnes*.

Additional evidence of the hypersensitivity of sarcoid patients to *P. acnes* was obtained in studies of BAL cells. When stimulated with a crude extract of *P. acnes* with pyridine, BAL cells from patients with sarcoidosis proliferated more than BAL cells from healthy subjects or from patients with lung cancer [36]. Interleukin-2 production and interleukin-2 receptor expression of BAL cells stimulated by the *P. acnes* antigen was greater in sarcoidosis patients than in healthy subjects or patients with other lung diseases [37]. *P. acnes* DNA was detected in BAL cells from 21 (70%) of 30 sarcoid patients and 7 (23%) of 30 control patients with other lung diseases [38]. In situ signals of *P. acnes* DNA were detected in the cytoplasm of a few alveolar macrophages among the BAL cells from sarcoid patients, but from no other kinds of BAL cells, including alveolar lymphocytes and neutrophils. Gallium-67 uptake by lung parenchyma was found in about half of the 30 sarcoid patients with *P. acnes* DNA, but in none of the other sarcoid patients [38].

6.2. NOD1 gene polymorphism

Mutations in the related NOD2 gene predispose patients to granulomatous diseases, including Crohn's disease [39], Blau syndrome [40], and early-onset sarcoidosis [41]. Although Blau syndrome and early-onset sarcoidosis are reported to share identical NOD2 mutations, no association has been reported between NOD2 and sarcoidosis [42]. NOD1 shares many structural and functional similarities with NOD2. Tanabe *et al* found that intracellular *P. acnes* activates NF-κB in both an NOD1- and NOD2-dependent manner [43]. A systematic search for NOD1 gene polymorphisms in Japanese sarcoidosis patients identified two alleles, 796G-haplotype (156C, 483C, 796G, 1722G) and 796A-haplotype (156G, 483T, 796A, 1722A). Allelic discrimination of 73 sarcoidosis patients and 215 healthy individuals showed that the frequency of the 796A-type allele is significantly higher in sarcoidosis patients and the odds ratios (ORs) are significantly elevated in NOD1-796G/A and 796A/A genotypes (OR [95% CI] = 2.250 [1.084, 4.670] and 3.243 [1.402, 7.502], respectively) as compared to the G/G genotype, showing an increasing trend across the 3 genotypes ($P = 0.006$ for trend). Functional studies indicated that the NOD1 796A-allele is associated with reduced expression leading to diminished NF-κB activation in response to intracellular *P. acnes* (Figure 17).

P. acnes has been studied for its role in immunomodulation with the conclusion that Toll-like receptor 2 (TLR2), TLR4, and TLR9 mediate the effects of *P. acnes* infection [44, 45]. These studies, however, only investigated non-invasive *P. acnes*. TLRs are likely to serve as first-line receptors for *P. acnes*, but NOD proteins might play a major role in a subsequent phase of intracellular infection. NOD1 was recently reported to be a critical regulator of beta-defensin-2

Western blot of Nod1 expression

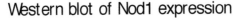

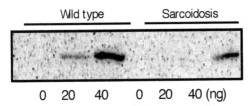

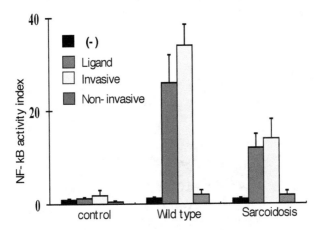

Figure 17. Functional studies (lower panel) revealed that intracellular *P. acnes* activates NF-κB in a NOD1-dependent manner and the NOD1 796A-allele predominant in sarcoidosis patients causes diminished NF-κB activation in response to intracellular *P. acnes*. Western blot analysis (upper panel) shows reduced expression of the NOD1 796A-allele.

during *Helicobacter pylori* infection [46]. It is possible that impaired expression of beta-defensin-2 through 796-A NOD1 due to a reduced ability to induce NF-κB enables *P. acnes* to survive and persist intracellularly, leading to the pathogenesis of sarcoidosis.

7. Experimental models

In experimental animals, granulomatous lesions can be induced by *P. acnes*. A single intravenous injection of *P. acnes* into mice leads to the development of many granulomas in the liver [47-49], but not in the lungs. Pulmonary granulomas can be induced, however, by an intravenous injection of *P. acnes* into sensitized rats [50] and rabbits [51]. In these two studies of experimental pulmonary granulomas, heat-killed *P. acnes* was used as a sensitizer, and a challenge by a single intravenous injection of the bacterium was essential for granulomas to form in the lungs.

7.1. Pulmonary granulomatosis caused by sensitization with *P. acnes* antigens

P. acnes trigger factor protein (RP35) or heat-killed *P. acnes* causes pulmonary granulomas in some (25%-57%) mice sensitized with the protein and complete Freund's adjuvant (CFA) [52]. An intravenous injection of *P. acnes* as a challenge was not essential for granulomas to form in the lungs. Granulomas were scattered throughout the lungs, especially in subpleural areas (Figure 18). The granulomas were composed of a core of epithelioid cells intermingled with a few and surrounded by many mononuclear cells. The detection frequency of pulmonary granulomas did not differ significantly between mice sensitized with the RP35 or heat-killed *P. acnes*.

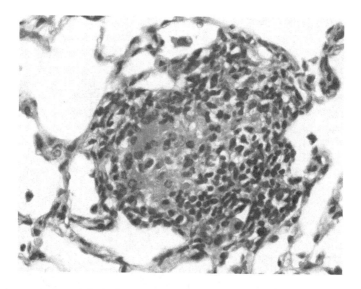

Figure 18. A non-caseating epithelioid cell granuloma observed in a mouse with experimental pulmonary granulomatosis induced by sensitization with *P. acnes* trigger factor protein and adjuvant.

This experimental protocol may provide a satisfactory model of sarcoidosis. First, hypersensitivity to *P. acnes* trigger factor, such as has been experimentally induced, has been reported in some patients with sarcoidosis. Second, situations resembling intravenous challenge with *P. acnes* are rare in humans, and sarcoidosis can start in asymptomatic persons without evidence of septicemia.

Experimental models of allergic diseases, such as encephalomyelitis [53], thyroiditis [54], and orchitis [55] have been produced by immunizing animals with self-antigens (myelin basic protein, thyroglobulin, and testicular homogenate, respectively) emulsified in CFA, which is essential for the experiment. Autoimmune inflammatory lesions are induced in this way only in the organs from which the self-antigens used for the sensitization originated. In the animal model of sarcoidosis, sensitization of mice with *P. acnes* trigger factor protein or heat-killed *P. acnes* in CFA induces granulomatous inflammation confined to the lungs. This finding suggests that such antigens from *P. acnes* exist in the lungs of mice even before the experiment.

Similar to the results obtained by bacterial culture of human samples from lung and lymph nodes, *P. acnes* was cultured from the lungs, liver, and lymph nodes from some of the untreated normal mice, and culture was most often successful with the lungs. There was an unexpected concordance in the rate (33%) of culture from normal lungs and the frequency of detection of pulmonary granulomas in mice sensitized with the trigger factor protein. The concordance suggests that mice without granulomas may have been free from *P. acnes* in the normal indigenous flora of their lungs before and during the experiment.

Using the same experimental protocol with rabbits bred in a conventional environment, rabbits sensitized with the *P. acnes* trigger factor antigen developed more severe and diffuse pulmonary granulomatosis than did sensitized mice. In fact, the severe granulomatous inflammation that developed could even be identified macroscopically (Figure 19, 20). Th1 immune response to the *P. acnes* trigger factor protein might have caused pulmonary granulomas at the sites of *P. acnes* infection. Indeed, the administration of antibiotics (azithromycin in mice and mino-cycline in rabbits) before and during the experiments prevented granuloma formation in these experimental models (Figure 21).

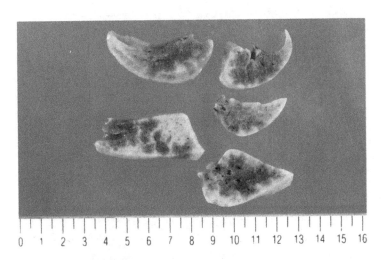

Figure 19. Cut sections of the lungs from a rabbit with experimental pulmonary granulomatosis induced by sensitization with *P. acnes* trigger factor protein and adjuvant. Whitish lesions are distributed throughout and are especially prominent in the subpleural and interlobular areas.

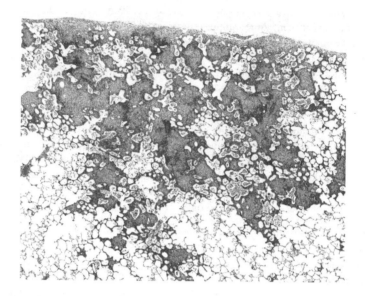

Figure 20. Histologic features of experimental pulmonary granulomatosis of the rabbit shown in Figure 19. Multiple non-caseating epithelioid cell granulomas are accompanied by surrounding lymphoid cell infiltration with alveolitis.

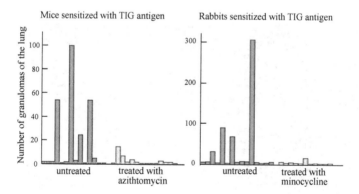

Figure 21. Prevention of pulmonary granulomatosis in mice and rabbits sensitized with *P. acnes* trigger factor (TIG) antigen by administration of antibiotics before and during the experiments.

7.2. Mechanism of granuloma formation in the experimental models

Nishiwaki *et al* further examined the mechanism of pulmonary granulomatosis caused by sensitization of heat-killed *P. acnes* [56], using a similar experimental protocol as used in a previous study [52]. In the study, *P. acnes* was identified in normal murine alveolar cells by immunostaining with a *P. acnes*-specific monoclonal antibody (PAB antibody). *P. acnes* was taken up by lung cells, and the *P. acnes*-bearing cells expressed F4/80 rather than CD11c or DEC205, consistent with the ability of macrophages to phagocytose and deliver antigens to dendritic cells in the lung. As far away as the end of the airway, airborne organisms are impacted and eliminated by mechanical defenses, including mucocilliary clearance and coughing. Nevertheless, a small number of *P. acnes* might escape this system and reside on the alveolar surface. *P. acnes* genomes were detected in normal pulmonary lymph nodes as well as the lungs, and lymphocytes from lymph nodes showed *P. acnes*-specific proliferation, suggesting that these cells had already been exposed to *P. acnes* by lung-derived antigen-presenting-cells and had established a memory response. Additionally, these results indicate that *P. acnes* were continuously transported to pulmonary regional lymph nodes in the steady state. Because of this constant delivery of antigens to the pulmonary lymph nodes for a long period, the small number of indigenous *P. acnes* in the normal lung would be enough to produce a specific immune response, but not for the formation of a steady-state granuloma. Although mycobacterial, atypical mycobacterial, and other propionibacterial antigens are potential candidate endogenous microorganisms that trigger pulmonary granuloma formation, genomic analyses revealed an absence of these organisms in the lungs of specific-pathogen-free C57BL/6 mice.

The adoptive transfer of *P. acnes*-sensitized lymph node CD4+ T cells into naïve mice resulted in granulomatous changes in the lung, indicating that extrapulmonary lymph node CD4+ T cells primed with *P. acnes* can interact with pulmonary resident cells via the circulation and induce granuloma formation in the normal lung. It was therefore hypothesized that a continuous supply of *P. acnes*-sensitized T cells should lead to chronic pulmonary granuloma formation, and consequently we performed continuous remote sensitization of normal mice with *P. acnes*. These mice exhibited distinct pulmonary granulomas, distributed in lymph-rich spaces such as the subpleural, peribronchial, and perivascular areas, and had typical cellular components of granuloma and preferential Th1 cytokine expression. These features are similar to those of pulmonary sarcoidosis. In addition, the ratio of CD4 to CD8 BAL lymphocytes was elevated in the group immunized twice, and serum calcium levels were also increased. Thus, the characteristics of this *P. acnes*-immunization model, without any direct exposure of antigen to the lung, showed several similarities to those of sarcoid patients.

That study also examined whether changes in the number of pre-existing *P. acnes* cells in the lung affected pulmonary granuloma formation. As expected, preloading of *P. acnes* exacerbated pulmonary disorders, whereas reduction of the *P. acnes* population by antimicrobial treatment reduced the pulmonary lesions. These findings suggest a pivotal role of normally localized *P. acnes* in the formation of pulmonary granuloma by extrapulmonary *P. acnes* sensitization, as well as the potential clinical usefulness of antimicrobial eradication targeting lung-indigenous *P. acnes* for the treatment of pulmonary granulomatosis induced by similar pathogenesis.

8. Etiology of sarcoidosis

In the past, once the germ theory of disease was accepted, microbes were considered to be pathogens if they met the stipulations of Koch's postulates. Although there are many microbes, however, most human infections are caused by only a few. Some microbes have been classified as pathogens although they do not cause disease in every host. In addition, some microbes have been classified as nonpathogenic although they cause disease in certain hosts. For these reasons, in a redefinition of the concepts of virulence and pathogenicity of microbes, Casadevall and Pirofski suggested a classification system for pathogens based on their ability to cause damage as a function of the host's immune response [57]. Koch's postulates for exogenous infection cannot be applied to diseases caused by endogenous bacteria. Endogenous infection is a disease caused by indigenous microorganisms. According to the classification system suggested by Casadevall and Pirofski, endogenous infection, which does not cause any lesions under normal immune conditions, can be classified into three major categories (Figure 22). Opportunistic infections, such as pneumocystis carinii pneumonia, are well known to be associated with immunodeficiency in AIDS patients. Combination type infections, such as Candida and Aspergillus, not only cause opportunistic infections, but may also cause hypersensitivity pneumonitis. The hypersensitivity type of endogenous infection does not cause any tissue damage until the hypersensitive immune response is triggered. *P. acnes* as a cause of sarcoidosis can therefore be classified within the group of endogenous diseases that results from hypersensitivity.

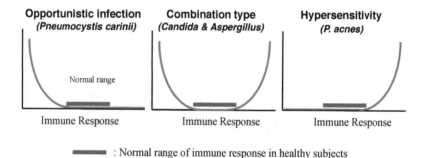

Figure 22. Three major categories of endogenous infection in the classification system of diseases caused by indigenous microorganisms.

8.1. Commensalism of *P. acnes* in the lungs and lymph nodes

P. acnes is the most common commensal bacterium in the lungs and lymph nodes from subjects without sarcoidosis [17]. Some *P. acnes* is found in 20% of non-sarcoid lymph nodes by bacterial culture [17], 15% of non-sarcoid lymph nodes by PCR [26], and 18% of non-sarcoid lung samples, and 22% of non-sarcoid lymph node samples by immunohistochemistry [28].

Occasional detection of intracellular *P. acnes* in non-granulomatous areas of the lungs and lymph nodes from non-sarcoid patients suggests that latent infection and endogenous reactivation of this indigenous bacterium occurs in these organs, even in patients without sarcoidosis. Sarcoidosis involves many organs, and the lungs and mediastinal lymph nodes are involved at the highest frequency [58]. Commensalism of *P. acnes* in these organs may explain why they are frequently involved in sarcoidosis.

8.2. Mechanism of granuloma formation in sarcoidosis

P. acnes, indigenous low-virulence bacterium, can cause latent infection in the lungs and lymph nodes and persist in a cell-wall-deficient form. This dormant form of *P. acnes* can be activated endogenously under certain environmental conditions and then proliferate in cells at the site of the latent infection. In patients hypersensitive to this endogenous bacterium, granulomatous inflammation is triggered by intracellular proliferation of the bacterium. Some proliferating bacteria may escape from isolation by the granuloma and spread to other organs via the lymph and blood streams. The spread of infective *P. acnes* might cause a new latent infection in systemic organs, such as eyes, skin, and heart. Latent infection established in certain systemic organs will be reactivated simultaneously by the next triggering event, resulting in the onset of systemic sarcoidosis (Figure 23).

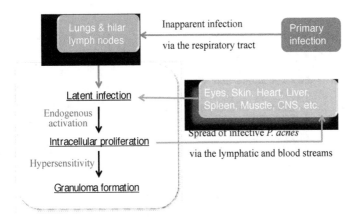

Figure 23. Hypothesized mechanism of systemic sarcoid granuloma formation caused by *P. acnes*.

Intracellular proliferation of *P. acnes* triggered by endogenous activation of latent infection might lead to the spread of the infectious *P. acnes*, giving rise to a new latent infection even within the same organ. As long as such latent infection is inadequately eradicated by the host defense mechanism of granuloma formation, the process will be repeated anytime reactivation occurs under the requisite environmental conditions. Relapsing sarcoidosis causes repetitive acute inflammation and post-inflammatory scars in the affected organs, which results in the progression of sarcoidosis through tissue damage and functional disorder in the affected organ.

Sarcoidosis is most likely the result of a complex interaction between infection, immunity, and allergic reaction (Figure 24). There are three conditions essential to the development of sarcoidosis caused by *P. acnes*: 1) latent infection with cell-wall-deficient *P. acnes*, 2) endogenous activation of dormant *P. acnes* triggered by certain environmental factors, and 3) a hypersensitive Th1 immune response towards the intracellular proliferation of *P. acnes*. The formation of sarcoid granulomas might be induced by a Th1 immune response to one or more antigens of *P. acnes* proliferating in the affected organ or tissue in an individual with a hereditary or acquired abnormality of the immune system.

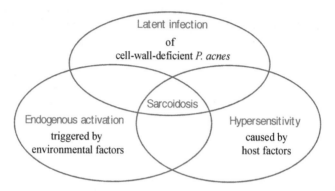

Figure 24. Sarcoidosis caused by *P. acnes* with a complex interaction of latent infection, endogenous activation, and host hypersensitivity.

8.3. Pathogenesis shared by sarcoidosis and tuberculosis

Tuberculosis shares many common features with sarcoidosis, not only their histopathologic features, but also aspects of their pathogenesis. Many tuberculosis cases arise from the endogenous activation of latent tuberculosis infection. Primary *M. tuberculosis* infection usually occurs in childhood and produces lesions termed the "primary complex", which is a combination of lesions in the lung and lung hilar lymph nodes. Around 90% of subjects with primary infection by *M. tuberculosis* exhibit a so-called "unapparent infection", i.e., they are asymptomatic. Latent infection by this pathogen is characterized by healed lesions comprising consolidated scar tissue or necrotic lesions that often becomes calcified. The persistent mycobacteria in this dormant phase are thought to be cell-wall-deficient. Active tuberculosis occurs when the latent mycobacterial infection is endogenously activated under certain environmental conditions, especially in older people. The risk for activation is also significantly increased by immunosuppressive triggers, such as HIV infection and diabetes. Recent immunologic data provide evidence of latent tuberculosis in about one-third of the global population, which corresponds to more than 2 billion individuals [59].

Endogenous reactivation of latent bacteria is well known to occur in tuberculosis, which shares many common features with sarcoidosis, not only the histopathologic features, but also the pathogenic features. Many cases of adult tuberculosis are caused by endogenous activation of latent tuberculosis infection [59, 60]. Tuberculosis and sarcoidosis are side effects of the anti-tumor necrosis factor-α drugs administered to patients with rheumatoid arthritis [61, 62]. Anti-tumor necrosis factor-α treatment is thought to reactivate latent tuberculosis infection [63]. In the same manner, latent *P. acnes* might be reactivated by anti- tumor necrosis factor-α treatment, resulting in sarcoidosis in certain susceptible subjects among these patients.

9. Treatment of sarcoidosis

Immunosuppressive, mainly corticosteroidal, therapy has been used for sarcoidosis for more than 50 years, but the long-term effects of steroidal treatment in chronic sarcoidosis are still disputed [3], Further, the high relapse rate after treatment and the side effects of long-term use are often a clinical challenge [64]. Steroids suppress the allergic reaction, thereby providing therapeutic effects. Interference of the inflammatory process by these immunosuppressive drugs, however, may impede the formation of granulomas, which function to curtail the spread of *P. acnes* infection.

9.1. Strategy for treating sarcoidosis caused by P. acnes

Antibiotics not only kill the bacteria proliferating in cells, but also prevent the endogenous activation of latent bacteria. Long-term administration of antibiotics may therefore be effective for patients with progressive sarcoidosis by preventing inflammatory relapses caused by reactivation of the latent bacteria (Figure 25). If latent bacterial infection persisting in organs can be eradicated by treatment with antibiotics, complete remission of sarcoidosis may be achieved. Complete eradication of latent bacteria might be difficult to achieve through the conventional use of antibiotics, however, as in the case of pulmonary tuberculosis.

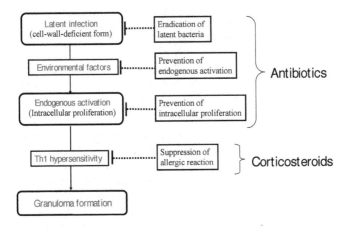

Figure 25. Strategy for treating sarcoidosis caused by *P. acnes*.

Another approach for treating sarcoidosis is specific suppression of the hypersensitivity to *P. acnes* antigens responsible for granuloma formation, such as the trigger factor protein. Recent advances in the modulation of epitope-specific immune responses by synthetic peptides might help to improve the treatment of sarcoidosis.

9.2. Tetracyclines for treating sarcoidosis

Minocycline is the first-choice antibiotic for patients with acne vulgaris caused by *P. acnes*. In an observational study, Bachelez and colleagues [65] reported the possible benefits of tetracyclines, to which *P. acnes* is sensitive, for the treatment of chronic forms of cutaneous sarcoidosis. The authors treated 12 patients with biopsy-proven cutaneous sarcoidosis with 200 mg daily minocycline over a median 12-month period. With a median follow-up of 26 months, the authors noted complete and partial responses to treatment in 8 and 2 patients, respectively. The mean time to reach a maximal response was 3.2 months. Of the 8 patients who had a complete response, minocycline could be withdrawn in 7 patients, 3 of whom experienced recurrent lesions and received further treatment with 200 mg daily doxycycline. Complete remission was maintained for a mean of 15.3 months. Regression of pulmonary infiltrates and mediastinal lymphadenopathy was noted in the 2 patients with concurrent pulmonary involvement.

The results of a nationwide questionnaire survey, performed by a Japanese research group in 2005 (reported in Japanese), indicated that antibiotic therapy was effective in 43% of 87 patients with sarcoidosis treated with many kinds of antibiotics, including minocycline, doxycycline, and clarithromycin. Baba and colleagues [66] used minocycline and clarithromycin for therapy against worsening of multiple endobronchial mass lesions, given the possible roles of *P. acnes* in the pathophysiology of sarcoidosis and the uncertainty of the long-term effects of corticosteroids. The lesions were worsening before the antibiotic therapy was initiated, so the improvements appeared to be due to the therapy. Park and colleagues [67] reported the first case of ocular and ocular adnexal sarcoidosis treated with minocycline. The patient in this report demonstrated a complete and recurrence-free response of lacrimal gland and choroidal lesions as well as parotid granulomas and pulmonary infiltrates after 3 months of minocycline therapy. Miyazaki and colleagues [68] reported the regression of nodular lesions of muscular sarcoidosis during minocycline treatment with decreased levels of angiotensin-converting enzyme, lysozyme, and soluble interleukin-2 receptor. The effectiveness of minocycline for muscular sarcoidosis in this case was confirmed when a prompt response to the minocycline therapy was repeatedly observed.

Based on the studies described in this section, the antimicrobial properties of tetracyclines are effective for treating sarcoidosis. Many researchers, have questioned the antimicrobial role of tetracyclines because tetracyclines also have anti-inflammatory properties, which were demonstrated by in vitro studies and corroborated by clinical trials. Tetracycline suppresses neutrophil migration and chemotaxis [69], and minocycline inhibits T-lymphocyte activation and proliferation [70]. Both minocycline and doxycycline obviate granuloma formation in vitro [71]. Although it remains controversial whether these antibiotics kill microbes or have only an anti-inflammatory effect, the mechanisms of sarcoid granuloma formation caused by *P.*

acnes proposed in this chapter suggest that these antibiotics have many roles in the process of granuloma formation, including the events triggering granuloma formation caused by intracellular proliferation of the bacterium.

9.3. Marshall protocol

The Marshall protocol [72] is an eradication therapy for intracellular bacteria established by Dr. Trevor Marshall. This therapeutic protocol is a combination of minocycline plus azithromycin or clindamycin, supported by the use of an angiotensin receptor blocker to prevent Herxheimer reactions. According to the results published by the Autoimmunity Research Foundation in 2006, this therapy is effective in 62% of patients with sarcoidosis. Information about the treatment can be found at the study site, marshallprotocol.com and also at autoimmunityresearch.org.

Author details

Yoshinobu Eishi*

Address all correspondence to: eishi.path@tmd.ac.jp

Department of Human Pathology, Division of Surgical Pathology, Tokyo Medical and Dental University, Japan

References

[1] Newman LS, Rose CS, Maier LA. Sarcoidosis. N Engl J Med 1997;336:1224-34.

[2] Hunninghake GW, Costabel U, Ando M, et al. ATS/ERS/WASOG statement on sarcoidosis. American Thoracic Society/European Respiratory Society/World Association of Sarcoidosis and other Granulomatous Disorders. Sarcoidosis, vasculitis, and diffuse lung diseases : official journal of WASOG / World Association of Sarcoidosis and Other Granulomatous Disorders 1999;16:149-73.

[3] Baughman RP, Lower EE, du Bois RM. Sarcoidosis. Lancet 2003;361:1111-8.

[4] Newman LS, Rose CS, Bresnitz EA, et al. A case control etiologic study of sarcoidosis: environmental and occupational risk factors. Am J Respir Crit Care Med 2004;170:1324-30.

[5] McGrath DS, Goh N, Foley PJ, et al. Sarcoidosis: genes and microbes--soil or seed? Sarcoidosis, vasculitis, and diffuse lung diseases : official journal of WASOG / World Association of Sarcoidosis and Other Granulomatous Disorders 2001;18:149-64.

[6]   du Bois RM, Goh N, McGrath D, et al. Is there a role for microorganisms in the pathogenesis of sarcoidosis? J Intern Med 2003;253:4-17.

[7]   Drake WP, Newman LS. Mycobacterial antigens may be important in sarcoidosis pathogenesis. Curr Opin Pulm Med 2006;12:359-63.

[8]   Eishi Y, Suga M, Ishige I, et al. Quantitative analysis of mycobacterial and propionibacterial DNA in lymph nodes of Japanese and European patients with sarcoidosis. J Clin Microbiol 2002;40:198-204.

[9]   Brownell I, Ramírez-Valle F, Sanchez M, et al. Evidence for Mycobacteria in Sarcoidosis. Am J Respir Cell Mol Biol 2011.

[10] Drake WP, Dhason MS, Nadaf M, et al. Cellular recognition of Mycobacterium tuberculosis ESAT-6 and KatG peptides in systemic sarcoidosis. Infect Immun 2007;75:527-30.

[11] Ebe Y, Ikushima S, Yamaguchi T, et al. Proliferative response of peripheral blood mononuclear cells and levels of antibody to recombinant protein from Propionibacterium acnes DNA expression library in Japanese patients with sarcoidosis. Sarcoidosis Vasc Diffuse Lung Dis 2000;17:256-65.

[12] Zumla A, James DG. Granulomatous infections: etiology and classification. Clin Infect Dis 1996;23:146-58.

[13] Homma JY, Abe C, Chosa H, et al. Bacteriological investigation on biopsy specimens from patients with sarcoidosis. Jpn J Exp Med 1978;48:251-5.

[14] Abe C, Iwai K, Mikami R, et al. Frequent isolation of Propionibacterium acnes from sarcoidosis lymph nodes. Zentralbl Bakteriol Mikrobiol Hyg A 1984;256:541-7.

[15] Conron M, Du Bois RM. Immunological mechanisms in sarcoidosis. Clin Exp Allergy 2001;31:543-54.

[16] Agostini C, Meneghin A, Semenzato G. T-lymphocytes and cytokines in sarcoidosis. Curr Opin Pulm Med 2002;8:435-40.

[17] Ishige I, Eishi Y, Takemura T, et al. Propionibacterium acnes is the most common bacterium commensal in peripheral lung tissue and mediastinal lymph nodes from subjects without sarcoidosis. Sarcoidosis Vasc Diffuse Lung Dis 2005;22:33-42.

[18] Furukawa A, Uchida K, Ishige Y, et al. Characterization of Propionibacterium acnes isolates from sarcoid and non-sarcoid tissues with special reference to cell invasiveness, serotype, and trigger factor gene polymorphism. Microb Pathog 2009;46:80-7.

[19] Cue DR, Cleary PP. High-frequency invasion of epithelial cells by Streptococcus pyogenes can be activated by fibrinogen and peptides containing the sequence RGD. Infect Immun 1997;65:2759-64.

[20] Fidler HM, Rook GA, Johnson NM, et al. Mycobacterium tuberculosis DNA in tissue affected by sarcoidosis. BMJ 1993;306:546-9.

[21] Popper HH, Winter E, Höfler G. DNA of Mycobacterium tuberculosis in formalin-fixed, paraffin-embedded tissue in tuberculosis and sarcoidosis detected by polymerase chain reaction. Am J Clin Pathol 1994;101:738-41.

[22] Saboor SA, Johnson NM, McFadden J. Detection of mycobacterial DNA in sarcoidosis and tuberculosis with polymerase chain reaction. Lancet 1992;339:1012-5.

[23] Bocart D, Lecossier D, De Lassence A, et al. A search for mycobacterial DNA in granulomatous tissues from patients with sarcoidosis using the polymerase chain reaction. Am Rev Respir Dis 1992;145:1142-8.

[24] Richter E, Greinert U, Kirsten D, et al. Assessment of mycobacterial DNA in cells and tissues of mycobacterial and sarcoid lesions. Am J Respir Crit Care Med 1996;153:375-80.

[25] Vokurka M, Lecossier D, du Bois RM, et al. Absence of DNA from mycobacteria of the M. tuberculosis complex in sarcoidosis. Am J Respir Crit Care Med 1997;156:1000-3.

[26] Ishige I, Usui Y, Takemura T, et al. Quantitative PCR of mycobacterial and propionibacterial DNA in lymph nodes of Japanese patients with sarcoidosis. Lancet 1999;354:120-3.

[27] Yamada T, Eishi Y, Ikeda S, et al. In situ localization of Propionibacterium acnes DNA in lymph nodes from sarcoidosis patients by signal amplification with catalysed reporter deposition. J Pathol 2002;198:541-7.

[28] Negi M, Takemura T, Guzman J, et al. Localization of Propionibacterium acnes in granulomas supports a possible etiologic link between sarcoidosis and the bacterium. Mod Pathol 2012;25:1287-97.

[29] Boyd JF, Valentine JC. Unidentified yellow bodies in human lymph-nodes. The Journal of pathology 1970;102:58-60.

[30] Doyle WF, Brahman HD, Burgess JH. The nature of yellow-brown bodies in peritoneal lymph nodes. Archives of pathology 1973;96:320-6.

[31] Moscovic EA. Sarcoidosis and mycobacterial L-forms. A critical reappraisal of pleomorphic chromogenic bodies (Hamazaki corpuscles) in lymph nodes. Pathology annual 1978;13 Pt 2:69-164.

[32] SILTZBACH LE. The Kveim test in sarcoidosis. A study of 750 patients. JAMA 1961;178:476-82.

[33] Hunninghake GW, Crystal RG. Pulmonary sarcoidosis: a disorder mediated by excess helper T-lymphocyte activity at sites of disease activity. N Engl J Med 1981;305:429-34.

[34] Moller DR, Forman JD, Liu MC, et al. Enhanced expression of IL-12 associated with Th1 cytokine profiles in active pulmonary sarcoidosis. J Immunol 1996;156:4952-60.

[35] Furusawa H, Suzuki Y, Miyazaki Y, et al. Th1 and Th17 immune responses to viable Propionibacterium acnes in patients with sarcoidosis. Respir Investig 2012;50:104-9.

[36] Nakata Y, Ejiri T, Kishi T, et al. Alveolar lymphocyte proliferation induced by Propionibacterium acnes in sarcoidosis patients. Acta Med Okayama 1986;40:257-64.

[37] Mori Y, Nakata Y, Kataoka M, et al. [Interleukin-2 production and receptor expression of alveolar lymphocytes stimulated by Propionibacterium acnes in sarcoidosis]. Nihon Kyobu Shikkan Gakkai Zasshi 1989;27:42-50.

[38] Hiramatsu J, Kataoka M, Nakata Y, et al. Propionibacterium acnes DNA detected in bronchoalveolar lavage cells from patients with sarcoidosis. Sarcoidosis, vasculitis, and diffuse lung diseases : official journal of WASOG / World Association of Sarcoidosis and Other Granulomatous Disorders 2003;20:197-203.

[39] Ogura Y, Bonen DK, Inohara N, et al. A frameshift mutation in NOD2 associated with susceptibility to Crohn's disease. Nature 2001;411:603-6.

[40] Miceli-Richard C, Lesage S, Rybojad M, et al. CARD15 mutations in Blau syndrome. Nat Genet 2001;29:19-20.

[41] Kanazawa N, Okafuji I, Kambe N, et al. Early-onset sarcoidosis and CARD15 mutations with constitutive nuclear factor-kappaB activation: common genetic etiology with Blau syndrome. Blood 2005;105:1195-7.

[42] Schürmann M, Valentonyte R, Hampe J, et al. CARD15 gene mutations in sarcoidosis. Eur Respir J 2003;22:748-54.

[43] Tanabe T, Ishige I, Suzuki Y, et al. Sarcoidosis and NOD1 variation with impaired recognition of intracellular Propionibacterium acnes. Biochim Biophys Acta 2006;1762:794-801.

[44] Nagy I, Pivarcsi A, Koreck A, et al. Distinct strains of Propionibacterium acnes induce selective human beta-defensin-2 and interleukin-8 expression in human keratinocytes through toll-like receptors. J Invest Dermatol 2005;124:931-8.

[45] Kalis C, Gumenscheimer M, Freudenberg N, et al. Requirement for TLR9 in the immunomodulatory activity of Propionibacterium acnes. J Immunol 2005;174:4295-300.

[46] Boughan PK, Argent RH, Body-Malapel M, et al. Nucleotide-binding oligomerization domain-1 and epidermal growth factor receptor: critical regulators of beta-defensins during Helicobacter pylori infection. J Biol Chem 2006;281:11637-48.

[47] Senaldi G, Yin S, Shaklee CL, et al. Corynebacterium parvum- and Mycobacterium bovis bacillus Calmette-Guerin-induced granuloma formation is inhibited in TNF receptor I (TNF-RI) knockout mice and by treatment with soluble TNF-RI. J Immunol 1996;157:5022-6.

[48] Tsuji H, Harada A, Mukaida N, et al. Tumor necrosis factor receptor p55 is essential for intrahepatic granuloma formation and hepatocellular apoptosis in a murine model of bacterium-induced fulminant hepatitis. Infect Immun 1997;65:1892-8.

[49] Yoneyama H, Matsuno K, Zhang Y, et al. Regulation by chemokines of circulating dendritic cell precursors, and the formation of portal tract-associated lymphoid tissue, in a granulomatous liver disease. J Exp Med 2001;193:35-49.

[50] Yi ES, Lee H, Suh YK, et al. Experimental extrinsic allergic alveolitis and pulmonary angiitis induced by intratracheal or intravenous challenge with Corynebacterium parvum in sensitized rats. Am J Pathol 1996;149:1303-12.

[51] Ichiyasu H, Suga M, Iyonaga K, et al. Role of monocyte chemoattractant protein-1 in Propionibacterium acnes-induced pulmonary granulomatosis. Microsc Res Tech 2001;53:288-97.

[52] Minami J, Eishi Y, Ishige Y, et al. Pulmonary granulomas caused experimentally in mice by a recombinant trigger-factor protein of Propionibacterium acnes. J Med Dent Sci 2003;50:265-74.

[53] Swanborg RH. Experimental autoimmune encephalomyelitis in the rat: lessons in T-cell immunology and autoreactivity. Immunol Rev 2001;184:129-35.

[54] Goulvestre C, Batteux F, Charreire J. Chemokines modulate experimental autoimmune thyroiditis through attraction of autoreactive or regulatory T cells. Eur J Immunol 2002;32:3435-42.

[55] Teuscher C, Hickey WF, Grafer CM, et al. A common immunoregulatory locus controls susceptibility to actively induced experimental allergic encephalomyelitis and experimental allergic orchitis in BALB/c mice. J Immunol 1998;160:2751-6.

[56] Nishiwaki T, Yoneyama H, Eishi Y, et al. Indigenous pulmonary Propionibacterium acnes primes the host in the development of sarcoid-like pulmonary granulomatosis in mice. Am J Pathol 2004;165:631-9.

[57] Casadevall A, Pirofski LA. Host-pathogen interactions: redefining the basic concepts of virulence and pathogenicity. Infect Immun 1999;67:3703-13.

[58] Iwai K, Takemura T, Kitaichi M, et al. Pathological studies on sarcoidosis autopsy. II. Early change, mode of progression and death pattern. Acta Pathol Jpn 1993;43:377-85.

[59] Lin PL, Flynn JL. Understanding latent tuberculosis: a moving target. J Immunol 2010;185:15-22.

[60] Tufariello JM, Chan J, Flynn JL. Latent tuberculosis: mechanisms of host and bacillus that contribute to persistent infection. Lancet Infect Dis 2003;3:578-90.

[61] Keane J, Gershon S, Wise RP, et al. Tuberculosis associated with infliximab, a tumor necrosis factor alpha-neutralizing agent. N Engl J Med 2001;345:1098-104.

[62] Gifre L, Ruiz-Esquide V, Xaubet A, et al. Lung sarcoidosis induced by TNF antago-nists in rheumatoid arthritis: a case presentation and a literature review. Arch Bron-coneumol 2011;47:208-12.

[63] Keane J. TNF-blocking agents and tuberculosis: new drugs illuminate an old topic. Rheumatology (Oxford) 2005;44:714-20.

[64] Gottlieb JE, Israel HL, Steiner RM, et al. Outcome in sarcoidosis. The relationship of relapse to corticosteroid therapy. Chest 1997;111:623-31.

[65] Bachelez H, Senet P, Cadranel J, et al. The use of tetracyclines for the treatment of sarcoidosis. Arch Dermatol 2001;137:69-73.

[66] Baba K, Yamaguchi E, Matsui S, et al. A case of sarcoidosis with multiple endobron-chial mass lesions that disappeared with antibiotics. Sarcoidosis, vasculitis, and dif-fuse lung diseases : official journal of WASOG / World Association of Sarcoidosis and Other Granulomatous Disorders 2006;23:78-9.

[67] Park DJ, Woog JJ, Pulido JS, et al. Minocycline for the treatment of ocular and ocular adnexal sarcoidosis. Arch Ophthalmol 2007;125:705-9.

[68] Miyazaki E, Ando M, Fukami T, et al. Minocycline for the treatment of sarcoidosis: is the mechanism of action immunomodulating or antimicrobial effect? Clin Rheumatol 2008;27:1195-7.

[69] Esterly NB, Koransky JS, Furey NL, et al. Neutrophil chemotaxis in patients with acne receiving oral tetracycline therapy. Arch Dermatol 1984;120:1308-13.

[70] Kloppenburg M, Verweij CL, Miltenburg AM, et al. The influence of tetracyclines on T cell activation. Clin Exp Immunol 1995;102:635-41.

[71] Webster GF, Toso SM, Hegemann L. Inhibition of a model of in vitro granuloma for-mation by tetracyclines and ciprofloxacin. Involvement of protein kinase C. Arch Dermatol 1994;130:748-52.

[72] Marshall TG, Marshall FE. Sarcoidosis succumbs to antibiotics--implications for auto-immune disease. Autoimmun Rev 2004;3:295-300.

Chapter 2

The Role of Type I IFN and TNF-α in the Pathogenesis of Sarcoidosis

Mitsuteru Akahoshi

Additional information is available at the end of the chapter

1. Introduction

Sarcoidosis is a chronic systemic disorder of an unknown etiology and it is characterized by the presence of noncaseating granulomas in multiple organs. The granulomatous leison affected by sarcoidosis is marked by the accumulation and activation of CD4+ helper T (Th) cells with the Th1 phenotype and monocytes/macrophages, which suggest that a Th1-type immune response plays a dominant role in the disease pathogenesis [1]. For example, the important roles for IFN-γ and IL-12 were found in sarcoid lung [2], and a genome-wide gene expression analysis of sarcoid lund tissues identified signal transducer and activator of transcription-1 gene (*STAT1*) as one of the dominant network genes most highly expressed in the sarcoidosis group [3].

IFN-α is known to be a potent stimulator of Th1 immune response, and increased type I IFN signaling has been implicated in a number of autoimmune diseases such as systemic lupus erythematosus (SLE) [4]. On the other hand, type I IFN has been used to treat a variety of diseases, including chronic hepatitis C (HCV) infection. However, due to its immunomedulatory effects, it has also been reported to induce several autoimmune and/or inflammatory disorders [5]. Notably, an increasing number of sarcoidosis has been reported in chronic HCV patients who received type I IFN therapy [6, 7]. In some cases, the sarcoid lesions improved following dose reduction or cessation of the therapy, suggesting the importance of type I IFN in the disease development. Moreover, from a genetic standpoint, we recently showed an association between polymorphisms in the *IFNA* gene and susceptibility to sarcoidosis [8]. Another recent study found that in an European-American population, serum type I IFN activity was higher in sarcodosis cases as compared to matched controls [9]. In addition, besides IFN-induced sarcoidosis, a dozen case reports of sarcidosis have also been reported in patients treated with tumor necrosis factor (TNF) antagonists [10]. A cross-regulation between type I IFN and TNF-α pathways has been proposed recently. This review focuses on a potential role of these cytokines, type I IFN and TNF-α, in the pathogenesis of sarcoidosis.

2. Cross-regulation between type I IFN and TNF-α

TNF is a pivotal pro-inflammatory cytokine produced by macrophages, activated T cells, natural killer cells and mast cells, it can also be produced by other non-immune cells such as endothelial cells or stromal cells [11]. Type I IFNs (IFN-α and IFN-β) can be produced by almost every cell type, including leukocytes, fibroblasts and endothelial cells and exert antiviral and multiple immunomodulatory activities [12].

It is well accepted that TNF plays a critical role in the pathogenesis of certain autoim-mune diseases such as rheumatoid arthritis (RA), whereas there is growing evidence that IFN-α plays a pivotal role in another set of autoimmune diseases such as SLE [13]. The elevated levels of type I IFN activity in SLE patient sera has been confirmed in the 1980s [14, 15], and it was subsequently shown that overexpression of type I IFN-induced genes, called IFN signature, was a common dominant pattern in human SLE [16]. The role of type I IFN in SLE was further confirmed in the studies demonstrating induction of lupus-like disease during IFN therapy [17].

Recently, anti-TNF agents are found to be associated with the development of drug-induced lupus (DIL) as well. Indeed, a titer of anti-dsDNA antibodies has been found up to 15% of RA patients on anti-TNF therapy [18]. Postmarketing studies on the three anti-TNF drugs have suggested an estimated incidence of DIL of 0.1-0.4% (about 0.2%) [19, 20]. Another intriguing side effect of TNF blockade is the induction of psoriasis-like disease in 3 to 5% of arthritis patients without pre-existing psoriasis, which was also unexpected and paradoxical adverse effect considering the excellent clinical response of psoriasis to TNF blockade [21]. This side effect and the lupus-like syndrome observed in a part of patients undergoing therapy with TNF antagonists led to us hypothesize that TNF might actually act as an antagonist of the type I IFN pathway, further proposing cross-regulation between TNF-α and type I IFN [13].

What is the mechanism of cross-regulation between IFN-α and TNF-α pathways? Recent study demonstrated that TNF regulates IFN-α production either by inhibiting the generation of plasmacytoid dendritic cells (pDCs), a major producer of type I IFN, from CD34+ hematopoietic progenitors in vitro or by inhibiting virus-induced IFN-α release by PBMCs. In addition, neutralization of endogenous TNF sustained IFN-α secretion by pDCs [13]. Also, TNF can induce the differentiation of the potent IFN-α-secreting immature pDCs to become mature pDCs [22], which may cause downregulation of IFN-α production [23, 24]. These might explain why a deficiency in TNF related to treatment with anti-TNF inhibitors can trigger a syndrome that shares a number of features with SLE.

The relative balance between IFN-α and TNF-α has been also studied genetically and ethni-cally. In the study showing serum levels of TNF-α and IFN-α in sarocoidosis, significant differences in cytokine levels were found between sarcoidosis patients of different ancestral backgrounds [9]. In this study, African-Americans had higher TNF-α levels than European-American patients or matched controls, and patients with neurologic disease had significantly higher TNF-α than patients lacking this manifestation. In a European-American population, serum type I IFN activity was higher in sarcoidosis cases as compared to matched controls, and patients with extra-pulmonary disease represented a high serum IFN group [9]. This study demonstrated ancestral and subphenotype correlations with serum cytokine levels in patients with sarcoidosis. On the other hand, however, in patients with SLE, serum TNF-α levels were high in many SLE patients, and the high serum TNF-α levels were positively correlated with high serum IFN-α levels across different ancestral backgrounds [25]. A genetic association study demonstrated that the PTPN polymorphism was associated with skewing of cytokine profiles toward higher IFN-α activity and lower TNF-α levels in vivo in patients with SLE. Moreover, in untreated patients with juvenile dermatomyositis (JDM), serum IFN-α levels was shown to be associated with the TNF-α G-308A promoter polymorphism [26]. In sarcoidosis, the presence of a TNF-α -308A variant allele was also reported to be associated with the susceptibility to and risk of sarcoidosis [27, 28].

While some studies suggest cross-regulation between IFN-α and TNF-α, not all studies of autoimmune diseases fit this model. As in the example above, a positive correlation between serum IFN-α and TNF-α in SLE was observed [25]. In JDM, the TNF-α -308A allele that has been linked to higher TNF-α production [29] was associated with increased serum IFN-α levels [26, 30]. In addition, besides known up-regulation of TNF-α in RA synovium, the increased expression of type I IFN has been also reported in the synovium of patients with RA [31]. Therefore, it is likely that cross-regulation of IFN-α and TNF-α in humans may be more complex.

In clinical settings, systemic juvenile arthritis treated with TNF antagonists display increased transcription of IFN-α-regulated genes in their blood leukocytes compared with untreated patients [13]. Further analysis revealed that infliximab (IFX) treatment induced an upregulation of the type I IFN genes in RA compared with untreated patients, whereas type I IFN response genes were not affected in patients with a good response to TNF-α blockade [32]. In addition, TNF-α blockade with etanercept (ETN), but not IFX, induced a persistent upregulation of type I IFN serum activity from 4 to 12 weeks of treatment in spondyloarthritis [33]. Similarly, in patients with Sjögren's syndrome, a significant increase in IFN-α activity was detected after treatment with ETN [34]. Meanwhile, in patients with inflammatory myopathies, there was a significant increase in the type I IFN serum activity after IFX treatment without any clinical improvement [35]. However, the relationship between type I IFN and TNF-α appears to be complex and may be influenced by timing and disease progression.

Collectively, although there may exist the trend of a reciprocal regulation between type I IFN and TNF-α in human autoimmunity, these studies as well as the cellular studies and experimental data indicate that the effect of TNF-α blockade on type I IFN is not universal and may depend on the disease, the type of TNF-α blocker, as well as the clinical response to treatment [11]. There are several hypothesis regarding cross-regulation between type I IFN and TNF-α. The original hypothesis proposes that both cytokines can be regarded as opposite vectors and both vectors are normally in balance. A shift towards the one arm may create a permissive environment for TNF-mediated inflammation (RA) or IFN-driven autoimmunity (SLE) [11]. Alternatively, type I IFN and IFN-α are influencing each other but the balance will be lost in a pathological condition. In addition, an alternative hypothesis proposes that type I IFN plays an important role in the initiation of autoimmunity, while the role of TNF-α increases during the secondary effector phase of the disease [11].

3. Interferon-induced sarcoidosis

A cardinal feature of sarcoidosis is the presence of CD4+ T cells that interact with antigen-presenting cells to initiate the formation and maintenance of glanulomas [36]. Activated CD4+ cells differentiate into Th1-like cells and secrete predominantly IL-2 and IFN-γ. Such cytokines maintain the activation of antigen-presenting cells such as macrophages and amplify the local cellular immune response, establishing a vicious cycle that ultimately leads to the formation of granulomas.

The first case of interferon-induced sarcoidosis (IIS) was reported in a patient treated with IFN-β for advanced renal cell carcinoma in 1987 [37]. Since then, there has been an increasing number of reports that supports a possible association between IFN therapy and the development or recurrence of sarcoidosis. Although the incidence of IIS is not known, the prevalence of sarcoidosis in IFN-treated HCV patients has been reported to be rare range from 0.09% to 0.44% [38, 39]. The precise prevalence of IIS, however, may be underestimated and difficult to assess because its clinical presentation mimics the constitutional IFN-related adverse effects [6]. Actually, Hoffman et al. found a 5% incidence of sarcoidosis in a cohort of 60 patients who participated in a randomized trial of IFN-α therapy for chronic HCV [40]

Basically the clinical presentation of IIS resembles that of its idiopathic counterpart. The most commonly affected sites of involvement in IIS are skin and lungs, though many other organ systems have also been involved such as liver, joints and heart. The lungs are the most frequent organ affected in IIS (70%), similar but not as high as the incidence reported in typical sarcoidosis (90%). The most frequent symptoms are dry cough and dyspnea. The second major organ is the skin. The incidence of skin involvement appears to be much higher that reported in natural sarcoidosis (60% versus 25%) [6, 38, 41]. The most common skin manifestation is subcutaneous nodules, whereas erythema nodosum, reported to be the most common cutaneous manifestation in typical sarcoidosis, is less frequently observed in IIS. On the basis of the reported cases, IIS with cutaneous involvement can be expected to resolve within approximately 6 months of treatment discontinuation. Its onset may vary from 2 weeks to 3 years after beginning of treatment. Men and women are equally affected [42, 43], and the mean age of patients was approximately 50 years [39]. The majority (roughly two-thirds) of cases of IIS arise during the first 6 months of IFN therapy, but clinical manifestations may also appear after discontinuation of the antiviral treatment [38].

The pathophysiology of IIS is still unclear, but enhancement of Th1 immune response by type I IFNs may play a crucial role. IFN-α has been shown to promote overexpression of MHC class II antigens as well as upregulation of pro-inflammatory cytokines release by APCs and to stimulate monocytes to release IL-12. Furthermore, IFN-α, together with IL-12, can induce the expression of the IL-12 receptor (IL-12R) β2 chain after antigen triggering [44]. In contrast to asthma, T cells in bronchoalveolar lavage fluid in sarcoid lungs express a functional IL-12 receptor composed of both the β1 and β2 subunits [45], suggesting a role of IFN-α in sarcoid pathogenesis. So, type I IFN stimulates the differentiation of Th1-type lymphocytes and reduction of the activation of Th2 lymphocytes, favoring the formation of granuloma in susceptible patients. However, among IIS, when compared to IFN-α therapy, IFN-β-accosiated sarcoidosis is relatively rare [46].

The causal link between type I IFN and sarcoidosis is strengthened by the temporal relationship between IFN therapy and appearance of sarcoidosis, by the remission with therapy cessation, and by the recurrence of symptoms on rechallenge with IFN. The occurrence of sarcoidosis during monotherapy for diseases other than chronic hepatitis also supports this relationship. Another recent study found that in an European American population, serum IFN-α activity was higher in sarcoidosis cases as compared to matched controls [9].

Of patients with IIS, the majority of individuals (approximately 80%) received therapy for chronic HCV infection, while sarcoidosis has also developed in association with the management of hepatitis B infection, multiple sclerosis, hematological and other malignant diseases. To date, more than 80 patients cases of sarcoidosis that occurred in association with IFN-α therapy for chronic HCV have been reported [47]. Similar to other species of viruses and bacteria implicated in the etiology of sarcoidosis [48], some reports have suggested a potential role for the HCV itself in the development of sarcoidosis [38, 49-51]. As chronic HCV infection is associated with induction/stimulation of type 1 cellular immune response causing chronic liver damage [52] as well as various immunological diseases [53-56], it is possible that the antigenicity and viral persistence can serve as a trigger factor for the development of clinical sarcoidosis in susceptible individuals [6]. IFN-α may act as an exacerbationg factor in this situation.

Peginterferon (plus ribavirin) has recently been used to treat HCV infection. Pegylated IFN-α is the result of adding a polyethylene glycol (Peg) moiety to the standard IFN-α molecule. This modification reduces the clearance rate of the protein from the blood and extends the half-time of IFN-α, providing a constant viral suppression which entails a more sustained virological response [57]. Ribavirin, a synthetic guanosine analogue, has been successfully used in conjunction with peginterferon in the treatment of chronic HCV infection due to its ability to inhibit RNA viral replication [58]. Although no cases of sarcoidosis that occurred with ribavirin monotherapy have been reported, ribavirin might be a contributory factor in the development of sarcoidosis via inhibiting Th2 cytokine response, and preserving or enhancing the Th1 immune reaction [59, 60]. This may explain why combination therapy with IFN-α and ribavirin is more efficacious in treating HCV and, conversely, why it also may further predispose patients to immunological disorders such as sarcoidosis [42]. Thus, enhanced clinical efficacy of peginterferon plus ribavirin possibly results from the skewing Th1 response, favoring the appearance of IIS with a greater likelihood than with conventional IFN-α (61).

Most patients with IIS had resolution of their disease without immunosuppressive treatment. Half of the cases in the literature report spontaneous remission, over the course of a few months, after stopping IFN without further therapy. There are even some reports of remission despite continuing IFN therapy. There was, however, a report showing that approximately 11% of cases, usually those with extracutaneous involvement, can have a chronic course and 6% may even reactivate after an initial improvement [38].

From a genetic stand of view, we previously showed an association between a polymorphism in the IFN-α gene (*IFNA*), namely *IFNA17*, and susceptibility to sarcoidosis in the Japanese population [8]. Then, we identified 2 major haplotype of the IFN-α gene and found that an *IFNA* allele, overrepresented in patients with sarcoidosis, was subsequently associated with increased IFN-α and IL-12 production *in vitro* [8]. Moreover, in a recent reported case of IIS, HLA typing was performed and revealed that the patient was positive for HLA-DRB1*03 and HLA-DQB1*02 [62], which have a correlation with the disease course or prognosis in sarcoidosis [63-65]. The authors hypothesized that this HLA profile predisposed the patient to IIS development [62].

In summary, the immunopathogenesis of sarcoidosis is not fully understood, but it is likely that the T cell response is biased toward a Th1 phenotype. To date, many cases of IIS have been reported, suggesting a relationship between sarcoidosis and IFN therapy in patients with a variety of diseases, especially chronic HCV infection. In addition to this, many lines of evidence support the idea that IFN-α appears to play a role in the pathogenesis of sarcoidosis by promoting Th1 immune response.

4. Anti-TNF-associated sarcoidosis

In the recent decades, TNF-α antagonists have made significant therapeutic milestones in the treatment of various inflammatory diseases such as RA, psoriasis, and inflammatory bowel disease. It has been suggested that CD4+ T-helper 1 cells and alveolar macrophages, which secrete IFN-γ and TNF-α, play a pivotal role in the induction and maintenance of sarcoid granuloma [66, 67]. Because of this, it has been postulated that TNF antagonists could be useful for the treatment of granulomatous diseases like sarcoidosis. Indeed, in a multicenter randomized double-blind placebo controlled study of IFX in 138 patients with chronic sarcoidosis, the efficacy of IFX was confirmed [68]. Moreover, case series with a total of 50 patients reported a positive treatment outcome with IFX in different type of sarcoidosis [69]. In contrast, the soluble TNF receptor ETN failed to show therapeutic efficacy in both an open-label trial in progressive pulmonary sarcoidosis and a double-blind randomized trial in refractory chronic ocular sarcoidosis [69-71].

On the other hand, there are increasing cases of acute sarcoidosis and sarcoid-like granulomatosis in patients treated with anti-TNF blocking agents have been reported. The frequency of this adverse effect was roughly estimated to be at least 0.04% (1/2800] [72], and this complication has been described in all three major anti-TNF blocking agents (IFX, ETN, and adalibumab), which suggests a class effect [10]. However, while ETN accounted for 27% of patient years of exposure to all three anti-TNF agents as of 2009, it represented 61% of case reports of anti-TNF-induced sarcoidosis at that time, suggesting some predilection for granuloma formation with this drug [73]. Other studies also suggest an increased risk of sarcoidosis in patients treated with ETN compared to the other two agents [74, 75]. Therefore, it is intriguing that ETN appeared to be more commonly associated with this complication than other anti-TNF drugs and, meanwhile, to be less efficacious in sarcoidosis treatment [70, 71].

The underlying diseases in cases of anti-TNF-associated sarcoidosis include RA, psoriasis/psoriatic arthritis, juvenile idiopathic arthritis, ankylosing spondylitis, and Crohn's disease [19, 76]. The time between initiation of therapy and the onset of signs and symptoms of sarcoidosis in highly variable, with a median duration of approximately 21 months, a range < 1 month to 4 years [76]. Like IIS cases, the clinical picture of this type of sarcoidosis included predominantly pulmonary and cutaneous features. Pulmonary involvement was found in 74% patients, and cutaneous involvement in 29% [76].

The prognosis of sarcoidosis occurring during TNF blockade is generally favorable since almost all patients showed clinical recovery after anti-TNF discontinuation with or without corticosteroid therapy [75, 76]. Therapy with TNF antagonist was discontinued, resulting in spontaneous resolution in some patients, whereas symptoms persisted in others, necessitating corticosteroid treatment (40-50%) [74, 75]. While in some patients recurrence or exacerbations of sarcoidosis after switching to a different TNF antagonist have been reported, other patients were able to switch to a different TNF inhibitor without experiencing recurrences or exacerbations [72, 76].

The pathogenic mechanisms involved in the appearance of sarcoid granulomatosis in patients treated with TNF antagonists are unclear. In addition, there could be notable differences regarding risk of this complication among anti-TNF drugs. Although all the anti-TNF drugs exert their action through blocking TNF-α, they have important differences in their structure and pharmacokinetics, which could explain, in part, the differences that can be observed in clinical efficacy as well as adverse effects, including the risk of granulomatous infections [77]. IFX and adalimumab (ADA) are monoclonal TNF-α antibodies whereas ETN is a TNF-α p75 soluble receptor. ETN binds mainly to soluble TNF-α molecules and interacts with transmembrane TNF with reduced avidity compared with IFX, which binds both transmembrane and soluble TNF. Clearance of ETN is 13 times greater than that of IFX and ADA. Therefore, suppression of TNF-α is greater and more prolonged with IFX and ADA. IFX, therefore, completely neutralizes TNF bioactivity, whereas freely diffusing ETN might be considered to redistribute bioavailable TNF from sites of production to other sites of lower concentration [77]. Also ETN, unlike IFX, does not produce cell lysis, therefore the inhibition of TNF would not be enough to preserve the formation of the granuloma.

Furthermore, a recent study suggested that regulatory T (T reg) cells isolated from patients with active RA were functionally defective in their ability to suppress cytokine production as well as to convey suppressive phenotype to CD4+ effector T cells [78]. Another study showed that sarcoidosis T reg cells, which is globally amplified in circulationg blood and BALF of patients, completely inhibit IL-2 production of CD4+CD25- cells, but not that of IFN-γ or TNF-α, suggesting the insufficient ability of sarcoid T reg cells to control local inflammation [79]. Treatment with IFX can restore the number and function of T reg cells [78]. Thus, treatment with IFX strongly inhibits TNF-α activity, leading to a restoration of T reg cell-mediated inflammatory suppression. In contrast, low levels of TNF-α can persist after treatment with ETN, hence T reg cells may remain down-regulated to some extent and can lead to an sustained Th1 response. Moreover, enhanced IL-17A expression in sarcoid granulomas and in circulating memory T cells from sarcoidosis patients was recently reported [80]. There is a report showing that Th17 responses were inhibited by T reg cells from RA patients responding to the anti-TNF antibody ADA, whereas there was no alteration in T reg number, function or phnotype in ETN treated patients [81].

As previously noted, physiological crosstalk between TNF-α and IFN-α pathways has been reported. There are some indications that type I IFN activity is upregulated during treatment with TNF antagonists in some patients with inflammatory or autoimmune disease [13, 34]. IFN-α can enhance the production of IFN-γ and IL-2, expression levels of both cytokines are elevated in sarcoid T cells [67]. As IFN-γ along with TNF-α is strongly implicated in granuloma formation, the increased production of IFN-γ seen in some patients undergoing anti-TNF therapy [76, 82, 83] may contribute to the development of sarcoid-like granulomatosis. Actually, monoclonal anti-TNF-α antibodies can raise the Th1/Th2 ratio in the peripheral blood [83, 84]. Thus, anti-TNF therapies can modulate the cytokine environment and may restore a Th1 response. IFX and ADA inhibit T cell activation and IFN-γ production, whereas ETN does not [85]. ETN even can enhance T cell production of IFN-γ [84, 86]. This fact could partially explain the greater incidence of sarcoidosis with ETN compared with monoclonal antibody.

It is interesting to note that sarcoid-like granulaoma preferentially developed in the skin and lungs, which are in direct contact with exogenous antigen. Several lines of evidence support the idea that sarcoidosis results from exposures to possible environmental agents such as *Mycobacterium tuberculosis* (*M. tuberculosis*) and *Propionibacterium acnes* (*P. acnes*) [87-89]. *M. tuberculosis* or *P. acnes* associated with anti-TNF treatment was also reported [90, 91]. Anti-TNF drugs are known to decrease antigenic clearance and increase infections. Then, mechanisms involved in granulomatosis development during anti-TNF therapy could include increased susceptibility to infection and modification of the cytokine environment and cellular recruit-ment within the tissues [72]. Among ant-TNF drugs, several studies indicate that infection with granulomatous pathogens such as *M. tuberculosis*, histoplasmosis, and coccidioidomycosis occur with 2-10-fold greater frequencies in patients treated with IFX than in those treated with ETN [85, 92-94]. Additionally, in most cases of *Listeria monocytogenes* infection during treatment with anti-TNF agent, IFX or ETN, patients had received IFX [95]. Both IFN-γ and TNF-α are essential for protection against tuberculosis. The higher risk of such intracellular granuloma-tous pathogens that IFX poses than does ETN is therefore possibly due to the simultaneous suppression of TNF-α and IFN-γ, and may as well explain why IFX, but not ETN, is effective in treatment of sarcoidosis, where the presense of both IFN-γ and TNF-α is necessary.

Together, the development of sarcoid-like granulomatosis during therapy with TNF antago-nist is paradoxical in view of the central role of TNF-α in the formation and maintenance of granulomas. There seems to be significant differences between the 2 classes of TNF antagonists in the risk of this complication with the greater incidence of a soluble TNF receptor ETN-associated sarcoidosis. Anti-TNF monoclonal antibody IFX or ADA can suppress TNF-α as well as IFN-γ and inhibit Th1 (and Th17) response partially through restoring the number and function of T reg cells. IFX and ADA may also eliminate activated T cells and monocyte/ macrophage directly either by cell lysis or by inducing apoptosis [96]. On the contrary, ETN therapy may result in an insufficient inhibition of TNF bioactivity and may enhance Th1 response with IFN-γ production causing the formation of the granuloma.

5. Conclusion

Type I IFN and TNF-α are cytokines with important roles in coordinating immune reactions and potentially appear to contribute to the local and systemic inflammatory processes underlying sarcoidosis pathogenesis. The increasing case reports of interferon-induced and TNF-associated sarcoidosis support this idea. A cross-regulation between type I IFN and TNF-α has been proposed in some autoimmune or inflammatory disorders. However, the studies in patients with sarcoidosis show that there is not necessarily a direct balance between the levels of type I IFN and TNF-α, and that the type of clinical manifestations, the disease phase, and patient heterogeneity may contribute to create a complex picture. Ancestral background as well as genetic polymorphisms may influence each cytokine level and clinical manifestations, which can cause heterogeneous phenotype of the disease. Further work regarding sarcoidosis induced by the cytokine/anti-cytokine therapy as well as clinical and *in vitro* studies in sarcoidosis will help evaluate and treat these patients properly depend on the disease phenotype and disease activity in the future.

Author details

Mitsuteru Akahoshi

Address all correspondence to: akahoshi@intmed1.med.kyushu-u.ac.jp

Department of Medicine and Biosystemic Science, Kyushu University Graduate School of Medical Sciences, Fukuoka, Japan

References

[1] Iannuzzi MC, Rybicki BA, Teirstein AS. Sarcoidosis. *N Engl J Med*. 2007;357(21): 2153-2165.

[2] Moller DR, et al. Enhanced expression of IL-12 associated with Th1 cytokine profiles in active pulmonary sarcoidosis. *J Immunol*. 1996;156(12):4952-4960.

[3] Crouser ED, et al. Gene expression profiling identifies MMP-12 and ADAMDEC1 as potential pathogenic mediators of pulmonary sarcoidosis. *Am J Respir Crit Care Med.* 2009;179(10):929-938.

[4] Niewold TB, Hua J, Lehman TJ, Harley JB, Crow MK. High serum IFN-α activity is a heritable risk factor for systemic lupus erythematosus. *Genes Immun.* 2007;8(6): 492-502.

[5] Raanani P, Ben-Bassat I. Immune-mediated complications during interferon therapy in hematological patients. *Acta Haematol.* 2002;107(3):133-144.

[6] Alazemi S, Campos MA. Interferon-induced sarcoidosis. *Int J Clin Pract.* 2006;60(2): 201-211.

[7] Doyle MK, Berggren R, Magnus JH. Interferon-induced sarcoidosis. *J Clin Rheumatol.* 2006;12(5):241-248.

[8] Akahoshi M, et al. Association between *IFNA* genotype and the risk of sarcoidosis. *Hum Genet.* 2004;114(5):503-509.

[9] Sweiss NJ, et al. Linkage of type I interferon activity and TNF-alpha levels in serum with sarcoidosis manifestations and ancestry. *PLoS One.* 2011;6(12):e29126.

[10] Massara A, Cavazzini L, La Corte R, Trotta F. Sarcoidosis appearing during anti-tumor necrosis factor α therapy: a new "class effect" paradoxical phenomenon. Two case reports and literature review. *Semin Arthritis Rheum.* 2010;39(4):313-319.

[11] Cantaert T, Baeten D, Tak PP, van Baarsen LG. Type I IFN and TNFα cross-regulation in immune-mediated inflammatory disease: basic concepts and clinical relevance. *Arthritis Res Ther.* 2010;12(5):219.

[12] Gonzalez-Navajas JM, Lee J, David M, Raz E. Immunomodulatory functions of type I interferons. *Nat Rev Immunol.* 2012;12(2):125-135.

[13] Palucka AK, Blanck JP, Bennett L, Pascual V, Banchereau J. Cross-regulation of TNF and IFN-α in autoimmune diseases. *Proc Natl Acad Sci U S A.* 2005;102(9):3372-3377.

[14] Preble OT, Black RJ, Friedman RM, Klippel JH, Vilcek J. Systemic lupus erythematosus: presence in human serum of an unusual acid-labile leukocyte interferon. *Science.* 1982;216(4544):429-431.

[15] Ytterberg SR, Schnitzer TJ. Serum interferon levels in patients with systemic lupus erythematosus. *Arthritis Rheum.* 1982;25(4):401-406.

[16] Niewold TB. Interferon alpha as a primary pathogenic factor in human lupus. *J Interferon Cytokine Res.* 2011;31(12):887-892.

[17] Niewold TB, Swedler WI. Systemic lupus erythematosus arising during interferon-alpha therapy for cryoglobulinemic vasculitis associated with hepatitis C. *Clin Rheumatol.* 2005;24(2):178-181.

[18] Feldmann M, Maini RN. Anti-TNFα therapy of rheumatoid arthritis: what have we learned? *Annu Rev Immunol.* 2001;19:163-196.

[19] Ramos-Casals M, Roberto Perez A, Diaz-Lagares C, Cuadrado MJ, Khamashta MA. Autoimmune diseases induced by biological agents: a double-edged sword? *Autoimmun Rev.* 2010;9(3):188-193.

[20] Katz U, Zandman-Goddard G. Drug-induced lupus: an update. *Autoimmun Rev.* 2010;10(1):46-50.

[21] Cuchacovich R, Espinoza CG, Virk Z, Espinoza LR. Biologic therapy (TNF-alpha antagonists)-induced psoriasis: a cytokine imbalance between TNF-alpha and IFN-alpha? *J Clin Rheumatol.* 2008;14(6):353-356.

[22] Lutz MB, et al. An advanced culture method for generating large quantities of highly pure dendritic cells from mouse bone marrow. *J Immunol Methods.* 1999;223(1):77-92.

[23] Bave U, Vallin H, Alm GV, Ronnblom L. Activation of natural interferon-α producing cells by apoptotic U937 cells combined with lupus IgG and its regulation by cytokines. *J Autoimmun.* 2001;17(1):71-80.

[24] Davis LS, Hutcheson J, Mohan C. The role of cytokines in the pathogenesis and treatment of systemic lupus erythematosus. *J Interferon Cytokine Res.* 2011;31(10):781-789.

[25] Weckerle CE, et al. Large-scale analysis of tumor necrosis factor α levels in systemic lupus erythematosus. *Arthritis Rheum.* 2012;64(9):2947-2952.

[26] Niewold TB, Kariuki SN, Morgan GA, Shrestha S, Pachman LM. Elevated serum interferon-α activity in juvenile dermatomyositis: associations with disease activity at diagnosis and after thirty-six months of therapy. *Arthritis Rheum.* 2009;60(6): 1815-1824.

[27] Medica I, Kastrin A, Maver A, Peterlin B. Role of genetic polymorphisms in ACE and TNF-α gene in sarcoidosis: a meta-analysis. *J Hum Genet.* 2007;52(10):836-847.

[28] Wijnen PA, Nelemans PJ, Verschakelen JA, Bekers O, Voorter CE, Drent M. The role of tumor necrosis factor alpha G-308A polymorphisms in the course of pulmonary sarcoidosis. *Tissue Antigens.* 2010;75(3):262-268.

[29] Pachman LM, et al. TNFα-308A allele in juvenile dermatomyositis: association with increased production of tumor necrosis factor α, disease duration, and pathologic calcifications. *Arthritis Rheum.* 2000;43(10):2368-2377.

[30] Niewold TB, Kariuki SN, Morgan GA, Shrestha S, Pachman LM. Gene-gene-sex interaction in cytokine gene polymorphisms revealed by serum interferon alpha phenotype in juvenile dermatomyositis. *J Pediatr.* 2010;157(4):653-657.

[31] van Holten J, Smeets TJ, Blankert P, Tak PP. Expression of interferon β in synovial tissue from patients with rheumatoid arthritis: comparison with patients with osteoarthritis and reactive arthritis. *Ann Rheum Dis.* 2005;64(12):1780-1782.

[32] van Baarsen LG, et al. Regulation of IFN response gene activity during infliximab treatment in rheumatoid arthritis is associated with clinical response to treatment. *Arthritis Res Ther*;12(1):R11.

[33] Cantaert T, et al. Exposure to nuclear antigens contributes to the induction of humoral autoimmunity during tumour necrosis factor alpha blockade. *Ann Rheum Dis.* 2009;68(6):1022-1029.

[34] Mavragani CP, Niewold TB, Moutsopoulos NM, Pillemer SR, Wahl SM, Crow MK. Augmented interferon-α pathway activation in patients with Sjogren's syndrome treated with etanercept. *Arthritis Rheum.* 2007;56(12):3995-4004.

[35] Dastmalchi M, et al. A high incidence of disease flares in an open pilot study of infliximab in patients with refractory inflammatory myopathies. *Ann Rheum Dis.* 2008;67(12):1670-1677.

[36] Agostini C, Adami F, Semenzato G. New pathogenetic insights into the sarcoid granuloma. *Curr Opin Rheumatol.* 2000;12(1):71-76.

[37] Abdi EA, Nguyen GK, Ludwig RN, Dickout WJ. Pulmonary sarcoidosis following interferon therapy for advanced renal cell carcinoma. *Cancer.* 1987;59(5):896-900.

[38] Ramos-Casals M, et al. Sarcoidosis in patients with chronic hepatitis C virus infection: analysis of 68 cases. *Medicine (Baltimore).* 2005;84(2):69-80.

[39] Goldberg HJ, Fiedler D, Webb A, Jagirdar J, Hoyumpa AM, Peters J. Sarcoidosis after treatment with interferon-α: a case series and review of the literature. *Respir Med.* 2006;100(11):2063-2068.

[40] Hoffmann RM, et al. Sarcoidosis associated with interferon-alpha therapy for chronic hepatitis C. *J Hepatol.* 1998;28(6):1058-1063.

[41] Adla M, Downey KK, Ahmad J. Hepatic sarcoidosis associated with pegylated interferon alfa therapy for chronic hepatitis C: case report and review of literature. *Dig Dis Sci.* 2008;53(10):2810-2812.

[42] Hurst EA, Mauro T. Sarcoidosis associated with pegylated interferon alfa and ribavirin treatment for chronic hepatitis C: a case report and review of the literature. *Arch Dermatol.* 2005;141(7):865-868.

[43] Cogrel O, Doutre MS, Marliere V, Beylot-Barry M, Couzigou P, Beylot C. Cutaneous sarcoidosis during interferon alfa and ribavirin treatment of hepatitis C virus infection: two cases. *Br J Dermatol.* 2002;146(2):320-324.

[44] Rogge L, et al. Selective expression of an interleukin-12 receptor component by human T helper 1 cells. *J Exp Med.* 1997;185(5):825-831.

[45] Rogge L, et al. Antibodies to the IL-12 receptor β2 chain mark human Th1 but not Th2 cells in vitro and in vivo. *J Immunol.* 1999;162(7):3926-3932.

[46]   Chakravarty SD, Harris ME, Schreiner AM, Crow MK. Sarcoidosis Triggered by In-
       terferon-Beta Treatment of Multiple Sclerosis: A Case Report and Focused Literature
       Review. *Semin Arthritis Rheum*. 2012.

[47]   Fantini F, Padalino C, Gualdi G, Monari P, Giannetti A. Cutaneous lesions as initial
       signs of interferon α-induced sarcoidosis: report of three new cases and review of the
       literature. *Dermatol Ther*. 2009;22 Suppl 1:S1-7.

[48]   Statement on sarcoidosis. Joint Statement of the American Thoracic Society (ATS),
       the European Respiratory Society (ERS) and the World Association of Sarcoidosis
       and Other Granulomatous Disorders (WASOG) adopted by the ATS Board of Direc-
       tors and by the ERS Executive Committee, February 1999. *Am J Respir Crit Care Med*.
       1999;160(2):736-755.

[49]   Bonnet F, et al. Sarcoidosis-associated hepatitis C virus infection. *Dig Dis Sci*.
       2002;47(4):794-796.

[50]   Tsimpoukas F, Goritsas C, Papadopoulos N, Trigidou R, Ferti A. Sarcoidosis in un-
       treated chronic hepatitis C virus infection. *Scand J Gastroenterol*. 2004;39(4):401-403.

[51]   Yamada S, Mine S, Fujisaki T, Ohnari N, Eto S, Tanaka Y. Hepatic sarcoidosis associ-
       ated with chronic hepatitis C. *J Gastroenterol*. 2002;37(7):564-570.

[52]   Bertoletti A, et al. Different cytokine profiles of intrahepatic T cells in chronic hepa-
       titis B and hepatitis C virus infections. *Gastroenterology*. 1997;112(1):193-199.

[53]   Agnello V, Chung RT, Kaplan LM. A role for hepatitis C virus infection in type II cry-
       oglobulinemia. *N Engl J Med*. 1992;327(21):1490-1495.

[54]   Eddy S, Wim R, Peter VE, Tanja R, Jan T, Werner VS. Myasthenia gravis: another au-
       toimmune disease associated with hepatitis C virus infection. *Dig Dis Sci*. 1999;44(1):
       186-189.

[55]   Haddad J, et al. Lymphocytic sialadenitis of Sjögren's syndrome associated with
       chronic hepatitis C virus liver disease. *Lancet*. 1992;339(8789):321-323.

[56]   Mayo MJ. Extrahepatic manifestations of hepatitis C infection. *Am J Med Sci*.
       2003;325(3):135-148.

[57]   Fried MW, et al. Peginterferon alfa-2a plus ribavirin for chronic hepatitis C virus in-
       fection. *N Engl J Med*. 2002;347(13):975-982.

[58]   Di Bisceglie AM, et al. Ribavirin as therapy for chronic hepatitis C. A randomized,
       double-blind, placebo-controlled trial. *Ann Intern Med*. 1995;123(12):897-903.

[59]   Ning Q, et al. Ribavirin inhibits viral-induced macrophage production of TNF, IL-1,
       the procoagulant fgl2 prothrombinase and preserves Th1 cytokine production but in-
       hibits Th2 cytokine response. *J Immunol*. 1998;160(7):3487-3493.

[60] Tam RC, et al. Ribavirin polarizes human T cell responses towards a Type 1 cytokine profile. *J Hepatol*. 1999;30(3):376-382.

[61] Guilabert A, Bosch X, Julia M, Iranzo P, Mascaro JM, Jr. Pegylated interferon alfa-induced sarcoidosis: two sides of the same coin. *Br J Dermatol*. 2005;152(2):377-379.

[62] Zampino MR, Corazza M, Borghi A, Marzola A, Virgili A. HLA typing in an IFN-α-induced scar sarcoidosis: possible pathogenetic and clinical implications. *Acta Derm Venereol*. 2009;89(6):661-662.

[63] Grunewald J, Eklund A, Olerup O. Human leukocyte antigen class I alleles and the disease course in sarcoidosis patients. *Am J Respir Crit Care Med*. 2004;169(6):696-702.

[64] Seitzer U, Gerdes J, Muller-Quernheim J. Genotyping in the MHC locus: potential for defining predictive markers in sarcoidosis. *Respir Res*. 2002;3:6.

[65] Sato H, et al. HLA-DQB1*0201: a marker for good prognosis in British and Dutch patients with sarcoidosis. *Am J Respir Cell Mol Biol*. 2002;27(4):406-412.

[66] Ziegenhagen MW, Muller-Quernheim J. The cytokine network in sarcoidosis and its clinical relevance. *J Intern Med*. 2003;253(1):18-30.

[67] Nunes H, Soler P, Valeyre D. Pulmonary sarcoidosis. *Allergy*. 2005;60(5):565-582.

[68] Baughman RP, et al. Infliximab therapy in patients with chronic sarcoidosis and pulmonary involvement. *Am J Respir Crit Care Med*. 2006;174(7):795-802.

[69] Baeten D, van Hagen PM. Use of TNF blockers and other targeted therapies in rare refractory immune-mediated inflammatory diseases: evidence-based or rational? *Ann Rheum Dis*. 2010;69(12):2067-2073.

[70] Utz JP, et al. Etanercept for the treatment of stage II and III progressive pulmonary sarcoidosis. *Chest*. 2003;124(1):177-185.

[71] Baughman RP, Lower EE, Bradley DA, Raymond LA, Kaufman A. Etanercept for refractory ocular sarcoidosis: results of a double-blind randomized trial. *Chest*. 2005;128(2):1062-1047.

[72] Daien CI, et al. Sarcoid-like granulomatosis in patients treated with tumor necrosis factor blockers: 10 cases. *Rheumatology (Oxford)*. 2009;48(8):883-886.

[73] Skoie IM, Wildhagen K, Omdal R. Development of sarcoidosis following etanercept treatment: a report of three cases. *Rheumatol Int*. 2012;32(4):1049-1053.

[74] Gifre L, Ruiz-Esquide V, Xaubet A, Gomez-Puerta JA, Hernandez MV, Sanmarti R. Lung sarcoidosis induced by TNF antagonists in rheumatoid arthritis: a case presentation and a literature review. *Arch Bronconeumol*. 2011;47(4):208-212.

[75] Kanellopoulou T, Filiotou A, Kranidioti H, Dourakis SP. Sarcoid-like granulomatosis in patients treated with anti-TNFα factors. A case report and review of the literature. *Clin Rheumatol*. 2011;30(4):581-583.

[76] Borchers AT, Leibushor N, Cheema GS, Naguwa SM, Gershwin ME. Immune-mediated adverse effects of biologicals used in the treatment of rheumatic diseases. *J Autoimmun.* 2011;37(4):273-288.

[77] Wallis RS, Ehlers S. Tumor necrosis factor and granuloma biology: explaining the differential infection risk of etanercept and infliximab. *Semin Arthritis Rheum.* 2005;34(5 Suppl1):34-38.

[78] Ehrenstein MR, et al. Compromised function of regulatory T cells in rheumatoid arthritis and reversal by anti-TNFα therapy. *J Exp Med.* 2004;200(3):277-285.

[79] Miyara M, et al. The immune paradox of sarcoidosis and regulatory T cells. *J Exp Med.* 2006;203(2):359-370.

[80] Ten Berge B, et al. Increased IL-17A expression in granulomas and in circulating memory T cells in sarcoidosis. *Rheumatology (Oxford).* 2012;51(1):37-46.

[81] McGovern JL, Nguyen DX, Notley CA, Mauri C, Isenberg DA, Ehrenstein MR. Th17 cells are restrained by regulatory T cells from patients responding to anti-TNF antibody therapy via inhibition of IL-6. *Arthritis Rheum.* 2012.

[82] Berg L, Lampa J, Rogberg S, van Vollenhoven R, Klareskog L. Increased peripheral T cell reactivity to microbial antigens and collagen type II in rheumatoid arthritis after treatment with soluble TNFalpha receptors. *Ann Rheum Dis.* 2001;60(2):133-139.

[83] Baeten D, et al. Impaired Th1 cytokine production in spondyloarthropathy is restored by anti-TNFα. *Ann Rheum Dis.* 2001;60(8):750-755.

[84] Maurice MM, van der Graaff WL, Leow A, Breedveld FC, van Lier RA, Verweij CL. Treatment with monoclonal anti-tumor necrosis factor α antibody results in an accumulation of Th1 CD4+ T cells in the peripheral blood of patients with rheumatoid arthritis. *Arthritis Rheum.* 1999;42(10):2166-2173.

[85] Saliu OY, Sofer C, Stein DS, Schwander SK, Wallis RS. Tumor-necrosis-factor blockers: differential effects on mycobacterial immunity. *J Infect Dis.* 2006;194(4):486-492.

[86] Kawashima M, Miossec P. Effect of treatment of rheumatoid arthritis with infliximab on IFNγ, IL4, T-bet, and GATA-3 expression: link with improvement of systemic inflammation and disease activity. *Ann Rheum Dis.* 2005;64(3):415-418.

[87] Ishige I, Usui Y, Takemura T, Eishi Y. Quantitative PCR of mycobacterial and propionibacterial DNA in lymph nodes of Japanese patients with sarcoidosis. *Lancet.* 1999;354(9173):120-123.

[88] Drake WP, Pei Z, Pride DT, Collins RD, Cover TL, Blaser MJ. Molecular analysis of sarcoidosis tissues for mycobacterium species DNA. *Emerg Infect Dis.* 2002;8(11): 1334-1341.

[89] Gazouli M, Ikonomopoulos J, Trigidou R, Foteinou M, Kittas C, Gorgoulis V. Assessment of mycobacterial, propionibacterial, and human herpesvirus 8 DNA in tissues of greek patients with sarcoidosis. *J Clin Microbiol*. 2002;40(8):3060-3063.

[90] Keane J, et al. Tuberculosis associated with infliximab, a tumor necrosis factor α-neutralizing agent. *N Engl J Med*. 2001;345(15):1098-1104.

[91] Bassi E, Poli F, Charachon A, Claudepierre P, Revuz J. Infliximab-induced acne: report of two cases. *Br J Dermatol*. 2007;156(2):402-403.

[92] Wallis RS, Broder M, Wong J, Lee A, Hoq L. Reactivation of latent granulomatous infections by infliximab. *Clin Infect Dis*. 2005;41 Suppl 3:S194-198.

[93] Bergstrom L, et al. Increased risk of coccidioidomycosis in patients treated with tumor necrosis factor α antagonists. *Arthritis Rheum*. 2004;50(6):1959-1966.

[94] Lee JH, et al. Life-threatening histoplasmosis complicating immunotherapy with tumor necrosis factor α antagonists infliximab and etanercept. *Arthritis Rheum*. 2002;46(10):2565-2570.

[95] Slifman NR, Gershon SK, Lee JH, Edwards ET, Braun MM. Listeria monocytogenes infection as a complication of treatment with tumor necrosis factor α-neutralizing agents. *Arthritis Rheum*. 2003;48(2):319-324.

[96] Furst DE, Wallis R, Broder M, Beenhouwer DO. Tumor necrosis factor antagonists: different kinetics and/or mechanisms of action may explain differences in the risk for developing granulomatous infection. *Semin Arthritis Rheum*. 2006;36(3):159-167.

Genetic Factors

Chapter 3

Genetics of Sarcoidosis

Nabeel Y. Hamzeh and Lisa A. Maier

Additional information is available at the end of the chapter

1. Introduction

Sarcoidosis is a multi-system, T-helper 1 (Th1) cell biased granulomatous disorder. The current hypothesis is that sarcoidosis develops in a genetically predisposed individual who is exposed to a yet unknown environmental trigger(s) [1]. Antigen presentation in the context of major histocompatibility complex II (MHC-II) activates Th1 cells with subsequent production of various cytokines and chemokines including but not limited to IFN-γ, TNF-α, TGF-β, IL-2, IL-12 and others leading to further immune cell recruitment and activation [2]. The immune response ultimately leads to the formation of granulomas which consist of a central core of mononuclear cells surrounded by CD4+ cells and a small number of CD8+ and B-cells [2]. A role for regulatory T-cells has been proposed but their exact role in sarcoidosis is yet unknown [3].

The disparity in prevalence and variability of organ involvement between ethnic groups [1] and the familial clustering of sarcoidosis strongly support a genetic basis for sarcoidosis [4]. Several genome wide associations studies (GWAS) have identified potential association between specific genetic loci and sarcoidosis [5-11] and several studies have also associated various human leukocyte antigen (HLA) markers and gene-specific single nucleotide polymorphisms (SNP) with the risk, disease course and organ involvement with sarcoidosis indicating that sarcoidosis is a polygenic disease. Adding to this complexity, certain genetic markers have shown an association based on ethnicity and gender and some have shown differential associations based on gender and ethnicity [34]. Genetic polymorphisms that are functional can potentially influence the immune system's recognition of an antigen and the subsequent immune response to the antigen thus dictating disease phenotype (Figure 1).

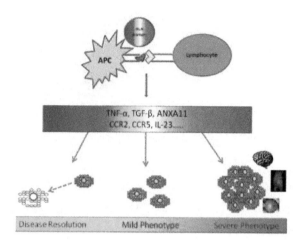

Figure 1. Functional genetic polymorphisms dictate immune response and disease phenotype

Genetic studies have played an important role in revealing new pathways and mechanisms involved in the pathogenesis of immune mediated diseases such as rheumatoid arthritis, inflammatory bowel disease, psoriasis, systemic lupus erythematosus, type 1 diabetes and others [12]. Genome-wide association studies investigate the potential association of a disease with genetic markers across the entire genome without a mechanistic hypothesis [13]. Thousands of representative SNPs (tagging SNPs) that span the whole genome are assayed for potential association with a specific disease. In contrast, a candidate-gene approach is hypothesis driven and investigates the potential association of disease with polymorphisms in a specific gene(s) that encode molecule(s) (receptor, cytokine, signal transduction…) that are involved in the pathogenesis of a disease [13]. Familial-genetic studies investigate the association of genetic markers with a rare disease. Family members of an affected individual are studied for genetic markers that are present in affected members but absent in others [13].

Several environmental and infectious agents have been proposed to be associated with sarcoidosis but none proven yet. The ACCESS (A Case Controlled Etiological Study in Sarcoidosis) study group identified 5 occupations and 5 exposures that were more prevalent in sarcoidosis patients [14]. These exposures included agricultural employment, physicians, jobs raising birds, jobs in automotive manufacturing and middle/secondary school teachers, insecticides, employment in pesticide-using industries, occupational exposure to mold and mildew, occupational exposure to musty odors and use of home central air-conditioning [14]. In contrast, smoking appears to be protective against sarcoidosis [14, 15]. Infectious agents, particularly Mycobateria, are re-emerging as a potential antigen in sarcoidosis with studies detecting Mycobacteria proteins in tissues from sarcoidosis patients and T-cells from sarcoidosis patients responding to stimulation by Mycobacterial antigens [16-23]. Recent studies have also demonstrated an interaction between genetic markers and in vitro immune responses to Mycobacterial antigens further supporting the gene-environment interaction theory. [22]

In this review, we will attempt to summarize the current literature on the association of genetic markers with sarcoidosis from a functional perspective and highlight differences that might exist between different racial groups.

Genetic markers and risk of disease (Table 1):

Gene	Polymorphism	Population	OR	CI	p	Ref
Lofgren's Syndrome						
HLA	DRB1*03	White UK/Dutch	7.97	4.16-15.26	<0.0001	[26]
	DRB1*0301	White Spanish	3.52	1.83-6.79	0.0004	[27]
	DRB1*0301	White Swedish	7.71	4.63-12.84	<0.0001	[27]
	DRB1*03	White Swedish	6.71	NR	<0.0001	[28]
	DRB1*03-DQB1*0201	White Dutch	12.5	5.69-27.52	<0.0001	[29]
	DRB1*0301	Finnish	2.46	1.11-5.45	0.044	[33]
	DRB1*1501	Finnish	2.16	1.06-4.41	0.037	[33]
MHC2TA	rs3087456G	White Swedish	1.31†	1.04-1.65†	.019	[31]
	rs11074932C	White Swedish	1.27†	1.02-1.58†	.026	[31]
BTNL2	rs3117099T	White UK/Dutch	3.05	2.01-4.62	<0.0001	[26]
CCR2	Haplotype 2*	White Dutch	4.4	1.9-9.7	<0.0001	[41]
	Haplotype 2*	Spanish	2.03	1.11-3.73	0.041	[27]
	Haplotype 2*	Swedish	3.02	1.65-5.52	0.0027	[27]
CCR5	rs2040388A	German/Female	1.93	1.35-2.77	0.0003	[53]
	rs2856757C	German/Female	1.65	1.17-2.33	0.004	[53]
TNF#	TNF-α 308AA rs1800629	US White	8.182	2.45-27.34	0.027	[73]
	TNF-α 308A rs1800629	Polish	2.3	1.23-4.32	<0.01	[77]
	TNF-α 308A	UK/Dutch	3.1†	1.33-7.20†	0.006	[78]
	TNF-α 308A	German	NR	NR	0.0078	[79]
	LTA-252G rs909253	Polish	2.98	1.67-5.29	<0.001	[77]
	LTA-252GG rs909253	US White females	11.33	3.18-40.37	0.027	[73]
ANXA11	rs1049550TT	Czech	0.31	0.11-0.84	0.02	[95]
Increased risk of non-Lofgren's						
HLA	DQB1*0602-DRB1*15	White Dutch	2.27	1.46-3.54†	0.0032	[32]
	DRB1*12	White UK/Dutch	2.5	1.26-4.96	0.003	[26]
	DRB1*12	UK	3.7	1.73-7.94	0.001	[29]
	DRB1*12	Japanese	2.5	1.17-5.21	0.03	[29]
	DRB1*1201	US White/AA	2.13	1.14-4.12	0.015	[34]
	DRB1*10	White UK/Dutch	2.4	1.00-5.88	0.01	[26]
	DRB1*14	White UK/Dutch	3.1	1.7-5.57	0.0003	[26]
	DRB1*14	White Swedish	1.79	NR	0.017	[28]
	DRB1*1401	US White/AA	2.29	1.21-4.34	0.011	[34]

Gene	Polymorphism	Population	OR	CI	p	Ref
	DRB1*14	UK	2.54	1.47-4.41	0.001	[29]
	DQB1*0503/4	Dutch	2.4	1.11-5.18	0.04	[29]
	DRB1*15	Finnish	1.67	1.12-2.5	0.011	[33]
	DRB1*1501	US White/AA	1.7	1.18-2.46	0.003	[34]
	DRB1*1101	US White/AA	1.98	1.37-2.9	<0.001	[34]
	DRB3*0101	US White/AA	1.6	1.16-2.2	0.004	[34]
	DRB1*1201	US AA	2.67	1.2-6.52	0.014	[34]
	DPB1*0101	US AA	1.72	1.14-2.62	0.008	[34]
	DRB1*0402	US white	2.57	1.02-7.28	0.043	[34]
	DRB1*1501	US White	2.08	1.39-3.15	<0.001	[34]
	DRB1*13	Czech	2.4	1.43-4.03	<0.02	[74]
BTNL-2	rs2076530A	German	2.31	1.27-4.23	<0.006	[37]
	rs2076530A	White UK/Dutch	1.49	1.20-1.86	0.002	[26]
	rs2076530A	White Dutch	1.85	1.19-2.88	0.007	[38]
	rs2076530A	White US	2.03	1.32-3.12	NR	[39]
	rs2294878C	White UK/Dutch	1.54	1.24-1.92	0.001	[26]
TNF	LTA-252G rs909253	Czech	2.63	1.63-4.25	<0.00001	[74]
	TNF-α 308A rs1800629	Polish	2.167	1.17-4.01	<0.05	[77]
	TNF-α -857T	UK/Dutch	NR	NR	0.002	[78]
TLR						
TLR-10	rs1109695C	Dutch	NR	NR	0.002	[68]
	rs7658893A	Dutch	NR	NR	0.001	[68]
TLR-1	rs5743604G	Dutch	NR	NR	0.003	[68]
	rs5743594G	Dutch	NR	NR	0.049	[68]
SLC11A1						
	Allele 2$^\varepsilon$	US AA	0.48	0.28-0.81	0.014	[69]
	Allele 3$^¥$	Polish	1.68	1.01-2.81	0.04	[71]
	Allele 3$^¥$	Turkish	2.69	1.61-4.47	<0.001	[70]
	Allele 3$^¥$	Greek	1.52	1.08-4.52	0.015	[72]
	INT4	Turkish	2.75	1.68-4.52	<0.001	[70]
ANXA11	rs1049550C	German	1.54	1.23-1.92	0.00014	[94]
	rs1049550T	Czech	0.77	NR	0.04	[95]
	rs2573346C	German	1.55	1.24-1.92	0.00008	[94]
Decreased risk						
HLA	DRB1*01	White Swedish	0.61	NR	0.003	[28]
	DRB1*01	White UK/Dutch	0.5	0.35-0.82	0.001	[26]
	DRB1*01	UK	0.5	0.34-0.76	0.001	[29]
	DRB1*01	Dutch	0.4	0.23-0.76	0.006	[29]
	DRB1*01	Japanese	0.12	0.03-0.52	0.001	[29]
	DRB1*01	Finnish	0.43	0.26-0.72	0.001	[109]
	DRB1*04	White UK/Dutch	0.6	0.46-0.92	0.02	[26]

Gene	Polymorphism	Population	OR	CI	p	Ref
	DRB1*0401	US White/AA	0.48	0.28-0.8	0.003	[34]
	DRB1*04	UK	0.54	0.35-0.84	0.008	[29]
	DQB1*0301	UK	0.69	0.51-0.94	0.02	[29]
	DQB1*0603	US Males	0.5	NR	NR	[34]
	DRB1*1503	US AA	0.56	0.3-0.99	0.44	[34]
	DRB1*0401	Us white	0.44	0.25-0.77	0.003	[34]
	DRB1*07	Czech	0.40†	0.21-0.76†	0.0031	[74]
CCR2						
	CCR2-64I	Japanese	0.37	0.21-0.67	0.0007	[43]

US: United States of America

UK: United Kingdom

AA: African American.

HLA: Human Leukocyte Antigen.

TLR: Toll-like receptor

NR: Not reported.

£Allele 2: $T(GT)_5AC(GT)_5AC(GT)_{10}$

¥Allele 3: $T(GT)_5AC(GT)_5AC(GT)_9$

*haplotype 2: (A at -6752,A at 3000, T at 3547 and T at 4385)

#TNF association with erythema nodosum

† Values calculated by authors from raw data provided in original manuscript.

Table 1. Association of genetic markers with risk of developing sarcoidosis.

Numerous studies have been published investigating the association of genetic markers with the risk of developing sarcoidosis or the risk of disease severity, disease course or specific organ involvement [5-11]. Genetic polymorphisms, that are functional, can influence the immune system's response or function leading to active, progressive disease or self-resolving, limited disease. Although it is yet unknown if, and how, many of the genetic polymorphisms detected can influence the immune response, they do provide new insight on pathways that are potentially involved in the pathogenesis of sarcoidosis and provide new potential therapeutic targets.

2. Receptors

2.1. HLA region

The HLA system plays an important role in the immune response and has been associated with various autoimmune diseases [24]. The HLA genes are encoded on chromosome 6 and consist of over 200 genes [25]. HLA class I molecules, HLA-A, B and C, are expressed by most somatic cells and are important in the immune response [25]. They are composed of an α polypeptide chain, which is coded by the class I genes, and a β chain which is coded by the β_2-microglobulin gene on chromosome 15 [25]. The HLA class II genes code for the α and β polypeptides of the class II molecule [25]. The HLA class II molecules are designated by 3 letters, the first (D) represents the class, the second (M,O,P,Q or R) represent the family and the third (A or B) represent the α or β chains [25]. The numbers that precedes the asterisk indicates the gene and the numbers following the asterisk represent the allelic variant of that gene [25]. HLA class II molecules are primarily expressed on immune cells. The HLA class II molecules play an important role in the immune response presenting antigens to the effector cells and induce activation of the immune cells [25].

Sarcoidosis can present insidiously (non-Lofgren's syndrome) or present acutely with systemic symptoms, acute arthritis, erythema nodosum and bilateral hilar lymphadenopathy, more commonly known as Lofgren's syndrome (LS) [1]. Several HLA alleles have been associated with LS. HLA-DRB1 is the most common and has been reported in a white Dutch and UK cohorts [26], Spanish and Swedish cohorts (HLA-DRB1*0301) [27], a Scandinavian cohort (HLA-DRB1*03) [28] and a Dutch cohort (HLA-DRB1*03-DQB1*0201) [29]. In addition, HLA-DQB1*0201 has been reported In White UK and Dutch cohorts [30]. HLA-DRB1*03 and HLA-DQB1*02 are in strong LD [30]. In addition, 2 SNPs (rs3087456 and rs11074932) in the major histocompatibility complex class II transactivator (MHC2TA) gene, which acts as a master regulator for the expression of MHC class II molecules, were found to be associated with LS independent of HLA-DRB1*03 [31].

Several HLA alleles have also been associated with increased risk of developing non-LS sarcoidosis. HLA-DQB1*0602 has been associated with increased risk of non-LS sarcoidosis in a Dutch cohort [32]. HLA-DRB1*14, *12 and *10 have been associated with increased risk of sarcoidosis in a white Dutch and British cohort [26], and HLA-DRB1*12 and DRB1*14 in cohorts from the UK, Netherlands and Japan [29] whereas HLA-DRB1*1501 was associated with risk of sarcoidosis in a Finnish cohort [33]. HLA-DRB1*1201, *1401, *1501, *1101 and HLA-DRB3*0101 were associated with sarcoidosis in the ACCESS cohort in the USA [34].

In contrast, HLA alleles that have been associated with decreased risk (protective) for sarcoidosis included HLA-DRB1*01 and *04 in white Dutch and UK cohorts [26] and HLA-DRB1*01 in cohorts from the UK, Netherlands and Japan [29] and HLA-DRB1*0101 was protective in a Finnish cohort [33]. In the ACCESS cohort, HLA-DRB1*0401 was protective for the overall cohort (African Americans and Caucasians) [34].

Some HLA markers are gender or ethnic specific in their association with sarcoidosis. In the ACCESS cohort, HLA-DRB1*1101 was associated with increased risk more in males than females whereas HLA-DRB1*0401 was associated with decreased risk more in males than females, [34] HLA-DQB1*0603 was a risk factor for females but a protective factor for males. [34] For blacks in the ACCESS cohort, HLA-DRB1*1201 and HLA-DPB1*1503 were associated with increased risk of sarcoidosis and HLA-DRB1*1503 was associated with decreased risk of sarcoidosis [34] whereas in whites, HLA-DRB1*0402 and DRB1*1501 were associated with increased risk whereas HLA-DRB1*0401 was protective against sarcoidosis [34].

Overall, HLA-DRB1 molecules appear to play an important role in the pathogenesis of sarcoidosis either by recognizing specific antigen(s) or mounting different immune responses to different antigen(s). A better understanding of the role of HLA molecules in the pathogenesis of sarcoidosis could move us a step closer to potentially identifying the antigen(s) that trigger sarcoidosis [35].

2.2. BTNL2

The butyrophilin like 2 gene (BTNL2) belongs to the immunoglobulin gene superfamily and is related to the CD80 and CD86 co-stimulatory receptors. [7] In a mouse model, it was shown that BTNL2 binds to activated T-cells and inhibits their proliferation. [36] BTNL-2 was first linked to sarcoidosis when a GWAS in 63 German families with sarcoidosis identified a linkage to chromosome 6p21. [5] Further investigation found an association between SNP rs2076530A in the BTNL2 gene and sarcoidosis. [7] rs2076530A produces an alternative splice site that results in an early stop codon and a truncated, non-functional protein as a final product. [7] These findings were replicated in another German sarcoidosis cohort [37]. In a white British and Dutch cohorts, the SNPs rs2076530A and rs2294878C both showed an association with increased risk of sarcoidosis whereas haplotype 4 (which included rs2076530G and rs2294878A) had a protective association [26]. The SNP rs2076530A was associated with non-Lofgren's sarcoidosis and a gene dose effect was detected (AG vs GG OR 1.98, AA vs GG OR 2.63) [26]. There was strong linkage disequilibrium (LD) between BTNL2 haplotype 2 and HLA-DRB1*03 and between BTNL2 haplotype 4 and HLA-DRB1*01. [26] When the association of rs2076530A with the risk of sarcoidosis was analyzed in the context of HLA-DRB1, the rs2076530A association no longer held whereas the association of HLA-DRB1*12 and *14 with the risk of sarcoidosis persisted. [26] In a Dutch cohort, BTNL2 rs2076530A was associated with increased risk of sarcoidosis and a strong LD was found with HLA-DRB1*15. [38] rs2076530A was also associated with an increased risk of sarcoidosis in an American Caucasian cohort whereas in an African American cohort, the BTNL2 gene risk and the HLA-DRB1 gene risk negated each other. [39] In the same cohort, BTNL2 rs3117099T was associated with Lofgren's syndrome, similar but stronger association was also detected for haplotype 2 which contains rs3117099T. [26] The association of both haplotype 2 and HLA-DRB1*03 with Lofgren's syndrome remained significant after adjusting for each other and was stronger when both were present and protective against sarcoidosis when both were absent [26].

2.3. CCR2

CCR2 is a receptor for the chemokines CCL5, CCL2 and CCL3 that play an important role in recruiting monocytes, T-cells and other inflammatory cells. [40, 41] The association of 8 SNPs in the CCR2 gene with sarcoidosis was investigated in a white Dutch sarcoidosis population, a haplotype that consisted of 4 unique alleles (A at -6752, A at 3000, T at 3547 and T at 4385) was associated with LS, this association remained significant after adjustment for HLA-DRB1*0301-DQB1*0201 and female gender (both of which have been associated with LS). [41] No difference was seen between non-LS and controls. [41] This association and independence from HLA-DRB1 was confirmed in Swedish and Spanish sarcoidosis cohorts. [27] Similar findings were found in a Czech cohort although the difference did not reach statistical significance. [40] No association was detected between 3 SNPs in CCR2 and sarcoidosis in a German cohort. [42] CCR2-64I mutation (A substitution mutation where isoleucine replaces valine in the transmembrane region) was found it to be protective against sarcoidosis in a Japanese cohort. [43]

2.4. CCR5

The CCR5 gene is located on the short arm of chromosome 3 [44] and codes for a receptor for several chemokines including CCL3, CCL4, CCL5 and CCL8. [45] These chemokines play an important role in lymphocyte and monocyte recruitment and activation in sarcoidosis. [46, 47] In Sarcoidosis, CCR5 expression is up-regulated in Bronchoalveolar lavage (BAL) macrophages and lymphocytes [48, 49] and levels of the CCR5 ligands, CCL3 and CCL5, correlate with risk of disease progression. [50-52] The CCR5Δ32 null allele results a 32bp deletion in the CCR5 gene and produces a non-functional receptor that is unable to bind to its ligand [53]. The A allele at position -5663 (rs2040388) and the C allele at position -3900 (rs2856757), both of which are part of the HHC haplotype, were associated with LS in a German cohort, particularly in females [53]. No association between 8 SNPs in the CCR5 gene and risk of sarcoidosis was detected in a white Dutch and UK cohorts but an association was noted with severity of lung disease. [54]

2.5. CARD15

CARD15/NOD2 is an intracellular molecule that is part of the innate immunity which recognizes muramyl dipeptide, a component of gram-positive and gram-negative bacteria cell wall [55]. It was first identified in association with the risk of Crohn's disease. [55] No significant association was detected between CARD15 polymorphisms and risk of sarcoidosis in German [56, 57], Japanese [58], Danish [59, 60] cohorts. In contrast, an association was noted with risk of disease in a Greek cohort [61].

2.6. Toll-Like receptors

Toll-like receptors (TLR) are transmembrane proteins that are critical in the innate immune system. [62] They are also known as pattern recognition receptors as they recognize specific microbial structures. [62] So far, 11 TLRs have been recognized. [62] Several studies in German and Dutch cohorts have investigated the potential association of polymorphisms in the TLR4, TLR2 and TLR9 genes with sarcoidosis but found no association with the risk of sarcoidosis. [63-67] One study in a German cohort suggested an association with chronic sarcoidosis. [63] In a Dutch cohort, SNPs rs1109695 and rs7658893 in the TLR-10 gene and rs57436004 and rs5743594 in the TLR-1 gene were associated with the risk of sarcoidosis. [68] None of the 4 SNPs were significantly different between remitting and chronic disease but they did differ significantly between healthy controls and sarcoidosis patients with chronic/progressive disease. [68]

2.7. SLC11A1 (NRAMP1, Natural Resistance-Associated Macrophage Protein Gene)

The SLC11A1 gene encodes a macrophage-specific, membrane protein whose function involves transport and appears to be important in the early stages of macrophage activation. [69] In US African Americans, a repeat polymorphism in 5' region (allele 2) of the gene was protective against sarcoidosis. [69] This finding was replicated in Polish, Turkish and Greek cohorts where the opposite polymorphism (allele 3) was associated with increased risk of sarcoidosis. [70-72] In the Turkish cohort, polymorphism in INT4 was also associated with increased risk of sarcoidosis but this association was not noted in the other cohorts. [70]

3. Cytokines/Chemokines

3.1. TNF-α and lymphotoxin-A (LTA, TNF-β)

TNF-α and LTA genes are located within the MHC class III region on chromosome 6p21.3 [73-75]. TNF-α plays a pivotal role in sarcoidosis [76]. It is produced by alveolar macrophages and high levels of spontaneous and stimulated release of TNF-α by macrophages from sarcoidosis patients correlates with disease severity. [76] Several Loci in the TNF-α gene have been studied including -307 (previously mislabeled as -308), -857, -863.

LTA-252G (rs909253) allele was associated with sarcoidosis in Czech and Polish cohorts [77] and TNF-α-308A (rs1800629) allele was associated with sarcoidosis in Polish and Czech sarcoidosis cohorts [77]. There was a strong LD between the TNF-α 308A, LTA252G alleles and HLA-DRB1*03 which has been associated with LS [74]. An association between TNF-α 308A (rs1800629) allele and LS and between TNF-α -857T allele and non-LS sarcoidosis was also found in a British and Dutch cohort [78] and German cohorts [79-81]. An association was found between the TNF-α -308 (rs1800629) and LTA252G(rs909253) SNPs and erythema nodosum in US white women [73] but no association between polymorphisms in the TNF-α gene and sarcoidosis in African Americans was detected. [82] There was also an increased frequency of the -857T allele in British and Dutch sarcoidosis patients compared to controls. [78]

The relationship between serum TNF-α levels and genotypes is unclear, one study found an increased serum TNF-α levels with the TNF-α-307(8)G and the TNF-α -238A alleles in a sarcoidosis population but not normal controls, [83] whereas another study did not detect any association in the spontaneous or stimulated release of TNF-α from BAL and PBMC cells with the TNF-α 308 and TNF-β (intron 1) genotypes. [84]

The TNF-α-863 position lies further upstream in the promoter region. It influences the binding of NF-kB p50-p50 to the promoter region and inhibiting TNF-α production. The A allele variant inhibits the binding of NF-kB p50-p50 and thus leading to a higher production of TNF-α. [85] There was a marginal association of the allele TNF-1031A with the risk of sarcoidosis and an association of TNF-1031A and TNF-α-863A with chronic disease in an Indian cohort. [83]

3.2. TGF-β

TGF-β is a growth factor with 3 isoforms: TGF-β1, TGF-β2 and TGF-β3. They have nearly identical biological properties but the functional properties are usually attributed to TGF-β1. [86] TGF-β induces the synthesis of extracellular matrix and decreases matrix degradation, has immunomodulatory properties acting as a mediator regulating chemotaxis and fibroblasts and has been implicated in pulmonary fibrosis. [86, 87] The variant allele C of -509T/C and C of codon 10 are associated with higher TGF-β1 protein levels in the serum and the codon 10 variant is associated with increased mRNA levels in PBMC. [88, 89] TGF-β1 levels in the BAL and alveolar macrophage supernatant are higher in patients with active sarcoidosis and especially in those with pulmonary function changes, [90] there was also a positive correlation with BAL lymphocytosis. [90]

No association was found between sarcoidosis and 2 polymorphisms (codon 10, T869C) in the TGF-β1 gene in a Japanese sarcoidosis cohort and no relationship with Scadding chest x-ray stage was found either. [91] Codon 10 was also not associated with sarcoidosis in a German cohort [92]. No association between polymorphisms in the TGF-β1, TGF-β2 and TGF-β3 genes and sarcoidosis was detected in a white Dutch cohort. [93]

4. Signaling molecules

4.1. Annexin A11

The ANXA11 gene plays a role in the apoptosis pathway and depletion or dysfunction of the Annexin A11 protein may impair cell apoptosis and the down-regulation of the immune response [8]. A GWAS analysis in a German sarcoidosis cohort found a strong association between several SNPs in the annexin A11 (ANXA11) gene on chromosome 10 (10q22.3) and the risk of sarcoidosis. [8] This association was confirmed in a separate German cohort were the C allele of both rs1049550 and rs2573346 were associated with the development of sarcoidosis. [94] The association of rs1049550 with risk of sarcoidosis was also confirmed in a Czech cohort [95].

5. Others

5.1. Angiotensin Converting Enzyme (ACE)

Serum ACE is one of the biochemical markers that reflect disease activity in sarcoidosis. [1] Serum ACE levels do correlate with ACE genotype, with genotype D/D having the highest levels and I/I the lowest. [96-100] Several studies have investigated the association of ACE genotypes with sarcoidosis. In an African American cohort, the DD genotype was associated with increased risk of sarcoidosis, but not extent or severity, and the association was stronger when a family history of sarcoidosis was taken into account. [101] This association was not noted in a later study in African Americans. [82] In a Japanese cohort, the DD genotype was associated with increased risk of sarcoidosis in their female patients. [96] No association was detected in a US Caucasian cohort [101]. Otherwise, no association between polymorphisms in the ACE gene and risk of sarcoidosis was detected in German, Dutch, Italian, British, Finnish and Czech sarcoidosis cohorts. [97-100, 102, 103]

The angiotensin II receptor 1 genotype AA and CC potentially increase the risk of sarcoidosis in males in a German cohort but these findings were not replicated in a Dutch cohort. [97, 98] No association existed between the angiotension II receptor 1 and 2 genotypes and sarcoidosis in a Japanese cohort. [104]

5.2. IL-10 and CD40

No association between polymorphisms in the IL-10 or the CD40 gene and risk of sarcoidosis in Japanese cohorts was detected. [105, 106]

Genetic markers and disease course / organ involvement (Table 2):

Gene	Polymorphism	Population	OR	CI	p	Ref
Progressive Pulmonary disease						
HLA	DQB1*0602	AA	NR	NR	0.032	[107]
	DRB1*07	Scandinavian	0.44	NR	0.009	[28]
	DRB1*14	Scandinavian	2.14	NR	0.005	[28]
	DRB1*15	Scandinavian	1.55	NR	0.011	[28]
	DRB1*01	Scandinavian	0.41	NR	<0.001	[28]
	DRB1*03	Scandinavian	5.42	NR	<0.001	[28]
	DRB1*03	Finnish	2.22	1.20-4.1	0.011	[33]
BTNL 2	rs2076530	Dutch	1.84	1.06-3.21	0.03	[38]
CCR5	HHC haplotype	British	6.8*	2.5-18.0	0.0045	[54]
	HHC haplotype	Dutch	9*	3.5-23.1	0.0009	[54]
CARD15/NOD2	rs2066844T	British	4.1	1.0-15.5	0.04	[110]
IL23	Rs11209026A	German	0.63	0.5-0.79	<0.001	[117]
TNF						
	TNF-α 308A	Dutch	0.43	0.31-0.61	<0.001	[75]

Gene	Polymorphism	Population	OR	CI	p	Ref
	TNF-α 308T	Italian	3.53	1.66-7.5	<0.001	[77]
TGF-β						
TGF-β1	rs1800469	US white	2.5	1.3-4.5	0.005	[118]
TGF-β3	rs3917165A	US White	7.9	2.1-30.9	P=0.01	[118]
TGF-β3	rs3917200C	US White	5.1	1.6-17.7	P=0.05	[118]
GREM1	rs1919364CC	Dutch	6.37	2.89-14.1	<0.001	[120]
ANXA11	rs1049550T	Czech	0.61	0.41-0.89	0.01	[95]
Ophthalmic						
HLA	DRB1*0401	AA/White	3.49	1.62-7.54	<0.0008	[34]
	DRB1*0401-DQB10301	UK	3.4	1.64-7.08	0.001	[29]
	DRB1*03-DQB1*0201	UK	0.21	0.08-0.54	<0.0001	[29]
Hypercalcemia	PBB1-0101	US white	4.28	1.45-12.6	0.005	[34]

* OR at 4 years

HLA : Human Leukocyte Antigen

Table 2. Association of genetic markers with sarcoidosis disease course, severity and/or organ invovlement.

6. Receptors

6.1. HLA region

HLA genetic markers were also investigated for their association with sarcoidosis disease course, severity and/or organ involvement. HLA-DQB1*0602 was associated with radiographic progression in an African American cohort [107], advanced pulmonary disease and uveitis in Dutch cohorts [30, 108] whereas in a Scandinavian cohort, HLA-DRB1*07,*14 and *15 were associated with progressive pulmonary disease whereas *01 and *03 were associated with non-progressive disease [28]. In a Finnish cohort, HLA-DRB1*03 was associated with resolving disease [109].

6.2. BTNL-2

In a Dutch cohort, BTNL2 16071A variant was associated with increased risk of progressive or persistent pulmonary sarcoidosis [38].

6.3. CCR5

CCR5Δ32 null allele was associated with the need for immunosuppressive therapy in a Czech cohort [40]. The haplotype HHC (-5663A, -3900C, -3458T, -2459G, -2135T, -2086G, -1835C, Δ32 wt) was strongly associated with the presence of parenchymal disease in British and Dutch cohorts at presentation, 2 and 4 years of follow up [54]. The haplotype HHC was also associated with lower forced expiratory volume in the first second (FEV1), forced vital capacity (FVC), bronchoalveolar lavage neutrophilia (>4%) but not other organ involvement with Sarcoidosis [54].

6.4. CARD15/NOD2

In a British cohort, there was an association between allele T at loci 2104 (rs2066844) and the risk of radiographic Scadding stage IV at year 4 of follow up and an association between the allele G at loci 1761 with better lung function, defined by DLCO, at presentation, 2 and 4 years of follow up. [110] Interestingly, in a study in Crohn's disease patients, variants in loci 2104, 2722 and 3020 were associated with decreased number of T-regulatory cells in the lamina propria. [111] T-regulatory cells have been implicated to have a role in the immune pathogenesis of sarcoidosis but their exact role is yet unknown. [3, 112, 113]

7. Cytokines/Chemokines

7.1. TNF-α 308, LTA252 (TNF-β)

A higher representation of the TNF-α308A allele was found in a Dutch cohort with non-persistent disease compared to persistent disease. [75] In a Polish cohort, TNF-α308 A/A was associated with disease remission. [77]

7.2. TGFβ

In a white Dutch cohort, there was an increased frequency of the A allele in rs3917165 in the TGF-β3 gene in the fibrotic group compared to the acute/chronic groups [93], in addition, the C allele in rs3917200 was more frequent in the fibrotic group compared to the acute/chronic groups. [93] In another study, white American sarcoidosis patients who had CC homozygosity at position -509 (rs1800469) were more likely to have parenchymal disease [118].

7.3. IL-23

IL-23 is a pro-inflammatory cytokine that stimulate Th-17 cells to produce IL-17 and other cytokines and has a role in a number of autoimmune diseases [114, 115]. Polymorphisms in rs11209026 can affect serum IL-17A levels in rheumatoid arthritis patients [116]. In a German cohort, rs11209026A was protective against chronic sarcoidosis [117].

8. Signaling

8.1. GREM1

Gremlin, encoded by GREM1, is a secreted glycoprotein and antagonizes bone morphogenetic protein (BMP) by forming heterodimers with BMP-2, BMP-4 and BMP-7 preventing BMP from interacting with its ligand and subsequent downstream signaling. [119] Dutch sarcoidosis patients with the CC genotype for rs1919364 in GREM1 had a 6 fold increased risk of developing fibrotic lung disease. [120]

8.2. Annexin A11

In a Czech cohort, rs1049550 T-allele was protective against parenchymal disease (Scadding stages II-IV) [95].

9. Other

9.1. COX2

In a Spanish cohort, there was an association between the CC genotype of the COX2.8473 polymorphism and increased risk of sarcoidosis [121] and an association of the C-allele of the COX2.3050 with systemic sarcoidosis versus non-systemic sarcoidosis [122].

9.2. IL-10 and CD40

There were no associations between polymorphisms in the IL-10 and CD40 gene in Japanese cohorts and the risk of sarcoidosis. [105, 106]

10. Organ involvement

A few genetic markers have also been associated with organ involvement in sarcoidosis. In the ACCESS study, HLA-DRB3 was associated with bone marrow involvement in blacks, HLA-DPB1*0101 with hypercalcemia in whites, HLA-DRB1*0401 with parotid and salivary gland involvement in blacks and HLA-DRB1*0401 was found to have possible association with eye involvement [34]. In a cohort from the UK, HLA-DRB1*0401-DQB1*0301 was associated with increased risk of uveitis whereas HLA-DRB1*03 and DQB1*0201 were protective for uveitis. [29] In a Japanese cohort, HLA-DRB1*15 and DQB1*0602 were associated with skin disease and HLA-DRB1*0803 with neurosarcoidosis. [29] In a Japanese cohort, polymorphisms in the CTLA-4 gene were associated with BAL lymphocytosis, ocular involvement and multi-organ involvement. [123, 124]

11. Conclusions

Sarcoidosis is a complex disease with variable presentations, course and organ involvement, as such, it is no surprise that research into the genetic basis of the disease yields complex and variable results. This is supported by the variability in presentation, course and organ involvement between various ethnic groups. To add to this complexity, linkage disequilibrium (LD) occurs when alleles at two loci are not independent of each other. As such, when one genetic marker is identified as associated with a disease or trait, then any allele in strong LD with that marker could be the actual link to the disease. For example, BTNL-2 has been associated with increased risk of sarcoidosis [5, 7, 8, 26, 37] but has also been shown to be in strong LD with HLA markers [26].

HLA molecules play an important role in antigen presentation and immune stimulation [24, 25]. The association of HLA markers with increased risk of sarcoidosis or specific organ involvement could potentially lead to identification of a causative agent(s), as seen in chronic beryllium disease [125], and a recent study has shown an interaction between genetics and immune response to certain environmental antigens [22]. Chronic beryllium disease, a granulomatous disorder that is caused by exposure to beryllium and resembles sarcoidosis, has been associated with HLA-DP-βGLu69 as a genetic risk factor [126]. Studies have shown that HLA-DP-βGlu69 interacts with beryllium with subsequent stimulation of the immune response [125]. In addition, the identification of genetic markers that are associated with sarcoidosis might uncover novel pathways not previously identified or suspected as contributors to disease pathogenesis, which could subsequently lead to identification of new therapeutic targets.

Further research is still needed to clarify the associations of the various genetic markers with risk and prognosis of disease and large validation studies will be needed to confirm these associations. Proper phenotyping of cases and stratification according to ethnicity and gender when analyzing genetic studies is extremely important. Several studies have shown opposite associations between gender and/or ethnicity and genetic markers when the analysis was stratified by gender and/or ethnicity [53]. In addition, the interaction between two or more distinct SNPs or haplotypes in sarcoidosis has yet to be studied [127].

So what role does genetic testing have in the clinical care of sarcoidosis patients? At this stage, genetic testing has no identifiable role in the clinical arena. The odds of a first or second degree relative of a sarcoidosis patient also having sarcoidosis are 4.6 and the familial relative risk was larger in sibs than in parents and higher in Whites than African Americans [4]. This said, the absolute risk and attributable risk for a sib or parent of a sarcoidosis patients is approximately 1% and as such, screening family members, clinically or genetically, is not recommended [4].

Potential future applications of genetic testing in the clinical arena include prognostication on disease course which will aid in determining intensity of follow up, prognostication on potential organ involvement which will influence frequency and intensity of screening for sarcoidosis involvement, and potentially a role for pharmacogenetics in guiding immunomodulatory therapy.

Author details

Nabeel Y. Hamzeh[1,2] and Lisa A. Maier[1,2]

1 Division of Environmental and Occupational Health Sciences, National Jewish Health, Denver, CO, USA

2 Division of Pulmonary and Critical Care Sciences, Department of Medicine, School of Medicine, University of Colorado, Aurora, CO, USA

References

[1] Statement on Sarcoidosis. Am J Respir Crit Care Med. 1999 August 1, 1999;160(2): 736-55.

[2] Gerke AK, Hunninghake G. The immunology of sarcoidosis. Clin Chest Med. 2008 Sep;29(3):379-90, vii.

[3] Miyara M, Amoura Z, Parizot C, Badoual C, Dorgham K, Trad S, et al. The immune paradox of sarcoidosis and regulatory T cells. The Journal of experimental medicine. 2006 Feb 20;203(2):359-70.

[4] Rybicki BA, Iannuzzi MC, Frederick MM, Thompson BW, Rossman MD, Bresnitz EA, et al. Familial aggregation of sarcoidosis. A case-control etiologic study of sarcoidosis (ACCESS). American journal of respiratory and critical care medicine. 2001 Dec 1;164(11):2085-91.

[5] Schurmann M, Reichel P, Muller-Myhsok B, Schlaak M, Muller-Quernheim J, Schwinger E. Results from a genome-wide search for predisposing genes in sarcoidosis. American journal of respiratory and critical care medicine. 2001 Sep 1;164(5): 840-6.

[6] Iannuzzi MC, Iyengar SK, Gray-McGuire C, Elston RC, Baughman RP, Donohue JF, et al. Genome-wide search for sarcoidosis susceptibility genes in African Americans. Genes and immunity. 2005 Sep;6(6):509-18.

[7] Valentonyte R, Hampe J, Huse K, Rosenstiel P, Albrecht M, Stenzel A, et al. Sarcoidosis is associated with a truncating splice site mutation in BTNL2. Nat Genet. 2005 Apr;37(4):357-64.

[8] Hofmann S, Franke A, Fischer A, Jacobs G, Nothnagel M, Gaede KI, et al. Genomewide association study identifies ANXA11 as a new susceptibility locus for sarcoidosis. Nat Genet. 2008;40(9):1103-6.

[9]   Franke A, Fischer A, Nothnagel M, Becker C, Grabe N, Till A, et al. Genome-wide association analysis in sarcoidosis and Crohn's disease unravels a common susceptibility locus on 10p12.2. Gastroenterology. 2008 Oct;135(4):1207-15.

[10] Rybicki BA, Levin AM, McKeigue P, Datta I, Gray-McGuire C, Colombo M, et al. A genome-wide admixture scan for ancestry-linked genes predisposing to sarcoidosis in African-Americans. Genes and immunity. 2010.

[11] Hofmann S, Fischer A, Till A, MÃ¼ller-Quernheim J, HÃ¤sler R, Franke A, et al. A genome-wide association study reveals evidence of association with sarcoidosis at 6p12.1. European Respiratory Journal. 2011 November 1, 2011;38(5):1127-35.

[12] Cho JH, Gregersen PK. Genomics and the multifactorial nature of human autoimmune disease. The New England journal of medicine. 2011 Oct 27;365(17):1612-23.

[13] Attia J, Ioannidis JP, Thakkinstian A, McEvoy M, Scott RJ, Minelli C, et al. How to use an article about genetic association: A: Background concepts. Jama. 2009 Jan 7;301(1):74-81.

[14] Newman LS, Rose CS, Bresnitz EA, Rossman MD, Barnard J, Frederick M, et al. A Case Control Etiologic Study of Sarcoidosis: Environmental and Occupational Risk Factors10.1164/rccm.200402-249OC. Am J Respir Crit Care Med. 2004 December 15, 2004;170(12):1324-30.

[15] Gerke AK, van Beek E, Hunninghake GW. Smoking Inhibits the Frequency of Bronchovascular Bundle Thickening in Sarcoidosis. Academic Radiology. 2011;18(7): 885-91.

[16] Song Z, Marzilli L, Greenlee BM, Chen ES, Silver RF, Askin FB, et al. Mycobacterial catalase-peroxidase is a tissue antigen and target of the adaptive immune response in systemic sarcoidosis. The Journal of Experimental Medicine. 2005 March 7, 2005;201(5):755-67.

[17] Dubaniewicz A, Dubaniewicz-Wybieralska M, Sternau A, Zwolska Z, Izycka-Swieszewska E, Augustynowicz-Kopec E, et al. Mycobacterium tuberculosis Complex and Mycobacterial Heat Shock Proteins in Lymph Node Tissue from Patients with Pulmonary Sarcoidosis. J Clin Microbiol. 2006;44:3448 - 51.

[18] Carlisle J, Evans W, Hajizadeh R, Nadaf M, Shepherd B, Ott RD, et al. Multiple Mycobacterium antigens induce interferon-gamma production from sarcoidosis peripheral blood mononuclear cells. Clinical & Experimental Immunology. 2007;150(3): 460-8.

[19] Carlisle J, Evans W, Hajizadeh R, Richter K, Drake WP. "Immune recognition of multiple mycobacterial antigens by sarcoidosis subjects." J Clin Exp Immunol. 2007;150:460 - 8.

[20] Drake WP, Dhason MS, Nadaf M, Shepherd BE, Vadivelu S, Hajizadeh R, et al. Cellular Recognition of Mycobacterium tuberculosis ESAT-6 and KatG Peptides in Systemic Sarcoidosis. Infect Immun. 2007 January 1, 2007;75(1):527-30.

[21] Allen S, Evans W, Carlisle J, Hajizadeh R, Nadaf M, Shepherd B, et al. Superoxide dismutase A antigens derived from molecular analysis of sarcoidosis granulomas elicit systemic Th-1 immune responses. Respiratory Research. 2008;9(1):36.

[22] Chen ES, Wahlstrom J, Song Z, Willett MH, Wiken M, Yung RC, et al. T Cell Responses to Mycobacterial Catalase-Peroxidase Profile a Pathogenic Antigen in Systemic Sarcoidosis. J Immunol. 2008 December 15, 2008;181(12):8784-96.

[23] Oswald-Richter KA, Culver DA, Hawkins C, Hajizadeh R, Abraham S, Shepherd BE, et al. Cellular Responses to Mycobacterial Antigens Are Present in Bronchoalveolar Lavage Fluid Used in the Diagnosis of Sarcoidosis. Infect Immun. 2009 September 1, 2009;77(9):3740-8.

[24] Klein J, Sato A. The HLA system. Second of two parts. The New England journal of medicine. 2000 Sep 14;343(11):782-6.

[25] Klein J, Sato A. The HLA system. First of two parts. The New England journal of medicine. 2000 Sep 7;343(10):702-9.

[26] Spagnolo P, Sato H, Grutters JC, Renzoni EA, Marshall SE, Ruven HJ, et al. Analysis of BTNL2 genetic polymorphisms in British and Dutch patients with sarcoidosis. Tissue Antigens. 2007 Sep;70(3):219-27.

[27] Spagnolo P, Sato H, Grunewald J, Brynedal B, Hillert J, Mana J, et al. A common haplotype of the C-C chemokine receptor 2 gene and HLA-DRB1*0301 are independent genetic risk factors for Lofgren's syndrome. J Intern Med. 2008 Nov;264(5):433-41.

[28] Grunewald J, Brynedal B, Darlington P, Nisell M, Cederlund K, Hillert J, et al. Different HLA-DRB1 allele distributions in distinct clinical subgroups of sarcoidosis patients. Respiratory research. 2010;11(26):25.

[29] Sato H, Woodhead FA, Ahmad T, Grutters JC, Spagnolo P, van den Bosch JM, et al. Sarcoidosis HLA class II genotyping distinguishes differences of clinical phenotype across ethnic groups. Human molecular genetics. 2010 Oct 15;19(20):4100-11.

[30] Sato H, Grutters JC, Pantelidis P, Mizzon AN, Ahmad T, Van Houte AJ, et al. HLA-DQB1*0201: a marker for good prognosis in British and Dutch patients with sarcoidosis. American journal of respiratory cell and molecular biology. 2002 Oct;27(4):406-12.

[31] Grunewald J, Idali F, Kockum I, Seddighzadeh M, Nisell M, Eklund A, et al. Major histocompatibility complex class II transactivator gene polymorphism: associations with Löfgren's syndrome. Tissue Antigens. 2010;76(2):96-101.

[32] Voörter CEM, Drent M, van den Berg-Loonen EM. Severe Pulmonary Sarcoidosis Is Strongly Associated With the Haplotype HLA-DQB1*0602-DRB1*150101. Human immunology. 2005;66(7):826-35.

[33] Wennerstrom A, Pietinalho A, Vauhkonen H, Lahtela L, Palikhe A, Hedman J, et al. HLA-DRB1 allele frequencies and C4 copy number variation in Finnish sarcoidosis patients and associations with disease prognosis. Human immunology. 2012;73(1): 93-100.

[34] Rossman MD, Thompson B, Frederick M, Maliarik M, Iannuzzi MC, Rybicki BA, et al. HLA-DRB1*1101: A Significant Risk Factor for Sarcoidosis in Blacks and Whites. Am J Hum Genet. 2003 Aug 20;73(4).

[35] Dai S, Murphy GA, Crawford F, Mack DG, Falta MT, Marrack P, et al. Crystal structure of HLA-DP2 and implications for chronic beryllium disease. Proceedings of the National Academy of Sciences of the United States of America. 2010 Apr 20;107(16): 7425-30.

[36] Nguyen T, Liu XK, Zhang Y, Dong C. BTNL2, a Butyrophilin-Like Molecule That Functions to Inhibit T Cell Activation. J Immunol. 2006 June 15, 2006;176(12):7354-60.

[37] Li Y, Wollnik B, Pabst S, Lennarz M, Rohmann E, Gillissen A, et al. BTNL2 gene variant and sarcoidosis. Thorax. 2006 Mar;61(3):273-4.

[38] Wijnen PA, Voorter CE, Nelemans PJ, Verschakelen JA, Bekers O, Drent M. Butyrophilin-like 2 in pulmonary sarcoidosis: a factor for susceptibility and progression? Human immunology. 2011 Jan 20.

[39] Rybicki BA, Walewski JL, Maliarik MJ, Kian H, Iannuzzi MC. The BTNL2 gene and sarcoidosis susceptibility in African Americans and Whites. Am J Hum Genet. 2005 Sep;77(3):491-9.

[40] Petrek M, Drabek J, Kolek V, Zlamal J, Welsh KI, Bunce M, et al. CC chemokine receptor gene polymorphisms in Czech patients with pulmonary sarcoidosis. American journal of respiratory and critical care medicine. 2000 Sep;162(3 Pt 1):1000-3.

[41] Spagnolo P, Renzoni EA, Wells AU, Sato H, Grutters JC, Sestini P, et al. C-C Chemokine Receptor 2 and Sarcoidosis: Association with Lofgren's Syndrome. Am J Respir Crit Care Med. 2003 November 15, 2003;168(10):1162-6.

[42] Valentonyte R, Hampe J, Croucher PJP, Muller-Quernheim J, Schwinger E, Schreiber S, et al. Study of C-C Chemokine Receptor 2 Alleles in Sarcoidosis, with Emphasis on Family-based Analysis. Am J Respir Crit Care Med. 2005 May 15, 2005;171(10): 1136-41.

[43] Hizawa N, Yamaguchi E, Furuya KEN, Jinushi E, Ito A, Kawakami Y. The Role of the C-C Chemokine Receptor 2 Gene Polymorphism V64I (CCR2-64I) in Sarcoidosis in a Japanese Population. Am J Respir Crit Care Med. 1999 June 1, 1999;159(6):2021-3.

[44] Samson M, Soularue P, Vassart G, Parmentier M. The genes encoding the human CC-chemokine receptors CC-CKR1 to CC-CKR5 (CMKBR1-CMKBR5) are clustered in the p21.3-p24 region of chromosome 3. Genomics. 1996 Sep 15;36(3):522-6.

[45] Blanpain C, Migeotte I, Lee B, Vakili J, Doranz BJ, Govaerts C, et al. CCR5 binds multiple CC-chemokines: MCP-3 acts as a natural antagonist. Blood. 1999 Sep 15;94(6): 1899-905.

[46] Baggiolini M, Loetscher P. Chemokines in inflammation and immunity. Immunology today. 2000 Sep;21(9):418-20.

[47] Ziegenhagen MW, Schrum S, Zissel G, Zipfel PF, Schlaak M, Muller-Quernheim J. Increased expression of proinflammatory chemokines in bronchoalveolar lavage cells of patients with progressing idiopathic pulmonary fibrosis and sarcoidosis. J Investig Med. 1998 Jun;46(5):223-31.

[48] Capelli A, Di Stefano A, Lusuardi M, Gnemmi I, Donner CF. Increased macrophage inflammatory protein-1alpha and macrophage inflammatory protein-1beta levels in bronchoalveolar lavage fluid of patients affected by different stages of pulmonary sarcoidosis. American journal of respiratory and critical care medicine. 2002 Jan 15;165(2):236-41.

[49] Katchar K, Eklund A, Grunewald J. Expression of Th1 markers by lung accumulated T cells in pulmonary sarcoidosis. J Intern Med. 2003 Dec;254(6):564-71.

[50] Iida K, Kadota J, Kawakami K, Matsubara Y, Shirai R, Kohno S. Analysis of T cell subsets and beta chemokines in patients with pulmonary sarcoidosis. Thorax. 1997 May;52(5):431-7.

[51] Keane MP, Standiford TJ, Strieter RM. Chemokines are important cytokines in the pathogenesis of interstitial lung disease. Eur Respir J. 1997 Jun;10(6):1199-202.

[52] Petrek M, Pantelidis P, Southcott AM, Lympany P, Safranek P, Black CM, et al. The source and role of RANTES in interstitial lung disease. Eur Respir J. 1997 Jun;10(6): 1207-16.

[53] Fischer A, Valentonyte R, Nebel A, Nothnagel M, Muller-Quernheim J, Schurmann M, et al. Female-specific association of C-C chemokine receptor 5 gene polymorphisms with Lofgren's syndrome. Journal of molecular medicine (Berlin, Germany). 2008 May;86(5):553-61.

[54] Spagnolo P, Renzoni EA, Wells AU, Copley SJ, Desai SR, Sato H, et al. C-C chemokine receptor 5 gene variants in relation to lung disease in sarcoidosis. American journal of respiratory and critical care medicine. 2005 Sep 15;172(6):721-8.

[55] Hugot JP, Chamaillard M, Zouali H, Lesage S, Cezard JP, Belaiche J, et al. Association of NOD2 leucine-rich repeat variants with susceptibility to Crohn's disease. Nature. 2001 May 31;411(6837):599-603.

[56] Schurmann M, Valentonyte R, Hampe J, Muller-Quernheim J, Schwinger E, Schreiber S. CARD15 gene mutations in sarcoidosis. Eur Respir J. 2003 Nov;22(5):748-54.

[57] Pabst S, Golebiewski M, Herms S, Karpushova A, Díaz-Lacava A, Walier M, et al. Caspase recruitment domain 15 gene haplotypes in sarcoidosis. Tissue Antigens. 2011;77(4):333-7.

[58] Akahoshi M, Ishihara M, Namba K, Kitaichi N, Ando Y, Takenaka S, et al. Mutation screening of the CARD15 gene in sarcoidosis. Tissue Antigens. 2008;71(6):564-7.

[59] Milman N, Nielsen FC, Hviid TV, Hansen TO. Blau syndrome-associated mutations in exon 4 of the caspase activating recruitment domain 15 (CARD 15) gene are not found in ethnic Danes with sarcoidosis. The clinical respiratory journal. 2007 Dec; 1(2):74-9.

[60] Milman N, Nielsen OH, Hviid TV, Fenger K. CARD15 single nucleotide polymorphisms 8, 12 and 13 are not increased in ethnic Danes with sarcoidosis. Respiration; international review of thoracic diseases. 2007;74(1):76-9.

[61] Gazouli M, Koundourakis A, Ikonomopoulos J, Gialafos EJ, Rapti A, Gorgoulis VG, et al. CARD15/NOD2, CD14, and toll-like receptor 4 gene polymorphisms in Greek patients with sarcoidosis. Sarcoidosis Vasc Diffuse Lung Dis. 2006 Mar;23(1):23-9.

[62] West AP, Koblansky AA, Ghosh S. Recognition and signaling by toll-like receptors. Annual review of cell and developmental biology. 2006;22:409-37.

[63] Pabst S, Baumgarten G, Stremmel A, Lennarz M, Knufermann P, Gillissen A, et al. Toll-like receptor (TLR) 4 polymorphisms are associated with a chronic course of sarcoidosis. Clinical and experimental immunology. 2006 Mar;143(3):420-6.

[64] Schurmann M, Kwiatkowski R, Albrecht M, Fischer A, Hampe J, Muller-Quernheim J, et al. Study of Toll-like receptor gene loci in sarcoidosis. Clinical and experimental immunology. 2008 Jun;152(3):423-31.

[65] Veltkamp M, Grutters JC, van Moorsel CH, Ruven HJ, van den Bosch JM. Toll-like receptor (TLR) 4 polymorphism Asp299Gly is not associated with disease course in Dutch sarcoidosis patients. Clinical and experimental immunology. 2006 Aug;145(2): 215-8.

[66] Veltkamp M, Van Moorsel CH, Rijkers GT, Ruven HJ, Van Den Bosch JM, Grutters JC. Toll-like receptor (TLR)-9 genetics and function in sarcoidosis. Clinical and experimental immunology. 2010 Oct;162(1):68-74.

[67] Veltkamp M, Wijnen PA, van Moorsel CH, Rijkers GT, Ruven HJ, Heron M, et al. Linkage between Toll-like receptor (TLR) 2 promotor and intron polymorphisms: functional effects and relevance to sarcoidosis. Clinical and experimental immunology. 2007 Sep;149(3):453-62.

[68] Veltkamp M, van Moorsel CH, Rijkers GT, Ruven HJ, Grutters JC. Genetic variation in the Toll-like receptor gene cluster (TLR10-TLR1-TLR6) influences disease course in sarcoidosis. Tissue Antigens. 2011 Jan;79(1):25-32.

[69] Maliarik MJ, Chen KM, Sheffer RG, Rybicki BA, Major ML, Popovich J, et al. The Natural Resistance-Associated Macrophage Protein Gene in African Americans with Sarcoidosis. American journal of respiratory cell and molecular biology. 2000 June 1, 2000;22(6):672-5.

[70] Akcakaya P, Azeroglu B, Even I, Ates O, Turker H, Ongen G, et al. The functional SLC11A1 gene polymorphisms are associated with sarcoidosis in Turkish population. Molecular biology reports. 2012 Apr;39(4):5009-16.

[71] Dubaniewicz A, Jamieson SE, Dubaniewicz-Wybieralska M, Fakiola M, Nancy Miller E, Blackwell JM. Association between SLC11A1 (formerly NRAMP1) and the risk of sarcoidosis in Poland. Eur J Hum Genet. 2005;13(7):829-34.

[72] Gazouli M, Koundourakis A, Ikonomopoulos J, Gialafos EJ, Papaconstantinou I, Nasioulas G, et al. The functional polymorphisms of NRAMP1 gene in Greeks with sarcoidosis. Sarcoidosis Vasc Diffuse Lung Dis. 2007 Sep;24(2):153-4.

[73] McDougal KE, Fallin MD, Moller DR, Song Z, Cutler DJ, Steiner LL, et al. Variation in the lymphotoxin-alpha/tumor necrosis factor locus modifies risk of erythema nodosum in sarcoidosis. The Journal of investigative dermatology. 2009 Aug;129(8): 1921-6.

[74] Mrazek F, Holla LI, Hutyrova B, Znojil V, Vasku A, Kolek V, et al. Association of tumour necrosis factor-alpha, lymphotoxin-alpha and HLA-DRB1 gene polymorphisms with Lofgren's syndrome in Czech patients with sarcoidosis. Tissue Antigens. 2005 Feb;65(2):163-71.

[75] Wijnen PA, Nelemans PJ, Verschakelen JA, Bekers O, Voorter CE, Drent M. The role of tumor necrosis factor alpha G-308A polymorphisms in the course of pulmonary sarcoidosis. Tissue Antigens.9999(9999).

[76] Ziegenhagen MW, Benner UK, Zissel G, Zabel P, Schlaak M, Muller-Quernheim J. Sarcoidosis: TNF-alpha release from alveolar macrophages and serum level of sIL-2R are prognostic markers. Am J Respir Crit Care Med. 1997 Nov;156(5):1586-92.

[77] Kieszko R, Krawczyk P, Chocholska S, Dmoszynska A, Milanowski J. TNF-alpha and TNF-beta gene polymorphisms in Polish patients with sarcoidosis. Connection with the susceptibility and prognosis. Sarcoidosis Vasc Diffuse Lung Dis. 2010 Jul;27(2): 131-7.

[78] Grutters JC, Sato H, Pantelidis P, Lagan AL, McGrath DS, Lammers J-WJ, et al. Increased Frequency of the Uncommon Tumor Necrosis Factor -857T Allele in British and Dutch Patients with Sarcoidosis. Am J Respir Crit Care Med. 2002 April 15, 2002;165(8):1119-24.

[79] Seitzer U, Swider C, Stuber F, Suchnicki K, Lange A, Richter E, et al. Tumour necrosis factor alpha promoter gene polymorphism in sarcoidosis. Cytokine. 1997 Oct;9(10): 787-90.

[80] Swider C, Schnittger L, Bogunia-Kubik K, Gerdes J, Flad H, Lange A, et al. TNF-alpha and HLA-DR genotyping as potential prognostic markers in pulmonary sarcoidosis. European cytokine network. 1999 Jun;10(2):143-6.

[81] Labunski S, Posern G, Ludwig S, Kundt G, BrÃcker E-B, Kunz M. Tumour Necrosis Factor-a Promoter Polymorphism in Erythema Nodosum. Acta Dermato-Venereologica. 2001;81(1):18 - 21.

[82] Rybicki BA, Maliarik MJ, Poisson LM, Iannuzzi MC. Sarcoidosis and granuloma genes: a family-based study in African-Americans. Eur Respir J. 2004 Aug;24(2): 251-7.

[83] Sharma S, Ghosh B, Sharma SK. Association of TNF polymorphisms with sarcoidosis, its prognosis and tumour necrosis factor (TNF)-alpha levels in Asian Indians. Clinical & Experimental Immunology. 2008;151(2):251-9.

[84] Somoskovi A, Zissel G, Seitzer U, Gerdes J, Schlaak M, Muller Quernheim J. Polymorphisms at position -308 in the promoter region of the TNF-alpha and in the first intron of the TNF-beta genes and spontaneous and lipopolysaccharide-induced TNF-alpha release in sarcoidosis. Cytokine. 1999 Nov;11(11):882-7.

[85] Udalova IA, Richardson A, Denys A, Smith C, Ackerman H, Foxwell B, et al. Functional consequences of a polymorphism affecting NF-kappaB p50-p50 binding to the TNF promoter region. Molecular and cellular biology. 2000 Dec;20(24):9113-9.

[86] Border WA, Noble NA. Transforming growth factor beta in tissue fibrosis. The New England journal of medicine. 1994 Nov 10;331(19):1286-92.

[87] Moses HL, Yang EY, Pietenpol JA. TGF-beta stimulation and inhibition of cell proliferation: new mechanistic insights. Cell. 1990 Oct 19;63(2):245-7.

[88] Grainger DJ, Heathcote K, Chiano M, Snieder H, Kemp PR, Metcalfe JC, et al. Genetic control of the circulating concentration of transforming growth factor type beta1. Human molecular genetics. 1999 Jan;8(1):93-7.

[89] Yamada Y, Miyauchi A, Goto J, Takagi Y, Okuizumi H, Kanematsu M, et al. Association of a polymorphism of the transforming growth factor-beta1 gene with genetic susceptibility to osteoporosis in postmenopausal Japanese women. J Bone Miner Res. 1998 Oct;13(10):1569-76.

[90] Salez F, Gosset P, Copin MC, Lamblin Degros C, Tonnel AB, Wallaert B. Transforming growth factor-beta1 in sarcoidosis. Eur Respir J. 1998 October 1, 1998;12(4):913-9.

[91] Niimi T, Sato S, Sugiura Y, Yoshinouchi T, Akita K, Maeda H, et al. Transforming growth factor-beta gene polymorphism in sarcoidosis and tuberculosis patients. The International Journal of Tuberculosis and Lung Disease. 2002;6:510-5.

[92] Murakozy G, Gaede KI, Zissel G, Schlaak M, Muller-Quernheim J. Analysis of gene polymorphisms in interleukin-10 and transforming growth factor-beta 1 in sarcoidosis. Sarcoidosis Vasc Diffuse Lung Dis. 2001 Jun;18(2):165-9.

[93] Kruit A, Grutters JC, Ruven HJT, van Moorsel CHM, Weiskirchen R, Mengsteab S, et al. Transforming Growth Factor-Î² Gene Polymorphisms in Sarcoidosis Patients With and Without Fibrosis*. Chest. 2006 June 2006;129(6):1584-91.

[94] Liu Y, Helms C, Liao W, Zaba LC, Duan S, Gardner J, et al. A genome-wide association study of psoriasis and psoriatic arthritis identifies new disease loci. PLoS Genet. 2008;4:e1000041.

[95] Mrazek F, Stahelova A, Kriegova E, Fillerova R, Zurkova M, Kolek V, et al. Functional variant ANXA11 R230C: true marker of protection and candidate disease modifier in sarcoidosis. Genes and immunity. 2011;12(6):490-4.

[96] Furuya K, Yamaguchi E, Itoh A, Hizawa N, Ohnuma N, Kojima J, et al. Deletion polymorphism in the angiotensin I converting enzyme (ACE) gene as a genetic risk factor for sarcoidosis. Thorax. 1996 Aug;51(8):777-80.

[97] A. Kruit HJTR, J.C. Grutters, J.M.M. van den Bosch. Angiotensin II Receptor Type 1 1166 A/C and Angiotensin Converting Enzyme I/D gene polymorphisms in a Dutch sarcoidosis cohor. SARCOIDOSIS VASCULITIS AND DIFFUSE LUNG DISEASES. 2010;27(2):147-52.

[98] Biller H, Ruprecht B, Gaede KI, Muller-Quernheim J, Zissel G. Gene polymorphisms of ACE and the angiotensin receptor AT2R1 influence serum ACE levels in sarcoidosis. Sarcoidosis Vasc Diffuse Lung Dis. 2009 Jul;26(2):139-46.

[99] Arbustini E, Grasso M, Leo G, Tinelli C, Fasani R, Diegoli M, et al. Polymorphism of angiotensin-converting enzyme gene in sarcoidosis. American journal of respiratory and critical care medicine. 1996 Feb;153(2):851-4.

[100] Tomita H, Ina Y, Sugiura Y, Sato S, Kawaguchi H, Morishita M, et al. Polymorphism in the angiotensin-converting enzyme (ACE) gene and sarcoidosis. American journal of respiratory and critical care medicine. 1997 Jul;156(1):255-9.

[101] Maliarik MJ, Rybicki BA, Malvitz E, Sheffer RG, Major M, Popovich J, Jr., et al. Angiotensin-converting enzyme gene polymorphism and risk of sarcoidosis. American journal of respiratory and critical care medicine. 1998 Nov;158(5 Pt 1):1566-70.

[102] McGrath DS, Foley PJ, Petrek M, Izakovicova-Holla L, Kolek V, Veeraraghavan S, et al. Ace gene I/D polymorphism and sarcoidosis pulmonary disease severity. American journal of respiratory and critical care medicine. 2001 Jul 15;164(2):197-201.

[103] Pietinalho A, Furuya K, Yamaguchi E, Kawakami Y, Selroos O. The angiotensin-converting enzyme DD gene is associated with poor prognosis in Finnish sarcoidosis patients. Eur Respir J. 1999 Apr;13(4):723-6.

[104] Takemoto Y, Sakatani M, Takami S, Tachibana T, Higaki J, Ogihara T, et al. Association between angiotensin II receptor gene polymorphism and serum angiotensin converting enzyme (SACE) activity in patients with sarcoidosis. Thorax. 1998 Jun;53(6): 459-62.

[105] Sakuyama K, Meguro A, Ota M, Ishihara M, Uemoto R, Ito H, et al. Lack of association between IL10 polymorphisms and sarcoidosis in Japanese patients. Molecular vision. 2012;18:512-8.

[106] Tanizawa K, Handa T, Nagai S, Ito I, Kubo T, Ito Y, et al. A CD40 single-nucleotide polymorphism affects the lymphocyte profiles in the bronchoalveolar lavage of Japanese patients with sarcoidosis. Tissue Antigens. 2011 Dec;78(6):442-5.

[107] Iannuzzi MC, Maliarik MJ, Poisson LM, Rybicki BA. Sarcoidosis susceptibility and resistance HLA-DQB1 alleles in African Americans. American journal of respiratory and critical care medicine. 2003 May 1;167(9):1225-31.

[108] van den Berg-Loonen EM, Voorter CEM, Drent M. Strong association of severe pulmonary sarcoidosis with HLA DQB1*0602. Human immunology. 2004;65(9-10, Supplement 1):S34-S.

[109] Wennerstrom A, Pietinalho A, Vauhkonen H, Lahtela L, Palikhe A, Hedman J, et al. HLA-DRB1 allele frequencies and C4 copy number variation in Finnish sarcoidosis patients and associations with disease prognosis. Human immunology. 2011(0).

[110] Sato H, Williams HRT, Spagnolo P, Abdallah A, Ahmad T, Orchard TR, et al. CARD15/NOD2 polymorphisms are associated with severe pulmonary sarcoidosis. Eur Respir J. 2009 August 13, 2009:09031936.0010209.

[111] Rahman MK, Midtling EH, Svingen PA, Xiong Y, Bell MP, Tung J, et al. The pathogen recognition receptor NOD2 regulates human FOXP3+ T cell survival. J Immunol. Jun 15;184(12):7247-56.

[112] Idali F, Wahlstrom J, Muller-Suur C, Eklund A, Grunewald J. Analysis of regulatory T cell associated forkhead box P3 expression in the lungs of patients with sarcoidosis. Clinical and experimental immunology. 2008 Apr;152(1):127-37.

[113] Taflin C, Miyara M, Nochy D, Valeyre D, Naccache J-M, Altare F, et al. FoxP3+ Regulatory T Cells Suppress Early Stages of Granuloma Formation but Have Little Impact on Sarcoidosis Lesions. Am J Pathol. 2009 January 15, 2009:ajpath.2009.080580.

[114] Weaver CT, Harrington LE, Mangan PR, Gavrieli M, Murphy KM. Th17: an effector CD4 T cell lineage with regulatory T cell ties. Immunity. 2006 Jun;24(6):677-88.

[115] Marieke A. Hoeve Nigel DLSTdBDennis MLLRde Waal MTom HMOFrank AWV. Divergent effects of IL-12 and IL-23 on the production of IL-17 by human T cells. European Journal of Immunology. 2006;36(3):661-70.

[116] Hazlett J, Stamp LK, Merriman T, Highton J, Hessian PA. IL-23R rs11209026 polymorphism modulates IL-17A expression in patients with rheumatoid arthritis. Genes and immunity. 2012 Apr;13(3):282-7.

[117] Fischer A, Nothnagel M, Franke A, Jacobs G, Saadati HR, Gaede KI, et al. Association of inflammatory bowel disease risk loci with sarcoidosis, and its acute and chronic subphenotypes. Eur Respir J. 2011 Mar;37(3):610-6.

[118] Jonth AC, Silveira L, Fingerlin TE, Sato H, Luby JC, Welsh KI, et al. TGF-beta1 Variants in Chronic Beryllium Disease and Sarcoidosis. J Immunol. 2007 September 15, 2007;179(6):4255-62.

[119] Hsu DR, Economides AN, Wang X, Eimon PM, Harland RM. The Xenopus dorsalizing factor Gremlin identifies a novel family of secreted proteins that antagonize BMP activities. Molecular cell. 1998 Apr;1(5):673-83.

[120] Heron M, van Moorsel CHM, Grutters JC, Huizinga TWJ, van der Helm-van Mil AHM, Nagtegaal MM, et al. Genetic variation in GREM1 is a risk factor for fibrosis in pulmonary sarcoidosis. Tissue Antigens. 2010;77(2):112-7.

[121] Lopez-Campos JL, Rodriguez-Rodriguez D, Rodriguez-Becerra E, Alfageme Michavila I, Guerra JF, Hernandez FJ, et al. Cyclooxygenase-2 polymorphisms confer susceptibility to sarcoidosis but are not related to prognosis. Respir Med. 2009 Mar; 103(3):427-33.

[122] Lopez-Campos JL, Rodriguez-Rodriguez D, Rodriguez-Becerra E, Michavila IA, Guerra JF, Hernandez FJ, et al. Association of the 3050G>C polymorphism in the cyclooxygenase 2 gene with systemic sarcoidosis. Archives of medical research. 2008 Jul;39(5):525-30.

[123] Handa T, Nagai S, Ito I, Shigematsu M, Hamada K, Kitaichi M, et al. Cytotoxic T-lymphocyte antigen-4 (CTLA-4) exon 1 polymorphism affects lymphocyte profiles in bronchoalveolar lavage of patients with sarcoidosis. Sarcoidosis Vasc Diffuse Lung Dis. 2003 Oct;20(3):190-6.

[124] Hattori N, Niimi T, Sato S, Achiwa H, Maeda H, Oguri T, et al. Cytotoxic T-lymphocyte antigen 4 gene polymorphisms in sarcoidosis patients. Sarcoidosis Vasc Diffuse Lung Dis. 2005 Mar;22(1):27-32.

[125] Falta MT, Bowerman NA, Dai S, Kappler JW, Fontenot AP. Linking Genetic Susceptibility and T Cell Activation in Beryllium-induced Disease. Proc Am Thorac Soc. May 1, 2010;7(2):126-9.

[126] Newman LS. Beryllium disease and sarcoidosis: clinical and laboratory links. Sarcoidosis. 1995 Mar;12(1):7-19.

[127] Zhang L, Liu R, wang z, Culver D, Wu R. Modeling Haplotype-Haplotype Interactions in Case-Control Genetic Association Studies. Frontiers in Genetics. 2012 2012-January-18;3.

Chapter 4

Genetic Factors Involved in Sarcoidosis

Birendra P. Sah and Michael C. Iannuzzi

Additional information is available at the end of the chapter

1. Introduction

Sarcoidosis is an immune mediated disease thought to be caused by complex interaction between genetic and environmental factors. Involvement of genetic factors in sarcoidosis is supported by familial clustering, increased concordance in monozygotic twins and varying incidence and disease presentation among different ethnic groups. Studies have revealed several human leukocyte antigen (HLA) and non-HLA alleles consistently associated with sarcoidosis susceptibility. Two genome scans have been reported in sarcoidosis: one in African Americans reporting linkage to chromosome 5 and the other in German families reporting linkage to chromosome 6. Follow-up studies on chromosome 6 identified the BTNL2 gene, a B7 family costimulatory molecule to be associated with sarcoidosis. Recent genome-wide association studies have found annexin A11 and RAB23 genes associated with sarcoidosis. The ongoing refinement of genetic marker maps, genotyping technology, and statistical analyses makes genomic exploration for sarcoidosis genes appealing.

2. Evidence for genetic predisposition to sarcoidosis

Familial sarcoidosis was first noted in Germany in 1923 by Martenstein, who reported two affected sisters [1]. After that several familial cases were reported across Europe and USA. Worldwide surveys revealed that familial sarcoidosis occurred in 10.3% cases from the Netherlands [2], 7.5% from Germany [3], 5.9% from the United Kingdom [4], 4.7% from Finland [5], 4.3% from Japan [5], 9.6% from Ireland[6] and 6.9 % from Sweden[7]. A family history survey of Detroit clinic–based population in USA showed that 17% of African Americans and 3.8% of white American reported a family history in first- and second degree relatives[8]. In African Americans, the sibling recurrence risk ratio, which compares disease risk among siblings with the disease prevalence in the general population, is about 2.2 (95% confidence interval [CI], 1.03–3.68) [9].

The main limitation of these familial reports is the lack of a comparison group, and therefore it was unclear whether variation in familial sarcoidosis is due to variation in familial aggregation of disease risk, disease prevalence, or both. This question was addressed in the multicenter Case-Control Etiologic Study of Sarcoidosis (ACCESS) which evaluated 706 cases and matched controls [10]. It showed that the siblings of the affected patients had the highest relative risk (odds ratio =5.8 and 95% confidence interval=2.1–15.9). The odds ratio for the parents was 3.8 (95% CI=1.2–11.3) [10]. White cases had a markedly higher familial relative risk compared with African-American cases (18.0 versus 2.8; p=0.098).

A registry-based twin study in the Danish and the Finnish population showed an 80-fold increased risk of developing sarcoidosis in monozygotic co-twins and 7-fold increased risk in dizygotic twins [11].

Differences in disease incidence among different ethnic and racial groups exist worldwide. In the United States, African Americans have about a threefold higher age-adjusted annual incidence; 35.5 per 100,000 compared with Caucasians, 10.9 per 100,000. African American females aged 30 to 39 years were found at greatest risk at 107/100,000.The lifetime risk was calculated to be 2.4% for African Americans and 0.85% for Caucasian Americans [12]. In the United Kingdom, prevalence of sarcoidosis was found to be three times higher in the Irish living in London than in native Londoners [14]. It was eight time more common in natives of Martinique living in France than in the indigenous French populations [14]. In London the annual incidence of sarcoidosis has been reported as 1.5 per 100, 000 for Caucasians, 16.8 per 100, 000 for Asians and 19.8 per 100, 000 for Africans [15]. A study of a Swedish urban population reported a lifetime risk of 1.0% and 1.3% for men and women, respectively [16]. In addition to differences in the incidence, the clinical presentation of sarcoidosis also shows characteristic variability between ethnic groups. In both Blacks and Asians the disease has been reported to be more common, more severe and more extensive than in Caucasians [13, 15].

3. Genetics of other granulomatous disease

Blau syndrome and Crohn's disease

Among the granulomatous diseases with a putative genetic component, perhaps the most intriguing are Blau syndrome and Crohn's disease. Blau syndrome is an autosomal dominant granulomatous disease which is characterized by an early onset (before age 20) and involvement of skin, eye, and joints, similar to sarcoidosis. The factors that distinguish Blau syndrome from sarcoidosis are a lack of pulmonary involvement and absence of Kveim reactivity [17]. Crohn's disease is a familial granulomatous inflammatory bowel disease which, like sarcoidosis, may present with uveitis, arthritis and skin rash. Crohn's disease may involve the lung however the pattern of lung involvement differs from sarcoidosis.

Mutation in CARD (caspase activating recruitment domain) 15 gene, located on chromosome 16, is responsible for Blau syndrome [17, 18] and Crohn's disease [19]. The nucleotide oligomerization domain protein-2 (NOD2), encoded by CARD15, recognizes peptidoglycan, a component of bacterial cell walls, and is expressed mainly by antigen-presenting cells and epithelial cells [20]. Activation of NOD2 leads to nuclear factor (NF)-κB activation [20]. Rybicki and colleagues tested 35 African American affected sib pairs by using exclusion mapping and showed that the Blau syndrome/IBD1 locus did not confer risk for sarcoidosis [21]. Schurmann and coworkers [22] evaluated four main coding CARD15 polymorphisms associated with increased risk of Crohn's disease in both case–control and family-based sarcoidosis samples and concluded that CARD15 mutations play no role in sarcoidosis. Kanazawa and colleagues using a small sample analyzed 10 patients with early-onset sarcoidosis who had disease onset ranging from 6 months to 4 year of age and found that 9 of the 10 cases had heterozygous missense mutations in the CARD15 gene [23]. In conclusion, while an attractive candidate, no firm evidence exists to support a role for CARD 15 in sarcoidosis risk.

Chronic beryllium disease

Chronic beryllium disease (CBD), a chronic granulomatous lung disease caused by exposure to beryllium, shares similar histological and clinical findings with sarcoidsois. Glu69, carried by allele HLADPB1* 0201, was found not to be associated with sarcoidosis [24, 25]. In a study of 33 cases and 44 exposed persons without CBD (controls), Richeldi and colleagues found Glu69 in 97% of cases and in 30% of control subjects [26]. This HLA-DPB1 Glu69 association in beryllium disease has been widely supported [27] but is not associated with sarcoidosis.

Tuberculosis and leprosy

Polymorphic variants of the natural resistance–associated macrophage protein-1 gene (NRAMP1), now named SLC11A1, have been found to be associated with tuberculosis and leprosy susceptibility in endemic areas of disease [28, 29]. SLC11A1 is expressed primarily in macrophages and polymorphonuclear leukocytes and immunolocalization studies demonstrate the presence of NRAMP1 in lysosomes [30]. SLC11A1, an attractive candidate, was found not to increase the risk of sarcoidosis among African Americans [31], although a more recent article has noted an association in Polish patients (OR, 1.68; 95% CI, 1.01–2.81) [32].

4. Genetic associatiation studies in sarcoidosis

Genetic studies in sarcoidosis have gone through three phases – candidate gene studies, genome scanning using affected sib pair (ASP) linkage analysis and most recently, genome wide association studies (GWAS).

4.1. Candidate gene approach

The search for sarcoidosis susceptibility genes has generally relied on the candidate gene approach [33]. Investigators have selected genes for study that fit into the prevailing disease model. Sarcoidosis is thought to be a dysregulated response to an inhaled antigen that involves antigen-presenting cells, T cells (primarily a helper T-cell type 1 polar response), and cytokine and chemokine release resulting in cell recruitment and the formation of granulomas in involved organs.

4.1.1. Association with Human Leukocyte Antigens (HLA)

HLA genes have been the best studied candidate genes in sarcoidosis. HLA genes are involved in presenting antigen to T cells and are grouped into three classes: class I, II and III. HLA association studies in sarcoidosis began over thirty years ago. A summary of the most consistent HLA associations in sarcoidosis is shown in Table 1. In 1977 Brewerton and colleague [34] first revealed an association of acute sarcoidosis with the HLA class I antigen HLA-B8 which was later confirmed by other groups [35, 36]. Hedfors and co-workers [35] also noted that HLA-B8/DR3 genes were inherited as a sarcoidosis risk haplotype in whites. In white HLA-B8/DR3 haplotype is associated with wide variety of autoimmune diseases [37]. These earlier studies of class I HLA antigens directed to the studies focused on HLA class II. A recent report by Grunewald and colleagues [38] suggests that HLA class I and II genes work together in sarcoidosis pathophysiology.

HLA gene	HLA class	Chromosome location	Risk Alleles	Putative Functional Significance
HLA-A	Class I	30,018, 309- 30, 021, 041 bp	A*1	Susceptibility
HLA-B	Class I	31, 431, 922- 31, 432, 914 bp	B*8	Susceptibility in several populations
HLA-DQB1	Class II	32, 735, 918- 32, 742, 420 bp	*0201 *0602	Protection, Lofgren's syndrome, mild disease in several populations Susceptibility/disease progression in several groups
HLA-DRB1	Class II	32, 654, 526- 32, 665, 559 bp	*0301 *01, *04 *1101	Acute onset/good prognosis in several groups Protection in several populations Susceptibility in whites and African Americans. Stage II/III chest X-ray
HLA-DRB3	Class II	32, 654, 526- 32, 665, 540 bp	*1501 *0101	Associated with Lofgren's syndrome Susceptibility/disease progression in whites
BTNL2	Class II	32, 470, 490- 32, 482, 878 bp	rs2076530	BTNL2 rs2076530 G → A is associated with sarcoidosis risk in white patients but not in black patients.

Table 1. Summary of the most consistent HLA association studies in Sarcoidosis.

Among the HLA class II antigens, HLA-DRB1 have been the most studied antigen associated with sarcoidosis. The variation in the HLA-DRB1 gene affects both susceptibility and prognosis in sarcoidosis [39, 40]. In the ACCESS study, the HLA-DRB1* 1101 allele was associated with sarcoidosis both in blacks and whites (p<0.01) and had a population attributable risk of 16% in blacks and 9% in whites [41]. In addition susceptibility markers, the ACCESS study also found that HLA class II alleles might be markers for different phenotypes of sarcoidosis such as RB1*0401 for eye involvement in blacks and whites, DRB3 for bone marrow involvement in blacks, and DPB1*0101 for hypercalcemia in whites [41]. Another consistent finding across populations has been the HLA-DQB1*0201 allele association with decreased risk and lack of disease progression [42]. Other reports strongly support the notion that several different HLA class II genes acting either in concert or independently predispose to sarcoidosis [42-44]. Linkage disequilibrium (LD) within the major histocompatibility complex (MHC) region limits the ability to precisely identify the involved HLA genes. LD exists when alleles at two distinctive loci occur in gametes more frequently than expected. Grunewald and colleagues showed that the HLA-DRB1*03 associated with resolved disease and HLA-DRB1*15 with persistent disease were synonymous with HLA-DQB1*0201 with resolved disease and HLA DQB1*0602 with persistent disease [38]. Consequently, determining the effects of HLA-DQB1 on sarcoidosis risk apart from DRB1 or dissecting out other gene effects from closely linked haplotypes in the MHC region may be an intractable problem in whites. In African Americans, HLA-DRB1/DQB1 LD may not be as strong as in Caucasians [45].

HLA alleles have been consistently associated with disease course which suggests that HLA may play greater role in determining phenotype. Furthermore, the discrepant findings in HLA association among susceptibility studies could be explained by the phenotype variation in composition of the sarcoidosis patient groups studied.

4.1.2. Association with Non-HLA candidate genes

Genes that influence antigen processing, antigen presentation, macrophage and T-cell activation, and cell recruitment and injury repair may be considered sarcoidosis candidate genes. A summary of non-HLA candidate genes reported to date is shown in Table 2.

Angiotensin-Converting Enzyme

Angiotensin-converting enzyme (ACE) is produced by sarcoidal granulomas and its serum level can be elevated in sarcoidosis. Serum ACE levels are thought to reflect granuloma burden. The ACE gene insertion (I)/deletion (D) polymorphism partially accounts for the serum ACE level variation, and investigators have proposed that this genotype should be used to adjust serum ACE reference values [46]. Studies to support a role for ACE gene polymorphisms in susceptibility or severity have been inconsistent. While only a few case control studies have suggested that ACE gene polymorphism is associated with sarcoidosis susceptibility and disease severity [47, 48], most of the studies does not support that findings [50-53].

Candidate Gene	Chromosome Location	Association*†	Putative Functional Significance
Angiotensin-converting enzyme (ACE)	17q23	C	Increased risk for ID and DD genotypes. Moderate association between II genotype and radiographic progression.
C-C chemokine receptor 2	3p21.3	C+/-	Protection/Lofgren's syndrome association
C-C chemokine receptor 5	3p21.3	C-	Association of CCR5Delta32 allele more common in patients needing corticosteroid therapy. Refuted with haplotype analysis and larger sample.
Clara cell 10 kD protein	11q 12-13	C	An allele associated with sarcoidosis and with progressive disease at 3 year follow-up.
Complement receptor 1	1q32	A	The GG genotype for the Pro1827Arg (C (5,507) G) polymorphism was significantly associated with sarcoidosis.
Cystic fibrosis trans-membrane regulator	7q31.2	A+/-	R75Q increases risk.
HSPA1L heat shock protein 70 1 like	6p21.3	c	HSP(+2437)CC associated with susceptibility and LS
Inhibitor kβ-α	14q13	C	Association with -297T allele. Association of haplotype GTT at -881, -826, and -297, respectively. Allele -827T in Stage II.
Interleukin -1α	2q14	A	The IL-1α -889 1.1 genotype increased risk.
Interleukin -4 receptor	16p11.2		No association detected in 241 members of 62 families
Interleukin -18	11q22	A+/-	Genotype -607CA increased risk over AA. No association with organ involvement.
Interferon-γ	9p22	A	IFNA17 polymorphism (551T→G) and IFNA10 (60A) IFN-α 17 (551G) haplotype increased risk.
Toll-like receptor (TLR) 4 TLR10-TLR1-TLR6 cluster	9q32 4	B	Asp299Gly and Thre399Ile mutations associated with chronic disease Genetic variation in this cluster is associated with increased risk of chronic disease
Transforming growth factor (TGF)	19q13.2	B	TGF-β2 59941 allele, TGF-β3 4875 A and 17369 C alleles were associated with chest X-ray detection of fibrosis.
Tumor necrosis factor (TNF-α)	6p21.3	C+/-	Genotype -307A allele associated with Lofgren's syndrome and erythema nodosum and -857T allele with sarcoidosis. -307A not associated in African Americans.
Vascular endothelial growth factor(VEGF)	6p12	C	Protective effect of +813 CT and TT genotypes. Lower FEV1/FVC ratio observed with -627 GG genotype.
Vitamin D receptor	12q12-14	A-	B allele elevated in sarcoidosis patients

* Type of association: A = susceptibility; B = disease course; C = both.

† Association replicated (+); association refuted (-)

Table 2. A summary of Non-HLA candidate gene associated with Sarcoidosis

CC-Chemokine Receptor 2 (CCR2]

CCR 2, a receptor for monocyte chemoattractant protein, plays an important role in recruiting monocytes, T-cells, natural killer cells and dendritic cells [54]. CCR2 knockout mice die rapidly when challenged with mycobacteria [55] and display decreased IFN-γ production when challenged with *Leishmania donovani* or *Cryptococcus neoformans* [56, 57]. A single nucleotide polymorphism (SNP) in CCR2 gene (G190A, Val64Ile) is associated with protection in Japanese patients [58]. Evaluation of eight SNPs in the CCR2 gene in 304 Dutch patients showed that haplotype 2 was associated with Lofgren's syndrome [59]. Underrepresentation of the Val64Ile variant was observed in 65 Czech patients and in 80 control subjects but did not achieve statistical significance [60]. Despite using case control–based and family-based study designs and a sample much larger than the previous three studies, Valentonyte and colleagues could not replicate the CCR2 association [61].

C-C chemokine Receptor 5 (CCR5)

CCR5 serves as a receptor for CCL3 (macrophage inflammatory protein 1-α), CCL4 (macrophage inflammatory protein 1-β), CCL5 (RANTES [regulated upon activation, T-cell expressed and secreted]), and CCL8 (monocyte chemotactic protein 2) [62, 63]. A 32 bp deletion in the CCR5 gene results in a non-functional receptor unable to bind its ligands [64]. Petrek and colleagues reported that 32-bp deletion in CCR5 gene was significantly increased in Czech patients [60], whereas Spagnolo and colleagues, using haplotype analysis, found no association in evaluating 106 white British patients and 142 control subjects and 112 Dutch patients and 169 control subjects [65].

Clara cell 10 kD protein gene

Clara cells act as stem cells in bronchial epithelial repair, provides xenobiotic metabolism, and counter regulates inflammation [66]. Clara cell 10-kD protein (CC10) has been shown to inhibit IFN-γ, tumor necrosis factor (TNF)-α, and interleukin (IL)-1β. Murine and human CC10 gene promoter regions contain sites where inflammatory mediators, such as TNF-$\alpha$and INF-α, -β, and -γ, alter transcriptional activity [67]. Increased level of CC10 in serum and BAL has been found in sarcoidosis patients whose disease had resolved compared with those whose disease had progressed [68]. The CC10 gene consists of three short exons separated by a long first and short second intron. An adenine to guanine substitution at position 38 (A38G) downstream from the transcription initiation site within the noncoding region of exon 1 has been the most studied CC10 polymorphism. The A/A genotype is believed to result in decreased CC10 levels [69]. The CC10A allele was found to be associated with sarcoidosis by Ohchi and colleague [70]. However association with the CC10 A38G polymorphism was not replicated in Dutch population or in Japanese subjects by Janssen and colleagues [71].

Complement receptor 1

Complement receptor 1 (CR1; CD35) is present on polymorphonuclear leukocytes, macrophages, B lymphocytes, some T lymphocytes, dendritic cells, and erythrocytes [71]. Immune complexes bound to CR1 are transferred to phagocytes as erythrocytes traverse the liver and spleen [72]. Immune complex clearance rates correlate with CR1 density. Low expression of erythrocyte CR1 is associated with impaired immune complex clearance and deposition outside the reticuloendothelial system [73]. These extrareticuloendothelial immune complex deposits incite local inflammatory responses and presumably granuloma formation. That immune complexes may be involved in sarcoidosis was suggested in the early 1970s. In a series involving 3,676 patients from 11 cities around the world, James and coworkers [74] reported elevated serum γ-globulin levels above 3.5 g/100 ml in 23 to 96% of patients, with IgG being the most consistently and persistently elevated [75]. The different sensitivities of the techniques used explain in part the wide range in γ-globulin levels. It is generally accepted that immune complexes are always present in sarcoidosis depending on when and how they are detected. Zorzetto and colleagues have been the only group to report a CR1 gene association with sarcoidosis [76]. The GG genotype for the Pro1827Arg (C507G) polymorphism was associated with sarcoidosis versus healthy control subjects (odds ratio [OR], 3.13; 95% CI, 1.49–6.69) and versus control subjects with chronic obstructive pulmonary disease (OR, 2.82; 95% CI, 1.27–6.39). The GG genotype was most strongly associated with disease in female patients (OR, 7.05; 95% CI, 3.10–1.61) versus healthy control subjects. No relationship with clinical variables was found.

Cystic fibrosis transmembrane conductance regulator

The R75Q mutation in the cystic fibrosis transmembrane conductance regulator (CFTR) occurs in high frequency in patients with atypical mild cystic fibrosis [77], bronchiectasis, and allergic bronchopulmonary aspergillosis [78]. Bombieri and colleagues reported a R75Q association with sarcoidosis [79], but in followup using complete cystic fibrosis gene mutation screening they could not replicate their findings [80]. Schurmann and colleagues could not demonstrate a CFTR association with sarcoidosis [81].

Heat shock protein A1L

Heat shock proteins (HSPs) comprise a conserved group of proteins with an average weight of 70 kD. Intracellular HSPs serve as molecular chaperones [82], whereas extracellular HSPs induce cellular immune responses [83]. HSPs may also act as carrier molecules for the immunogenic peptides presented on antigen-presenting cells [84]. Polymorphisms in the HSPA1L (alias HSP70-hom) have been associated with susceptibility to rheumatoid arthritis [85]. Antibodies to HSP70 in sarcoidosis have been reported [86, 87]. To further evaluate the role of HSPs in sarcoidosis, the HSP70 +2437 C allele was evaluated and found to be associated with sarcoidosis and Lo° fgren's syndrome in Polish patients [88] but not in Japanese patients [89].

Inhibitor κB-α

Inhibitor κB (IκB) masks the nuclear factor (NF)- κB nuclear localization sequence, thus retaining NF-κB in the cytoplasm and preventing DNA binding. On phosphorylation, IκB degrades, allowing NF-kB's nuclear localization and initiation of transcription [90]. Terminating the NF-κB response requires IκB-α. IκB-α knockout mice die 7 to 10 days after birth with increased levels of TNF-α mRNA in the skin and severe dermatitis [91]. NF-κB–dependent signaling in alveolar macrophage makes NF-κB and thus IκB central to sarcoid pathophysiology [92]. Abdallah and colleagues found the promoter -297T allele associated with sarcoidosis [93]. No other IκB studies in sarcoidosis have been reported.

Interlukin-1(IL-1)

IL-1β produced mainly by macrophages maintains T-cell alveolitis and granuloma formation. Hunninghake and colleagues also demonstrated higher IL-1β activity in the BALF of patients with sarcoidosis compared with normal subjects [94]. Mikuniya and colleagues suggested that the ratio of IL-1 receptor antagonist to IL-1β in sarcoidal alveolar macrophage culture supernatants could predict disease chronicity [95]. The IL-1α 5′ flanking −889 C allele was found nearly two times more commonly among Czech patients with sarcoidosis compared with control subjects [96].

Interleukin Receptor- 4 (IL-4R)

The inflammatory response in sarcoidosis is primarily Th1 mediated. IL-4 drives Th2 differentiation [97]. To test whether variation in the IL-4R gene confers susceptibility to sarcoidosis, Bohnert and colleagues typed 241 members of 62 families with 136 affected siblings and 304 healthy control subjects for three functional SNPs within the IL-4R gene and found no evidence for linkage or association, thus excluding a significant role for IL-4R [98].

Interlukin-18 (IL-18)

IL-18 produced by monocytes/macrophages induces IFN-γ and drives the Th1 response. BALF and serum IL-18 levels are increased in sarcoidosis [99]. An association between IL-18607 (A/ C) polymorphism and sarcoidosis has been reported and refuted in Japanese [100, 101] and white subjects [102, 103].

Interferon–α (IFN-α)

The increasing number of reported cases of IFN-α–induced sarcoidosis supports that IFN-α is important in sarcoidosis [104]. Akahoshi and colleagues found an IFN-α T551G (Ile184Arg) polymorphism associated with sarcoidosis susceptibility (OR, 3.27; 95% CI, 1.44–7.46; p=0.004) [105]. This allele is also associated with high IFN-α production and subsequent strong Th1 polarization.

Transforming Growth Factor-β (TGF-β)

Polymorphisms for all three isoforms of transforming growth factor (TGF) – β (TGF- β1, TGF-β2, and TGF-β3) have been associated with protein expression variation or functionality changes [106]. TGF-β1 levels are increased in patients with sarcoidosis who have impaired pulmonary function [107]. Kruit and colleagues reported that the TGF-β2 59941Gallele and the TGF-β3 4875 A and 17369 C alleles were associated with chest X-ray evidence of pulmonary fibrosis [85]. The TFG-β3 15101 G allele was lower in patients with fibrosis [108].

Toll-like receptor 4 (TLR4) and TLR10-TLR1-TLR6 cluster

Toll-like receptor 4 (TLR4), the first and best described of the many TLRs, plays a crucial role in detecting infection and inducing inflammatory and adaptive immune responses [109]. Pabst and colleagues examined 141 white German patients and control subjects for the TLR4 polymorphisms Asp299Gly and Thre399Ile and found no association with disease presence but did find a significant correlation with chronic disease [110].

Recently Veltcamp and colleague found that genetic variation in TLR10-TLR1-TLR6 cluster is associated with increased risk of chronic disease [111].

Tumor Necrosis Factor–α (TNF-α)

TNF-α has a broad range of inflammatory and immunostimulatory actions, including orchestrating granuloma formation. TNF-α stimulates cytokine production, enhances expression of adhesion molecules, and acts as a costimulator of T-cell activation. Alveolar macrophages from patients with active sarcoidosis secrete more TNF-α than those with inactive disease [112]. TNF-α has been considered a target for therapy in sarcoidosis [113].

Although it is unclear whether TNF-α promoter polymorphisms are functionally significant, studies suggest that a small but significant effect of the TNF-α promoter -307 A/G polymorphism may exist, with the A allele being associated with slightly greater levels of TNF-α transcription [114, 115]. A higher frequency of TNF-307A allele has been found in patients presenting with Lofgren's syndrome and erythema nodosum [116–118]. In evaluating five promoter polymorphisms, Grutters and colleagues found a significant increase in TNF -857T allele in white British and Dutch patients and confirmed the TNF -307A allele association with Lo° fgren's syndrome [119]. In these studies, it is not clear whether TNF-307A confers independent risk from HLA-DRB1 because TNF is in tight LD with HLA-DRBI [120]. Using a family-based approach, TNF-α was not found to be significantly associated with sarcoidosis [49].

Vascular endothelial growth factor

Dysregulated vascular endothelial growth factor (VEGF) expression has been implicated in several inflammatory diseases, such as rheumatoid arthritis and inflammatory bowel diseases [121, 122]. VEGF modulates angiogenesis, enhances monocyte migration, a key event in granuloma formation [123]. Tolnay and colleagues reported increased VEGF transcription and protein production in activated alveolar macrophages in epithelioid cells and multinuclear giant cells of pulmonary sarcoidal granulomas [124]. Several polymorphisms have been associated with VEGF protein production [125, 126]. Morohashi and colleagues found that the VEGF+813T allele was underrepresented (associated with decreased risk) in patients with sarcoidosis. The +813 site is predicted to lie within a potential transcription factor binding site and could potentially reduce VEGF expression [126].

Vitamin D receptors

The active form of vitamin D, 1,25-dihydroxy vitamin D3, modulates the immune response through control of cytokine expression, including IFN-γ and IL-2 [127]. Increased expression of vitamin D receptors (VDRs) on sarcoidal BAL T cells and alveolar macrophage production of 1,25-dihydroxy vitamin D3 have been reported [128, 129]. Niimi and colleagues reported a VDR Bsm1 restriction site polymorphism in intron 8 to be associated with sarcoidosis [130]. Guleva and Seitzer examined a VDR Taq1 polymorphism in linkage disequilibrium with the BsmI polymorphism in 85 patients and 80 control subjects and could not confirm Niimi and colleagues' findings [131]. Rybicki and colleagues also could not confirm VDRs as candidate genes in sarcoidosis [49].

CD80 and CD86

The B7 family of costimulatory molecules (CD80 and CD86) regulate T-cell activation. T-cell activation requires two signals: one mediated by T-cell receptor interaction with specific antigen in association with HLA molecules and an antigen-independent costimulatory signal provided by interaction between CD28 on T-cell surface and its ligands CD80 (B7-1) and CD86 (B7-2) on the antigen-presenting cells [146]. Handa and colleagues investigated CD80 and CD86 SNPs for sarcoidosis susceptibility in 146 Japanese patients and found no significant difference compared with 157 control subjects [147].

Unfortunately none of candidate gene chosen based on its likely function in sarcoidosis pathophysiology has been confirmed using the family-based study design. Limitation to many of these studies likely resides in the case-control study design's susceptibility to a form of confounding known as population stratification which can be overcome by using a family-based design that involves recruiting patients 'siblings and parents if available. In this design, parental alleles not transmitted to affected offspring are used as the control alleles and thus control for genetic background. The transmission disequilibrium test, one of the statistical methods used, counts the number of parental gene variants transmitted to affected offspring. Deviation from expected transmission supports a predisposing effect of the more frequently transmitted allele.

4.2. Genome scanning: Affected sib pair linkage analysis

Sarcoidosis genome scan in Germans

The first genome scan study related to sarcoidosis was conducted by Schurmann and colleagues, in which they used 225 microsatellite markers spanning the genome in 63 German families to identify a linkage signal (D6S1666) on chromosome 6p21 [132]. This group then used a three-stage single-nucleotide polymorphism (SNP) scan of the 16-MB region surrounding D6S1666 [133] and identified a single SNP, rs2076530, in the BTNL2 gene associated with sarcoidosis. This SNP (G/A) was found at the 3' boundary of the exon 5 coding region. The A allele at this position has been proposed to introduce an alternative splice site at the exon 5–3' intron boundary of the BTNL2 transcript that results in a premature truncation of the protein.

BTNL2, also known as "butyrophilin-like 2" and "BTL-2," is a butyrophilin gene that belongs to the immunoglobulin gene superfamily related to the B7 family [134, 135]. Butyrophilin was initially cloned from cattle mammary epithelial cells [136]. This gene was localized to the MHC class II region in humans. To determine the consistency of the BTNL2 gene as a sarcoidosis risk factor across different populations, Rybicki and colleagues characterized variation in the BTNL2 exon/intron 5 region in an African-American family sample that consisted of 219 nuclear families (686 individuals) and in 2 case–control samples (295 African-American matched pairs and 366 white American matched pairs) [137].They confirmed that BTNL2 somewhat was less associated with sarcoidosis in African Americans compared with whites. BTNL2 appears to have moderate influence on individual disease risk (odds ratio of 1.6 in heterozygotes and 2.8 in homozygotes). The population attributable risk of 23% for heterozygotes and homozygotes indicates a significant contribution at the population level.

Whether BTNL2 as a sarcoidosis risk factor is independent of HLA-DRB risk alleles or not, still remains a question. HLADRB and BTNL2 are in linkage disequilibrium. Linkage disequilibrium is the nonrandom association of alleles physically closes on a chromosome. HLA-DRB lies about 180 kb centromeric to BTNL2. On the basis of regression models, BTNL2 appears to be an independent risk factor [133, 137]. In the case of blacks, in whom the BTNL2-conferred sarcoidosis risk is less significant than for whites, a negative interaction with HLA-DR appears to exist [137]. In one study, BTNL2 was found not to be associated with Wegener's granulomatosis [138].

Most recently Hofmann and colleagues [139] conducted a Genome-Wide Linkage Analysis in 181 German sarcoidosis families using clustered biallelic markers. This study revealed one region of suggestive linkage on chromosome 12p13.31 at 20 cM (LOD= 2.53; local P value =. 0003) and another linkage on 9q33.1 at 134 cM (LOD =2.12; local P value =.0009). It is proposed that these regions might harbor yet-unidentified, possibly subphenotype-specific risk factors for the disease (e.g. immune-related functions like the tumor necrosis factor receptor 1).

Sarcoidosis genome scan in African Americans

Eleven centers joined together in an NHLBI-sponsored effort (Sarcoidosis Genetic Analysis Consortium [SAGA]) to perform a genome scan in African American siblings. This group performed a 380-microsatellite genomewide scan across 22 autosomes in 519 African American sib pairs. The significant findings included 15 markers with p values < 0.05 with the strongest linkage signal on chromosome 5 [140]. Fine mapping studies indicated a sarcoidosis susceptibility gene on chromosome 5q11.2 and a gene protective effect for sarcoidosis on 5p15.2 [141].

The reason why African Americans were chosen to uncover sarcoidosis susceptibility genes was that African Americans are more commonly and severely affected and have affected family members more often than whites. But the disadvantage of doing so is that African Americans are admixed with white and other populations to varying degrees with possible admixture among their participating centers ranging from 12% in South Carolina to 20% in New York [142]. To address the possibility that admixed subpopulations existed in the SAGA sample and affected the power to detect linkage, the sample was stratified by genetically determined ancestry using the data from the 380 microsatellite markers genotyped in the genome scan. The African-American families were clustered into subpopulations based on ancestry similarity. Evidence of two genetically distinct groups was found: Stratified linkage results suggest that one subpopulation of families contributed to previously identified linkage signals at 1p22, 3p21-14, 11p15, and 17q21 and that a second subpopulation of families contributed to those found at 5p15-13 and 20q13 [143]. These findings support the presence of sarcoidosis susceptibility genes in regions previously identified but indicate that these genes are likely to be specific to ancestral groups that have combined to form modern-day African Americans.

4.3. Genome-Wide Association Studies (GWAS)

In genome-wide association study high throughput genotyping methods are used to genotype a dense set of SNPs across the genome. A significant advantage of this approach is that association studies are more powerful than affected sib pair methods of linkage analysis. Hofmann and colleagues [144] conducted a genomewide association study of 499 German patients with sarcoidosis and 490 control subjects. The strongest signal mapped to the annexin A11 gene on chromosome 10q22.3. Validation in an independent sample confirmed the association. Annexin A11 has regulatory functions in calcium signaling, cell division, vesicle trafficking, and apoptosis. Depletion or dysfunction of annexin A11 may affect the apoptosis pathway in sarcoidosis. Later the same group [145] reported another associated locus 6p12.1 that comprises several genes, a likely candidate being RAB23. RAB23 is proposed to be involved in antibacterial defense processes and regulation of the sonic hedgehog signaling pathway.

5. Counseling and screening

In the context of genetic family counseling, this generally is perceived as a small risk by the clients and should lead to enhanced awareness but does not justify specific medical investigations in the absence of complaints.

6. Genetic testing

Genetic testing at present does not play a role in the diagnosis and treatment of sarcoidosis.

7. Future directions

The cause of sarcoidosis remains unknown. It is thought to be caused by interaction between environmental and genetic factors. Genetic studies have revealed the HLA and other candidate genes associated with sarcoidosis susceptibility. Association studies have been motivated by the hopes that identifying alleles that affect risk and phenotype will help in understanding disease etiology. Unfortunately, many of the reported associations have not been replicated. Two genome scans have been reported and one has yielded a likely candidate gene, BTNL2 that has been replicated in large studies. Emerging technologies and advances in genomics and proteomics will help find the causes sarcoidosis, better understanding of pathogenesis of sarcoidosis and to test new therapy. Gene expression profiling in BALF and blood carried out at the time of presentation will likely help to better predict disease resolution or progression.

Author details

Birendra P. Sah and Michael C. Iannuzzi

SUNY, Upstate Medical University, Syracuse, New York, USA

References

[1] Martenstein H Knochveranderungen bei lupus pernioZ Haut Geschlechtskr 7308, (1923).

[2] Wirnsberger, R. M, De Vries, J, Wouters, E. F, & Drent, M. Clinical presentation of sarcoidosis in The Netherlands an epidemiological study. Neth J Med. (1998). Aug; , 53(2), 53-60.

[3] Kristen, D. Sarcoidosis in Germany. Analysis of a questionnaire survey in 1992 of patients of the German Sarcoidosis Group. Pneumologie. (1995). Jun;, 49(6), 378-82.

[4] Mcgrath, D. S, Daniil, Z, & Foley, P. du Bois JL, Lympany PA, Cullinan P, du Bois RM. Epidemiology of familial sarcoidosis in the UK. Thorax. (2000). Sep; , 55(9), 751-4.

[5] Pietinalho, A, Ohmichi, M, Hirasawa, M, Hiraga, Y, Lofroos, A. B, & Selroos, O. Familial sarcoidosis in Finland and Hokkaido, Japan-a comparative study. *Respir Med* (1999). , 93, 408-412.

[6] Brennan, N. J, Crean, P, Long, J. P, & Fitzgerald, M. X. High prevalence of familial sarcoidosis in an Irish population. *Thorax* (1984). , 39, 14-18.

[7] Wiman, L. G. Familial occurrence of sarcoidosis. *Scand J Respir Dis Suppl* (1972). , 80, 115-119.

[8] Harrington, D, Major, M, & Rybicki, B. Popovich J Jr, Maliarik M, Iannuzzi MC. Familial analysis of 91 families. *Sarcoidosis* (1994). , 11, 240-243.

[9] Rybicki, B. A, Kirkey, K. L, Major, M, & Maliarik, M. J. Popovich J Jr, Chase GA, IannuzziMC. Familial risk ratio of sarcoidosis inAfrican-American sibs and parents. *Am J Epidemiol* (2001). , 153, 188-193.

[10] Rybicki, B. A, Iannuzzi, M. C, Frederick, M. M, Thompson, B. W, Rossman, M. D, Bresnitz, E. A, Terrin, M. L, Moller, D. R, Barnard, J, & Baughman, R. P. Familial aggregation of sarcoidosis: A Case-Control Etiologic Study of Sarcoidosis (ACCESS). *Am J Respir Crit Care Med* (2001). , 164, 2085-2091.

[11] Sverrild, A, Backer, V, Kyvik, K. O, Kaprio, J, Milman, N, Svendsen, C. B, & Thomsen, S. F. Heredity in sarcoidosis: a registry-based twin study. Thorax. (2008). Oct; Epub 2008 Jun 5., 63(10), 894-6.

[12] Rybicki, B. A, & Major, M. Popovich J Jr, Maliarik MJ, Iannuzzi MC. Racial differen-
      ces in sarcoidosis incidence: a 5-year study in a health maintenance organization. *Am
      J Epidemiol* (1997). , 145, 234-241.

[13] Rybicki, B. A, Maliarik, M. J, & Major, M. Popovich J Jr, Iannuzzi MC. Epidemiology,
      demographics, and genetics of sarcoidosis. Sem Respir Infect (1998). , 3, 166-173.

[14] James, D. G, Neville, E, & Siltzbach, L. E. A worldwide review of sarcoidosis. Ann N
      Y Acad Sci. (1976). , 278, 321-34.

[15] Edmondstone, W. M, & Wilson, A. G. Sarcoidosis in Caucasians, Blacks and Asians
      in London. Br J Dis Chest. (1985). Jan; , 79(1), 27-36.

[16] Hillerdal, G, No, u E, Osterman, K, et al. Sarcoidosis: epidemiology and prognosis. A
      15-year European study. Am Rev Respir Dis (1984). , 130, 29-32.

[17] Blau EB Familial granulomatous arthritisiritis, and rash. J Pediatr 107689493,(1985).

[18] Miceli-richard, C, Lesage, S, Rybojad, M, Prieur, A. M, Manouvrier-hanu, S, Hafner,
      R, Chamaillard, M, Zouali, H, Thomas, G, & Hugot, J. P. CARD15 mutations in Blau
      syndrome. *Nat Genet* (2001). , 29, 19-20.

[19] Hugot, J. P, Chamaillard, M, Zouali, H, Lesage, S, Cezard, J. P, Belaiche, J, Almer, S,
      Tysk, C, Morain, O, & Gassull, C. A. M, *et al.* Association of NOD2 leucine-rich re-
      peat variants with susceptibility to Crohn's disease.*Nature* (2001). , 411, 599-603.

[20] Strober, W, Murray, P. J, Kitani, A, & Watanabe, T. Signalling pathways and molecu-
      lar interactions of NOD1 and NOD2. *Nat Rev Immunol* (2006). , 6, 9-20.

[21] Rybicki, B. A, Maliarik, M. J, Bock, C. H, Elston, R. C, Baughman, R. P, Kimani, A. P,
      Sheffer, R. G, Chen, K. M, Major, M, & Popovich, J. The Blausyndrome gene is not a
      major risk factor for sarcoidosis. *Sarcoidosis Vasc Diffuse Lung Dis* (1999). , 16, 203-208.

[22] Schurmann, M, Valentonyte, R, Hampe, J, Muller-quernheim, J, Schwinger, E, &
      Schreiber, S. CARD15 gene mutations in sarcoidosis. *Eur Respir J* (2003). , 22, 748-754.

[23] Kanazawa, N, Okafuji, I, Kambe, N, Nishikomori, R, Nakata-hizume, M, Nagai, S,
      Fuji, A, Yuasa, T, Manki, A, & Sakurai, Y. Early-onset sarcoidosis and CARD15 muta-
      tions with constitutive nuclear factorkappaB activation: common genetic etiology
      with Blau syndrome. *Blood* (2005). , 105, 1195-1197.

[24] Maliarik, M. J, Chen, K. M, Major, M. L, & Sheffer, R. G. Popovich J Jr, Rybicki BA,
      Iannuzzi MC. Analysis of HLA-DPB1 polymorphisms in African-Americans with
      sarcoidosis. Am J Respir Crit Care Med (1998). , 158, 111-114.

[25] Schurmann, M, Bein, G, Kirsten, D, Schlaak, M, Muller-quernheim, J, & Schwinger, E.
      HLA-DQB1 and HLA-DPB1 genotypes in familial sarcoidosis. *Respir Med* (1998). , 92,
      649-652.

[26] Richeldi, L, Sorrentino, R, & Saltini, C. HLA-DPB1 glutamate 69: a genetic marker of beryllium disease. *Science* (1993)., 262, 242-244.

[27] Amicosante, M, Sanarico, N, Berretta, F, Arroyo, J, Lombardi, G, Lechler, R, Colizzi, V, & Saltini, C. Beryllium binding to HLA-DP molecule carrying the marker of susceptibility to berylliosis glutamate beta 69. *Hum Immunol* (2001)., 62, 686-693.

[28] Bellamy, R. Identifying genetic susceptibility factors for tuberculosis in Africans: a combined approach using a candidate gene study and a genome-wide screen. *Clin Sci (Lond)* (2000)., 98, 245-250.

[29] Abel, L, Sanchez, F. O, Oberti, J, Thuc, N. V, Hoa, L. V, Lap, V. D, Skamene, E, Lagrange, P. H, & Schurr, E. Susceptibility to leprosy is linked to the human NRAMP1 gene. *J Infect Dis* (1998)., 177, 133-145.

[30] Gruenheid, S, Pinner, E, Desjardins, M, & Gros, P. Natural resistance to infection with intracellular pathogens: the Nramp1 protein is recruited to the membrane of the phagosome. *J Exp Med* (1997)., 185, 717-730.

[31] Maliarik, M. J, Chen, K. M, Sheffer, R. G, Rybicki, B. A, & Major, M. L. Popovich J Jr, Iannuzzi MC. The natural resistance-associated macrophage protein gene in African Americans with sarcoidosis. *Am J Respir Cell Mol Biol* (2000)., 22, 672-675.

[32] Dubaniewicz, A, Jamieson, S. E, Dubaniewicz-wybieralska, M, & Fakiola, M. Nancy Miller E, Blackwell JM. Association between SLC11A1 (formerly NRAMP1) and the risk of sarcoidosis in Poland. *Eur J Hum Genet* (2005)., 13, 829-834.

[33] Iannuzzi, M. C, Rybicki, B. A, & Maliarik, M. Popovich J Jr. Finding disease genes: from cystic fibrosis to sarcoidosis [Thomas A. Neff Lecture].*Chest* (1997). S-73S

[34] Brewerton, D. A, Cockburn, C, James, D. C, James, D. G, & Neville, E. HLA antigens in sarcoidosis. *Clin Exp Immunol* (1977)., 27, 227-229.

[35] Hedfors, E, Lindstrom, F, & Hla-b, D. R. in sarcoidosis: correlation to acute onset disease with arthritis. *Tissue Antigens* (1983)., 22, 200-203.

[36] Smith, M. J, Turton, C. W, Mitchell, D. N, Turner-warwick, M, Morris, L. M, & Lawler, S. D. Association of HLA B8 with spontaneous resolution in sarcoidosis. *Thorax* (1981)., 36, 296-298.

[37] Lio, D, Candore, G, Romano, G. C, Anna, D, Gervasi, C, Di, F, Lorenzo, G, Modica, M. A, & Potestio, M. Caruso C. Modification of cytokine patterns in subjects bearing the HLA-B8,DR3 phenotype: implications for autoimmunity. *Cytokines Cell Mol Ther* (1997)., 3, 217-224.

[38] Grunewald, J, Eklund, A, & Olerup, O. Human leukocyte antigen class I alleles and the disease course in sarcoidosis patients. *Am J Respir Crit Care Med* (2004)., 169, 696-702.

[39] Rossman, M. D, Thompson, B, Frederick, M, Maliarik, M, Iannuzzi, M. C, Rybicki, B. A, Pandey, J. P, Newman, L. S, Magira, E, & Beznik-cizman, B. HLA-DRB1*1101: a

significant risk factor for sarcoidosis in blacks and whites. *Am J Hum Genet* (2003). , 73, 720-735.

[40] Ishihara, M, Ohno, S, Ishida, T, Ando, H, Naruse, T, Nose, Y, & Inoko, H. Molecular genetic studies ofHLA class II alleles in sarcoidosis. *Tissue Antigens* (1994). , 43, 238-241.

[41] Rossman, M. D, Thompson, B, Frederick, M, Maliarik, M, Iannuzzi, M. C, Rybicki, B. A, et al. HLA-DRB1*1101: a significant risk factor for sarcoidosis in blacks and whites. Am J Hum Genet (2003). , 73(4), 720-735.

[42] Iannuzzi, M. C, Maliarik, M. J, Poisson, L. M, & Rybicki, B. A. Sarcoidosis susceptibility and resistance HLA-DQB1 alleles in African Americans. *Am J Respir Crit Care Med* (2003). , 167, 1225-1231.

[43] Maliarik, M. J, Chen, K. M, Major, M. L, & Sheffer, R. G. Popovich J Jr, Rybicki BA, Iannuzzi MC. Analysis of HLA-DPB1 polymorphisms in African-Americans with sarcoidosis. *Am J Respir Crit Care Med* (1998). , 158, 111-114.

[44] 17. Rybicki, B. A, Maliarik, M. J, Poisson, L. M, Sheffer, R, Chen, K. M, Major, M, Chase, G. A, & Iannuzzi, M. C. The major histocompatibility complex gene region and sarcoidosis susceptibility in African Americans. *Am J Respir Crit Care Med* (2003). , 167, 444-449.

[45] Zachary, A. A, Bias, W. B, Johnson, A, Rose, S. M, & Leffell, M. S. Antigen, allele, and haplotype frequencies report of the ASHI minority antigens workshops: part 1, African-Americans. *Hum Immunol* (2001). , 62, 1127-1136.

[46] Sharma, P, Smith, I, Maguire, G, Stewart, S, Shneerson, J, & Brown, M. J. Clinical value of ACE genotyping in diagnosis of sarcoidosis. *Lancet* (1997). , 349, 1602-1603.

[47] Maliarik, M. J, Rybicki, B. A, Malvitz, E, Sheffer, R. G, & Major, M. Popovich J Jr, Iannuzzi MC. Angiotensin-converting enzyme gene polymorphism and risk of sarcoidosis. *Am J Respir Crit Care Med* (1998). , 158, 1566-1570.

[48] Pietinalho, A, Furuya, K, Yamaguchi, E, Kawakami, Y, & Selroos, O. The angiotensin converting enzyme DD gene is associated with poor prognosis in Finnish sarcoidosis patients.*Eur Resp J 1999137236*

[49] Rybicki, B. A, Maliarik, M. J, Poisson, L. M, & Iannuzzi, M. C. Sarcoidosis and granuloma genes: a family-based study in African-Americans. *Eur Respir J* (2004). , 24, 251-257.

[50] Planck, A, Eklund, A, Yamaguchi, E, & Grunewald, J. Angiotensin-converting enzyme gene polymorphism in relation to HLA-DR in sarcoidosis. J Intern Med. (2002). Mar; , 251(3), 217-22.

[51] Mcgrath, D. S, Foley, P. J, Petrek, M, & Izakovicova-holla, L. Du Bois RM. Ace gene I/D polymorphism and sarcoidosis pulmonary disease severity. Am J Respir Crit Care Med. (2001). Jul 15; , 164(2), 197-201.

[52] Schürmann, M, Reichel, P, Müller-myhsok, B, & Schwinger, E. Angiotensin-converting enzyme (ACE) gene polymorphisms and familial occurrence of sarcoidosis. J Intern Med. (2001). Jan; , 249(1), 77-83.

[53] Arbustini, E, Grasso, M, Leo, G, Tinelli, C, Fasani, R, Diegoli, M, Banchieri, N, Cipriani, A, Gorrini, M, & Semenzato, G. Polymorphism of angiotensin-converting enzyme gene in sarcoidosis. Am J Respir Crit Care Med (1996). , 153, 851-854.

[54] Boring, L, Gosling, J, Chensue, S. W, & Kunkel, S. L. Farese RV Jr, Broxmeyer HE, Charo IF. Impaired monocyte migration and reduced type 1 (Th1) cytokine responses in C-C chemokine receptor 2 knockout mice. J Clin Invest (1997). , 100, 2552-2561.

[55] Peters, W, Scott, H. M, Chambers, H. F, Flynn, J. L, Charo, I. F, & Ernst, J. D. Chemokine receptor 2 serves an early and essential role in resistance to Mycobacterium tuberculosis. Proc Natl Acad Sci USA (2001). , 98, 7958-7963.

[56] Traynor, T. R, Kuziel, W. A, Toews, G. B, & Huffnagle, G. B. CCR2 expression determines T1 versus T2 polarization during pulmonary Cryptococcus neoformans infection. J Immunol (2000). , 164, 2021-2027.

[57] Sato, N, Kuziel, W. A, Melby, P. C, Reddick, R. L, Kostecki, V, Zhao, W, Maeda, N, Ahuja, S. K, & Ahuja, S. S. Defects in the generation of IFN gamma are overcome to control infection with Leishmania donovani in CC chemokine receptor (CCR) 5-, macrophage inflammatory protein-1 alpha-, or CCR2-deficient mice. J Immunol (1999). , 163, 5519-5525.

[58] Hizawa, N, Yamaguchi, E, Furuya, K, Jinushi, E, Ito, A, & Kawakami, Y. The role of the C-C chemokine receptor 2 gene polymorphism CCR2- 64I) in sarcoidosis in a Japanese population. Am J Respir Crit Care Med (1999). , 64I

[59] Spagnolo, P, Renzoni, E. A, Wells, A. U, Sato, H, Grutters, J. C, Sestini, P, Abdallah, A, Gramiccioni, E, & Ruven, H. J. du Bois RM, et al. C-C chemokine receptor 2 and sarcoidosis: association with Lofgren's syndrome. Am J Respir Crit Care Med (2003). , 168, 1162-1166.

[60] Petrek, M, Drabek, J, Kolek, V, Zlamal, J, Welsh, K. I, Bunce, M, & Weigl, E. Du Bois R. CC chemokine receptor gene polymorphisms in Czech patients with pulmonary sarcoidosis. Am J Respir Crit Care Med (2000). , 162, 1000-1003.

[61] Valentonyte, R, Hampe, J, Croucher, P. J, Muller-quernheim, J, Schwinger, E, Schreiber, S, & Schurmann, M. Study of C-C chemokine receptor 2 alleles in sarcoidosis, with emphasis on family-based analysis. Am J Respir Crit Care Med (2005). , 171, 1136-1141.

[62] Blanpain, C, Migeotte, I, Lee, B, Vakili, J, Doranz, B. J, Govaerts, C, Vassart, G, Doms, R. W, & Parmentier, M. CCR5 binds multiple CC-chemokines: MCP-3 acts as a natural antagonist. *Blood* (1999). , 94, 1899-1905.

[63] Combadiere, C, Ahuja, S. K, Tiffany, H. L, & Murphy, P. M. Cloning and functional expression of CC CKR5, a human monocyte CC chemokine receptor selective for MIP-1(alpha), MIP-1(beta), and RANTES. *J Leukoc Biol* (1996). , 60, 147-152.

[64] Mantovani, A. The chemokine system: redundancy for robust outputs. Immunol Today. (1999). Jun;, 20(6), 254-7.

[65] Spagnolo, P, Renzoni, E. A, Wells, A. U, Copley, S. J, Desai, S. R, Sato, H, Grutters, J. C, Abdallah, A, & Taegtmeyer, A. du Bois RM, *et al.* C-C chemokine receptor 5 gene variants in relation to lung disease in sarcoidosis. *Am J Respir Crit Care Med* (2005). , 172, 721-728.

[66] Singh, G, & Katyal, S. L. Clara cells and Clara cell 10 kD protein (CC10). *Am J Respir Cell Mol Biol* (1997). , 17, 141-143.

[67] Cowan, M. J, Huang, X, Yao, X. L, & Shelhamer, J. H. Tumor necrosis factor alpha stimulation of human Clara cell secretory protein production by human airway epithelial cells. *Ann NY Acad Sci* (2000). , 923, 193-201.

[68] Shijubo, N, Itoh, Y, Shigehara, K, Yamaguchi, T, Itoh, K, Shibuya, Y, Takahashi, R, Ohchi, T, Ohmichi, M, & Hiraga, Y. Association of Clara cell 10-kDa protein, spontaneous regression and sarcoidosis. *Eur Respir J* (2000). , 16, 414-419.

[69] Laing, I. A, Hermans, C, Bernard, A, Burton, P. R, & Goldblatt, J. Le Souef PN. Association between plasma CC16 levels, the A38G polymorphism, and asthma. *Am J Respir Crit Care Med* (2000). , 161, 124-127.

[70] Ohchi, T, Shijubo, N, Kawabata, I, Ichimiya, S, Inomata, S, Yamaguchi, A, Umemori, Y, Itoh, Y, Abe, S, & Hiraga, Y. Polymorphism of Clara cell 10-kD protein gene of sarcoidosis. *Am J Respir Crit Care Med* (2004). , 169, 180-186.

[71] Janssen, R, Sato, H, Grutters, J. C, & Ruven, H. J. du Bois RM, Matsuura R, Yamazaki M, Kunimaru S, Izumi T, Welsh KI, *et al.* The Clara cell10 adenine38guanine polymorphism and sarcoidosis susceptibility in Dutch and Japanese subjects. *Am J Respir Crit Care Med* (2004). , 170, 1185-1187.

[72] Loegering, D. J, & Blumenstock, F. A. Depressing hepatic macrophage complement receptor function causes increased susceptibility to endotoxemia and infection. *Infect Immun* (1985). , 47, 659-664.

[73] Cornacoff, J. B, Hebert, L. A, Smead, W. L, Vanaman, M. E, Birmingham, D. J, & Waxman, F. J. Primate erythrocyte-immune complex-clearing mechanism. *J Clin Invest* (1983). , 71, 236-247.

[74] Schifferli, J. A, Ng, Y. C, Estreicher, J, & Walport, M. J. The clearance of tetanus toxoid/anti-tetanus toxoid immune complexes from the circulation of humans: comple-

ment- and erythrocyte complement receptor 1- dependent mechanisms. *J Immunol* (1988). , 140, 899-904.

[75] James, D. G, Neville, E, & Walker, A. Immunology of sarcoidosis. *Am JMed* (1975). , 59, 388-394.

[76] Zorzetto, M, Bombieri, C, Ferrarotti, I, Medaglia, S, Agostini, C, Tinelli, C, Malerba, G, Carrabino, N, Beretta, A, & Casali, L. Complement receptor 1 gene polymorphisms in sarcoidosis. *Am J Respir Cell Mol Biol* (2002). , 27, 17-23.

[77] Hughes, D, Dork, T, Stuhrmann, M, & Graham, C. Mutation and haplotype analysis of the CFTR gene in atypically mild cystic fibrosis patients from Northern Ireland. *J Med Genet* (2001). , 38, 136-139.

[78] Luisetti, M, & Pignatti, P. F. Genetics of idiopathic disseminated bronchiectasis. *Semin Respir Crit Care Med* (2003). , 24, 179-184.

[79] Bombieri, C, Luisetti, M, Belpinati, F, Zuliani, E, Beretta, A, Baccheschi, J, Casali, L, & Pignatti, P. F. Increased frequency of CFTR gene mutations in sarcoidosis: a case/control association study. *Eur J Hum Genet* (2000). , 8, 717-720.

[80] Bombieri, C, Belpinati, F, Pignatti, P. F, & Luisetti, M. Comment on 'CFTR gene mutations in sarcoidosis'. *Eur J Hum Genet* (2003). , 11, 553-554.

[81] Schurmann, M, Albrecht, M, Schwinger, E, & Stuhrmann, M. CFTR gene mutations in sarcoidosis. *Eur J Hum Genet* (2002). , 10, 729-732.

[82] Matouschek, A. Protein unfolding: an important process in vivo? *Curr Opin Struct Biol* (2003). , 13, 98-109.

[83] Asea, A, Kraeft, S. K, Kurt-jones, E. A, Stevenson, M. A, Chen, L. B, Finberg, R. W, Koo, G. C, & Calderwood, S. K. HSP70 stimulates cytokine production through a CD14-dependant pathway, demonstrating its dual role as a chaperone and cytokine. *Nat Med* (2000). , 6, 435-442.

[84] Srivastava, P. K, Udono, H, Blachere, N. E, & Li, Z. Heat shock proteins transfer peptides during antigen processing and CTL priming. *Immunogenetics* (1994). , 39, 93-98.

[85] Jenkins, S. C, March, R. E, Campbell, R. D, & Milner, C. M. A novel variant of the MHC-linked hsp70, hsp70-hom, is associated with rheumatoid arthritis. *Tissue Antigens* (2000). , 56, 38-44.

[86] De Smet, M. D, & Ramadan, A. Circulating antibodies to inducible heat shock protein 70 in patients with uveitis. *Ocul Immunol Inflamm* (2001). , 9, 85-92.

[87] Hrycaj, P, Wurm, K, Mennet, P, & Muller, W. Antibodies to heat shock proteins in patients with pulmonary sarcoidosis. *Sarcoidosis* (1995). , 12, 124-130.

[88] Bogunia-kubik, K, Koscinska, K, Suchnicki, K, & Lange, A. HSP70-hom gene single nucleotide (-2763 G/A and-2437 C/T) polymorphisms in sarcoidosis. *Int J Immunogenet* (2006)., 33, 135-140.

[89] Ishihara, M, Ohno, S, Ishida, T, Mizuki, N, Ando, H, Naruse, T, Ishihara, H, & Inoko, H. Genetic polymorphisms of the TNFB and HSP70 genes located in the human major histocompatibility complex in sarcoidosis. *Tissue Antigens* (1995)., 46, 59-62.

[90] Perkins, N. D. The Rel/NF-kappa B family: friend and foe. *Trends Biochem Sci* (2000)., 25, 434-440.

[91] Klement, J. F, Rice, N. R, Car, B. D, Abbondanzo, S. J, Powers, G. D, Bhatt, P. H, Chen, C. H, Rosen, C. A, & Stewart, C. L. IkappaBalpha deficiency results in a sustained NF-kappaB response and severe widespread dermatitis in mice. *Mol Cell Biol* (1996)., 16, 2341-2349.

[92] Conron, M, Bondeson, J, Pantelidis, P, Beynon, H. L, & Feldmann, M. duBois RM, Foxwell BM. Alveolar macrophages and T cells from sarcoid,but not normal lung, are permissive to adenovirus infection and allow analysis of NF-kappa b-dependent signaling pathways. *Am J Respir Cell Mol Biol* (2001)., 25, 141-149.

[93] Abdallah, A, Sato, H, Grutters, J. C, Veeraraghavan, S, Lympany, P. A, & Ruven, H. J. van den Bosch JM, Wells AU, du Bois RM, Welsh KI. Inhibitor kappa B-alpha (IkappaB-alpha) promoter polymorphisms in UK and Dutch sarcoidosis. *Genes Immun* (2003)., 4, 450-454.

[94] Hunninghake, G. W. Release of interleukin-1 by alveolar macrophages of patients with active pulmonary sarcoidosis. *Am Rev Respir Dis* (1984)., 129, 569-572.

[95] Mikuniya, T, Nagai, S, Takeuchi, M, Mio, T, Hoshino, Y, Miki, H, Shigematsu, M, Hamada, K, & Izumi, T. Significance of the interleukin-1 receptor antagonist/interleukin-1 beta ratio as a prognostic factor in patients with pulmonary sarcoidosis. *Respiration (Herrlisheim)* (2000)., 67, 389-396.

[96] Hutyrova, B, Pantelidis, P, Drabek, J, Zurkova, M, Kolek, V, Lenhart, K, & Welsh, K. I. Du Bois RM, Petrek M. Interleukin-1 gene cluster polymorphisms in sarcoidosis and idiopathic pulmonary fibrosis. *Am J Respir Crit Care Med* (2002)., 165, 148-151.

[97] Rengarajan, J, Szabo, S. J, & Glimcher, L. H. Transcriptional regulation of Th1/Th2 polarization. *Immunol Today* (2000)., 21, 479-483.

[98] Bohnert, A, Schurmann, M, Hartung, A, Hackstein, H, Muller-quernheim, J, & Bein, G. No linkage of the interleukin-4 receptor locus on chromosome 1611with sarcoidosis in German multiplex families. *Eur J Immunogenet* (2002).

[99] Shigehara, K, Shijubo, N, Ohmichi, M, Yamada, G, Takahashi, R, Okamura, H, Kurimoto, M, Hiraga, Y, Tatsuno, T, & Abe, S. Increased levels of interleukin-18 in patients with pulmonary sarcoidosis. *Am J Respir Crit Care Med* (2000)., 162, 1979-1982.

[100] Zhou, Y, Yamaguchi, E, Hizawa, N, & Nishimura, M. Roles of functional polymorphisms in the interleukin-18 gene promoter in sarcoidosis. *Sarcoidosis Vasc Diffuse Lung Dis* (2005). , 22, 105-113.

[101] Takada, T, Suzuki, E, Morohashi, K, & Gejyo, F. Association of single nucleotide polymorphisms in the IL-18 gene with sarcoidosis in a Japanese population. *Tissue Antigens* (2002). , 60, 36-42.

[102] Kelly, D. M, Greene, C. M, Meachery, G, Mahony, O, Gallagher, M, Taggart, P. M, Neill, C. C, O, & Mcelvaney, S. J. NG. Endotoxin up-regulates interleukin-18: potential role for gram-negative colonization in sarcoidosis. *Am J Respir Crit Care Med* (2005). , 172, 1299-1307.

[103] Janssen, R, Grutters, J. C, Ruven, H. J, Zanen, P, Sato, H, & Welsh, K. I. du Bois RM, van den Bosch JM. No association between interleukin-18 gene polymorphisms and haplotypes in Dutch sarcoidosis patients. *Tissue Antigens* (2004). , 63, 578-583.

[104] Goldberg, H. J, Fiedler, D, Webb, A, Jagirdar, J, Hoyumpa, A. M, & Peters, J. Sarcoidosis after treatment with interferon-alpha: A case series and review of the literature. *Respir Med* (2006). , 100, 2063-2068.

[105] Akahoshi, M, Ishihara, M, Remus, N, Uno, K, Miyake, K, Hirota, T, Nakashima, K, Matsuda, A, Kanda, M, & Enomoto, T. Association between IFNA genotype and the risk of sarcoidosis. *HumGenet* (2004). , 114, 503-509.

[106] Awad, M. R, Gamel, A, Hasleton, P, Turner, D. M, Sinnott, P. J, & Hutchinson, I. V. Genotypic variation in the transforming growth factor-beta1 gene: association with transforming growth factor-beta1 production, fibrotic lung disease, and graft fibrosis after lung transplantation. *Transplantation* (1998). , 66, 1014-1020.

[107] Salez, F, Gosset, P, & Copin, M. C. Lamblin Degros C, Tonnel AB, Wallaert B. Transforming growth factor-beta1 in sarcoidosis. *Eur Respir J* (1998). , 12, 913-919.

[108] Kruit, A, Grutters, J. C, Ruven, H. J, Van Moorsel, C. H, Weiskirchen, R, & Mengsteab, S. van den Bosch JM. Transforming growth factor-beta gene polymorphisms in sarcoidosis patients with and without fibrosis. *Chest* (2006). , 129, 1584-1591.

[109] Akira, S, Takeda, K, & Kaisho, T. Toll-like receptors: critical proteins linking innate and acquired immunity. *Nat Immunol* (2001). , 2, 675-680.

[110] Pabst, S, Baumgarten, G, Stremmel, A, & Lennarz, . . Toll-like receptor (TLR) 4 polymorphisms are associated with a chronic course of sarcoidosis. *Clin Exp Immunol* 2006; 143:420-426.

[111] Veltkamp, M, Van Moorsel, C. H, Rijkers, G. T, Ruven, H. J, Grutters, J. C, et al. Genetic variation in the Toll-like receptor gene cluster (TLR10-TLR1-TLR6) influences disease course in sarcoidosis. Tissue Antigens. (2012). Jan; , 79(1), 25-32.

[112] Zheng, L, Teschler, H, Guzman, J, Hubner, K, Striz, I, & Costabel, U. Alveolar macro-
      phage TNF-alpha release and BALcell phenotypes in sarcoidosis. *Am J Respir Crit
      Care Med* (1995). , 152, 1061-1066.

[113] Baughman, R. P, & Iannuzzi, M. Tumour necrosis factor in sarcoidosis and its poten-
      tial for targeted therapy. *BioDrugs* (2003). , 17, 425-431.

[114] Allen, R. D. Polymorphism of the human TNF-alpha promoter: random variation or
      functional diversity? *Mol Immunol* (1999). , 36, 1017-1027.

[115] Wilson, A. G. di Giovine FS, Blakemore AI, Duff GW. Single base polymorphism in
      the human tumour necrosis factor alpha (TNF alpha) gene detectable by NcoI restric-
      tion of PCR product. *Hum Mol Genet* (1992).

[116] Somoskovi, A, Zissel, G, Seitzer, U, Gerdes, J, & Schlaak, M. Muller Quernheim J.
      Polymorphisms at position-308 in the promoter region of the TNF-alpha and in the
      first intron of the TNF-beta genes and spontaneous and lipopolysaccharide-induced
      TNF alpha release in sarcoidosis. *Cytokine* (1999). , 11, 882-887.

[117] Seitzer, U, Swider, C, Stuber, F, Suchnicki, K, Lange, A, Richter, E, Zabel, P, Muller-
      quernheim, J, Flad, H. D, & Gerdes, J. Tumour necrosis factor alpha promoter gene
      polymorphism in sarcoidosis. *Cytokine* (1997). , 9, 787-790.

[118] Labunski, S, Posern, G, Ludwig, S, Kundt, G, Brocker, E. B, & Kunz, M. Tumour ne-
      crosis factor-alpha promoter polymorphism in erythema nodosum. *Acta Derm Vene-
      reol* (2001). , 81, 18-21.

[119] Grutters, J. C, Sato, H, Pantelidis, P, Lagan, A. L, Mcgrath, D. S, & Lammers, J. W.
      van den Bosch JM,Wells AU, du Bois RM, Welsh KI. Increased frequency of the un-
      common tumor necrosis factor-857T allele in British and Dutch patients with sarcoi-
      dosis. *Am J Respir Crit Care Med* (2002). , 165, 1119-1124.

[120] Wilson, A. G, De Vries, N, & Pociot, F. di Giovine FS, van der Putte LB, Duff GW. An
      allelic polymorphism within the human tumor necrosis factor alpha promoter region
      is strongly associated with HLA A1, B8, and DR3 alleles. *J Exp Med* (1993). , 177,
      557-560.

[121] Kanazawa, S, Tsunoda, T, Onuma, E, Majima, T, Kagiyama, M, & Kikuchi, K. VEGF,
      basic-FGF, and TGF-beta in Crohn's disease and ulcerative colitis: a novel mecha-
      nism of chronic intestinal inflammation. *Am J Gastroenterol* (2001). , 96, 822-828.

[122] Kasama, T, Shiozawa, F, Kobayashi, K, Yajima, N, Hanyuda, M, Takeuchi, H. T,
      Mori, Y, Negishi, M, Ide, H, & Adachi, M. Vascular endothelial growth factor expres-
      sion by activated synovial leukocytes in rheumatoid arthritis: critical involvement of
      the interaction with synovial fibroblasts. *Arthritis Rheum* (2001). , 44, 2512-2524.

[123] Flamme, I, Frolich, T, & Risau, W. Molecular mechanisms of vasculogenesis and em-
      bryonic angiogenesis. *J Cell Physiol* (1997). , 173, 206-210.

[124] Tolnay, E, Kuhnen, C, Voss, B, Wiethege, T, & Muller, K. M. Expression and localization of vascular endothelial growth factor and its receptor flt in pulmonary sarcoidosis. *Virchows Arch* (1998). , 432, 61-65.

[125] Watson, C. J, Webb, N. J, Bottomley, M. J, & Brenchley, P. E. Identification of polymorphisms within the vascular endothelial growth factor (VEGF) gene: correlation with variation in VEGF protein production. *Cytokine* (2000). , 12, 1232-1235.

[126] Renner, W, Kotschan, S, Hoffmann, C, Obermayer-pietsch, B, Pilger, E, & Common, C. T mutation in the gene for vascular endothelial growth factor is associated with vascular endothelial growth factor plasma levels. *J Vasc Res* (2000). , 37, 443-448.

[127] Hewison, M, & Vitamin, D. and the immune system. *J Endocrinol* (1992). , 132, 173-175.

[128] Biyoudi-vouenze, R, Cadranel, J, Valeyre, D, Milleron, B, Hance, A. J, & Soler, P. Expression of 1,25(OH)2D3 receptors on alveolar lymphocytes from patients with pulmonary granulomatous diseases. *Am Rev Respir Dis* (1991). , 143, 1376-1380.

[129] Adams, J. S, Singer, F. R, Gacad, M. A, Sharma, O. P, Hayes, M. J, Vouros, P, & Holick, M. F. Isolation and structural identification of 1, 25-dihydroxyvitamin D3 produced by cultured alveolar macrophages in sarcoidosis. *J Clin Endocrinol Metab* (1985). , 60, 960-966.

[130] Niimi, T, Tomita, H, Sato, S, Kawaguchi, H, Akita, K, Maeda, H, Sugiura, Y, & Ueda, R. Vitamin D receptor gene polymorphism in patients with sarcoidosis. *Am J Respir Crit Care Med* (1999). , 160, 1107-1109.

[131] Guleva, I, & Seitzer, U. Vitamin D receptor gene polymorphism in patients with sarcoidosis. *Am J Respir Crit Care Med* (2000). , 162, 760-761.

[132] Schurmann, M, Reichel, P, Muller-myhsok, B, Schlaak, M, Muller- Quernheim, J, & Schwinger, E. Results from a genome-wide search for predisposing genes in sarcoidosis. *Am J Respir Crit Care Med* (2001). , 164, 840-846.

[133] Valentonyte, R, Hampe, J, Huse, K, Rosenstiel, P, Albrecht, M, Stenzel, A, Nagy, M, Gaede, K. I, Franke, A, & Haesler, R. Sarcoidosis is associated with a truncating splice site mutation in BTNL2. *Nat Genet* (2005). , 37, 357-364.

[134] Rhodes, D. A, Stammers, M, Malcherek, G, Beck, S, & Trowsdale, J. The cluster of BTN genes in the extended major histocompatibility complex. *Genomics* (2001). , 71, 351-362.

[135] Sharpe, A. H, Freeman, G. J, & The, B. CD28 superfamily. *Nat Rev Immunol* (2002). , 2, 116-126.

[136] Jack, L. J, & Mather, I. H. Cloning and analysis of cDNA encoding bovine butyrophilin, an apical glycoprotein expressed in mammary tissue and secreted in association

with the milk-fat globule membrane during lactation. *J Biol Chem* (1990). , 265, 14481-14486.

[137] Rybicki, B. A, Walewski, J. L, Maliarik, M. J, Kian, H, & Iannuzzi, M. C. The BTNL2 gene and sarcoidosis susceptibility in African Americans and whites. *Am J Hum Genet* (2005). , 77, 491-499.

[138] Szyld, P, Jagiello, P, Csernok, E, Gross, W. L, & Epplen, J. T. On the Wegener granulomatosis associated region on chromosome 6*BMC Med Genet* (2006). , 21.

[139] Fischer, A, Hofmann, S, et al. A Genome-Wide Linkage Analysis in 181 German Sarcoidosis Families Using Clustered Biallelic Markers, *Chest 2010151157*

[140] Iannuzzi, M. C, & Iyengar, S. K. Gray-McGuire C, Elston RC, Baughman RP, Donohue JF, Hirst K, Judson MA, Kavuru MS, Maliarik MJ, *et al*. Genome-wide search for sarcoidosis susceptibility genes in African Americans. *Genes Immun* (2005). , 6, 509-518.

[141] Gray-McGuire C., Sinha R, Iyengar SK, Millard C, Rybicki BA, Elston RC, Iannuzzi MC. Genetic characterization and fine mapping of susceptibility genes for sarcoidosis in African Americans on chromosome 5. *Hum Genet* (2006). , 120, 420-430.

[142] Parra, E. J, Marcini, A, Akey, J, Martinson, J, Batzer, M. A, Cooper, R, Forrester, T, Allison, D. B, Deka, R, & Ferrell, R. E. Estimating African American admixture proportions by use of population-specific alleles. *Am J Hum Genet* (1998). , 63, 1839-1851.

[143] Thompson, C. L, Rybicki, B. A, Iannuzzi, M. C, Elston, R. C, & Iyengar, S. K. Gray-McGuire C. Stratified linkage analysis based on population substructure in a population of African-American sarcoidosis families. *Am J Hum Genet* (2006). , 79, 603-613.

[144] Hofmann, S, Franke, A, Fischer, A, et al. Genome-wide association study identifies ANXA11 as a new susceptibility locus for sarcoidosis. Nat Genet. (2008). , 40(9), 1103-1106.

[145] Hofmann, S, Fischer, A, et al. A genome-wide association study reveals evidence of association with sarcoidosis at 6Eur Respir J (2011). , 12.

[146] Sharpe, A. H, Freeman, G. J, & The, B. CD28 superfamily. *Nat Rev Immunol* (2002). , 2, 116-126.

[147] Handa, T, Nagai, S, Ito, I, Tabuena, R, Shigematsu, M, Hamada, K, Kitaichi, M, Izumi, T, Aoyama, T, & Toguchida, J. Polymorphisms of B7 (CD80 and CD86) genes do not affect disease susceptibility to sarcoidosis. *Respiration (Herrlisheim)* (2005). , 72, 243-248.

Clinical Features

Chapter 5

Airways Disease in Sarcoidosis

Adam S. Morgenthau

Additional information is available at the end of the chapter

1. Introduction

1.1. Nasal sarcoidosis

Lupus pernio was first described by Kreibich and Kraus in 1908. [6] Pathognomic for sarcoidosis, Lupus pernio is a plaque-like lesion that is usually swollen, scaly or shiny. Typically, it occurs on the nose, cheeks, lips or ears. [7] Lupus pernio is most commonly observed in African-American women [8] and approximately 20% of all sarcoidosis patients with the lesion have co-morbid upper respiratory tract disease. [9] The skin lesion often involves the nasal mucosa and sometimes the underlying cartilage and nasal bones are destroyed. [7]

Nasal disease is usually associated with sinus disease. [10, 11] However, the clinical manifestations of nasal granulomas differ from sinus granulomas. Nasal mucus membrane granulomas may cause nasal obstruction, [11] epistaxis, crusting, rhinorrhea, post-nasal drip, pain and anosmia. [3] Obstruction is usually the most common presenting symptom when polypoid granulomatous lesions involve the nasal septum and the inferior turbinate. Fergie and colleagues retrospectively reviewed eight patients with nasal sarcoidosis and found that epiphora was present in 4 patients. [12]

On examination, the nasal mucosa is usually hypertrophic, erythematous and granular. It may also contain polyps, masses and/or asymmetric crust-like patches. The nasal bones may demonstrate a variety of radiographic abnormalities. [9, 10] Septal perforation is rare but granulomatous inflammation of the nasal cartilage (figure 2) may result in the classic "saddle nose" deformity. [13] Occasionally, granulomatous lesions may erode through the hard or soft palate, creating intraoral lesions or oral-nasal fistulae. [14]

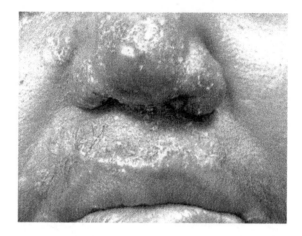

Figure 1. Sarcoidosis patient with Lupus Pernio.

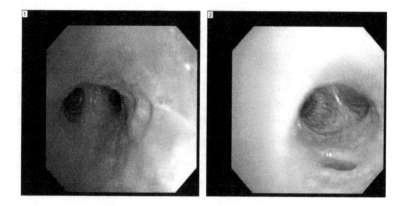

Figure 2. Bronchcoscopic appearance of endobronchial sarcoidosis demonstrating nodules and inflamed mucosa that narrows the right upper lobe bronchus.

2. Sinus sarcoidosis

The symptoms of nasal obstruction and chronic sinusitis often occur in patients concomitantly. [10, 11] The most common symptoms associated with sarcoidosis of the sinuses are recurrent infections, epistaxis, periorbital tenderness, post-nasal drip and headache. [15] Patients with sarcoidosis of the sinuses usually have involvement of multiple organ systems. [11] Sarcoidal lesions in the sinus mucosa are generally similar to those found in the nasal mucosa. Examination often demonstrates erythematous, friable, hypertrophied mucosa. Crusting, studding, plaque-like changes or polyps may also be visualized. Rarely, granulomatous lesions extend out of the sinuses and into the orbit, resulting in proptosis and/or decreased unilateral visual acuity. [16] Sarcoidosis of the sinuses is generally a chronic and recalcitrant form of the disease that requires prolonged systemic therapy. [6, 17, 18]

3. Laryngeal sarcoidosis

The epiglottis, aryepiglottic folds, arytenoids, false cords and subglottis are the most commonly affected regions in the larynx. The true vocal cords are relatively devoid of lymphatic tissue and are rarely ridden with disease. [19] Granulomatous involvement of the larynx may cause life-threatening stridor or dysphagia. [10] On examination, the involved laryngeal mucosa is typically pale pink, granular and edenomatous. Lesions vary in their size and shape. Localized submucosal induration, punctate nodules or polypoid masses may be present. In one review of 40 patients with laryngeal sarcoidosis, the presenting symptoms were: dysphagia (85%), hoarseness (63%), dyspnea or stridor (47%) and cough (13%). [20] Ulceration of the mucosa is rare. Patients also present with hoarseness, dysphonia, cough, dyspnea, a sensation of a lump in the throat and obstructive sleep apnea. [21]

Hoarseness is typically caused by granulomatous laryngitis. However, laryngeal sarcoidosis may cause hoarseness by two additional mechanisms. [22, 23] The first involves granulomatous infiltration of the vagus nerve, resulting in a polyneuropathy. Limited data suggests that vagal polyneuropathy is rare [24] and if present, is typically associated with other cranial neuropathies. [21] In rare cases, hoarseness may result from mediastinal lymphadenopathy that compresses the recurrent laryngeal nerve, resulting in vocal cord paralysis. The left recurrent laryngeal nerve is affected in more than 95% of cases. [21, 25] The predilection for left-sided injury results from the longer and more vulnerable course of the left recurrent laryngeal nerve through the mediastinum.

In one report, a young female presented with daytime hypersomnolence and snoring. [26]

Nasopharyngoscopy demonstrated an irregularly shaped and narrowed subglottis. Subsequent biopsy confirmed the presence of non-caseating granulomas. The patient was diagnosed with obstructive sleep apnea, secondary to laryngeal sarcoidosis. To determine the prevalence and risk factors for obstructive sleep apnea in sarcoidosis patients, 83 patients with sarcoidosis were prospectively evaluated. [27] The Epworth Sleepiness Scale was used to assess enrolled patients. A control group of 91 patients were similarly screened. Patients with a positive sleep questionnaire were referred for sleep studies. A total of 14 sarcoidosis patients (17%) were found to have sleep apnea, which was significantly higher than in the control group where 3/91 were found to have obstructive disease (3%, p < 0.001). [27] Lupus pernio was significantly more frequent in the sleep apnea group. [27] Although granulomatous laryngitis may be associated with obstructive sleep apnea, obstructive sleep apnea in patients with sarcoidosis usually results from obesity secondary to the administration of chronic corticosteroids.

4. Tracheal sarcoidosis

Sarcoidal involvement of the trachea is rare [28] and the literature on tracheal sarcodosis is sparse. Tracheal stenosis and dystonia are the primary manifestations that have been described. [28, 29] Brandstetter and associates [30] described a patient who complained of deteriorating voice strength for 30 years and eventually, stridulent breathing that was refractory to corticosteriods. In 1949, Lemoine described tracheal dystonia (tracheal collapse most pronounced on expiration) in sarcoidosis. Ellefsen detailed a 44-year-old female who complained of progressive dyspnea for 4 years prior to admission to the hospital. [29] She eventually developed wheezing and a severe nonproductive cough. Physical exam showed stridor and wheezing.

5. Bronchial sarcoidosis

Bronchial sarcoidosis was first described at autopsy by Bernstein and colleagues in 1929 and subsequently on bronchcoscopy by Benedict and Castleman in 1941. [31] Numerous case series have followed. [32-37] Granulomatous lesions typically occur in the bronchial submucosa. [37] The bronchial mucosa often appears inflamed with small or large nodules containing granulomas. [37] (Figure 2) Granulomatous involvement of the bronchi may cause edema and/or an endobronchial masses that results in reversible narrowing of the large airways. [33, 36, 37] Irreversible narrowing, especially of the right middle lobe bronchus, results from cicatricial stenosis. [33] Reversible or irreversible bronchial stenosis occurs more commonly in the presence of end-stage pulmonary fibrosis. But bronchostenosis may occur in milder stages of the disease. [33, 36, 37] Bronchial sarcoidosis may be isolated (one stenotic point) or diffuse (multiple stenotic points) involving the lobar or segmental bronchi. Compressive mediastinal and/or bronchopulmonary lymphadenopathy is rarely a cause of stenoses at these locations within the airway. [38, 39]

Patients with bronchial sarcoidosis present with dyspnea, cough and wheezing that is often misdiagnosed as asthma. [10] The symptoms generally progress and are refractory to bronchodilators and inhaled corticosteroids. Bronchial sarcoidosis is suggested by obstructive airways disease (a reduced ratio of forced expiratory volume in 1 second [FEV1] to forced vital capacity [FVC]) that may be accompanied by airways hyperreactivity on pulmonary function tests. Bronchoscopic inspection of the airways with or without biopsy of the parenchyma is the most efficient method to confirm the diagnosis. Endobronchial involvement is common in sarcoidosis. Endobronchial biopsy has a yield comparable to transbronchial biopsy and can safely increase the diagnostic value of fiberoptic bronchoscopy. Performance of endobronchial biopsies should routinely be considered in cases of suspected sarcoidosis.

6. Small airways sarcoidosis

Small airways disease is an underappreciated manifestation of pulmonary sarcoidosis. Regional air trapping, indicative of small airways disease, may be visualized on expiratory HRCT [40] and newer imaging modalities such as hyperpolarized 3-H MRI, [41, 42] in patients with pulmonary sarcoidosis who have obstructive airways disease. Peripheral airway obstruction with involvement of small airways may be caused by the formation of granulomas in a perilymphatic distribution along the bronchovascular bundles. [41, 43] Small airways dysfunction can be measured by forced expiratory flow during the middle half of the forced expiratory curve (MMEF$_{25-75\%}$), forced expiratory volume at 3 seconds (FEV$_3$) ratio of the residual volume to the total lung capacity (RV/TLC). In one study, the extent of air trapping on HRCT correlated significantly with RV/TLC and MMEF$_{25-75\%}$. [41, 43] In other studies, however, these physiologic measurements were highly variable and provided limited clinical information. [43-45]

Patients with small airways disease typically present with progressive dyspnea, cough and wheeze. They may also exhibit stridulent breathing. Lung auscultation demonstrates wheezing, stridor or squeaks.

Skin of the Nose (Lupus Pernio)
Nares
Nasal Septum
Sinuses
Larynx
Vocal Cords
Trachea
Bronchi
Bronchioles

Table 1. Airway Involvement in Sarcoidosis

INFECTIOUS	NON-INFECTIOUS
Tuberculosis	Sarcoidosis
Atypical Mycobacterial Disease	Wegener's Granulomatosis
Syphilis	Berylliosis
Leprosy	Silicosis
Aspergillosis	Hypersensitivity Pneumonitis
Histoplasmosis	Lymphoma
Rhinoscleroma	Cocaine
Coccidioidomycosis	Churg-Strauss Syndrome
Toxoplasmosis	Talc
Actinomycosis	Lymphoid Interstitial Pneumonia
Cryptoccosis	Rheumatoid Nodule

Table 2. Differential Diagnosis of Granulomatous Airways Diseases

6.1. Airway Hyperreactivity (AHR)

The incidence of airway hyperreactivity (AHR) in sarcoidosis is highly variable. Airway hyperreactivity has been observed in approximately 20%--50% of sarcoidosis patients. [46, 47] The statistical discrepancy probably results from different patient populations, study designs and different definitions of sarcoidosis and AHR.

Airway hyperreactivity has important clinical and prognostic implications in sarcoidosis. [47] Many patients with sarcoidosis exhibit normal pulmonary function and imaging but complain of cough, dyspnea and wheeze. The wall of the airway may be narrowed and thickened as a result of airway hyperreactivity or may collapse from an extrinsic pathologic process in the lung. Airway hyperreactivity in sarcoidosis may also cause chronic airflow obstruction, which has been associated with a poor prognosis. [47, 48] Fixed airway obstruction has been shown to nearly double the risk of mortality. [47]

The prevalence of AHR, as demonstrated by a positive methacholine challenge test, is significantly higher in sarcoidosis patients compared to normal controls. [1, 47] It is unclear whether AHR is a physiologic manifestation of endobronchial sarcoidosis or reversible airways disease in asthma. Rarely, asthma may be associated with sarcoidosis. [49] Airway hyperreactivity in sarcoidosis and reversible airways disease in asthma may often be distinguished by response to inhaled corticosteroids and/or beta-agonists. Asthmatic reactive airways disease usually improves with these medications. But AHR in sarcoidosis commonly requires treatment with oral corticosteroids. [33, 47] In many cases, AHR in sarcoidosis does not improve with systemic corticosteroids.

Importantly, cough and wheeze secondary to AHR (as demonstrated by positive methacholine challenge testing) should not be confused with cough and wheeze unrelated to AHR. *Sarcoidal cough and wheeze unrelated to AHR* responds favorably to inhaled corticosteroids and/or beta-agonists as does *asthmatic cough and wheeze related to AHR*. [47] Sarcoidal cough and wheeze associated with AHR, however, may require treatment with oral corticosteroids, which is often ineffective.

Several studies suggests that AHR in sarcoidosis correlates with both the degree of alveolitis and angiotensin converting enzyme (ACE) levels in bronchoalveolar lavage (BAL) fluid and serum. [50] In addition, higher serum ACE levels were found in sarcodosis patients with hyperreactivity. [47] Finally, patients with AHR were more likely to have a positive endobronchial biopsy (9/9, 100%) compared to individuals without hyperreactivity (15/33, 45.5%), which suggests that AHR is present in patients with more pronounced bronchial inflammation. [47]

6.2. Atelectasis

Lobar atelectasis may result from occlusion of a lobar bronchus. Bronchial obstruction may be caused by one of two mechanisms: endobronchial stenosis [37] or rarely, by extrinsic compression of the bronchus by enlarged lymph nodes. [51, 52] Atelectasis of the middle lobe is most common but atelectasis of the right upper lobe has also been reported. [53] The middle lobe is particularly susceptible to collapse because it has a small bronchial lumen, surrounded by many lymph nodes and emerges at a right angle from the bronchus intermedius. Collapse of the right upper lobe may result in the radiographic S-sign of Golden, which is commonly associated with cancer. Resolution of atelectasis is variable and it may occur even after several years. [54]

6.3. Fibrosis

Chronic, progressive, end-stage, pulmonary fibrosis with traction bronchiectasis, often referred to as "honeycomb lung", develops in approximately 25% of patients with chronic pulmonary sarcoidosis. [40, 55] The condition is characterized by parenchymal fibrosis, bronchiolectasis and enlarged, dilated air spaces. It usually occurs subpleurally within the upper regions of the lung [40, 56] (figure 3). Oxygenation and ventilatory function are impaired. Pulmonary function tests demonstrate severe restriction and gas transfer abnormalities. Importantly, fibrosis characterized by a stage IV radiographic pattern, rarely responds to treatment.

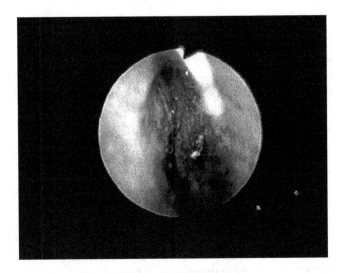

Figure 3. Sarcoidosis patient with granulomatous inflammation of the nasal cartilage

6.4. Bullous disease

Bullea (thin-walled air spaces in the lungs) may develop in patients with advanced pulmonary sarcoidosis. Most sarcoidosis patients with bullous disease do not exhibit an extensive smoking history and have airflow obstruction on pulmonary function tests. [10, 57] Dilatation and rupture of bullae probably results from granulomatous bronchostenosis. [58] Bullae may develop secondary to destruction of alveolar walls by alveolitis. [58] Bullous rupture may cause pneumothorax.

Giant bullous changes in sarcoidosis may rarely cause the Vanishing Lung Syndrome. [59] First described by Burke in 1937, the Vanishing Lung Syndrome describes an end stage of diffuse panacinar emphysema in which large air spaces develop, further impairing lung function. [59] Miller and associates reported two cases of the Vanishing Lung Syndrome. Postmortem analysis of the lungs demonstrated that the bullae were quite different from the localized air spaces frequently seen in chronic pulmonary sarcoidosis. [10, 60]

6.5. Cavitary lung disease, bronchiectasis and mycetomas

Although the terms cyst and cavity have overlapping meanings and may be used interchangeably, the technical definitions of these terms are different. Cysts are clearly defined air-containing space surrounded by a relatively thin (≤ 4 mm) wall. A cavity, in contrast, is meant to describe an air-containing lesion with a relatively thick (> 4 mm) wall or within an area of a surrounding infiltrate or mass. The distinction is useful because there is a different diagnostic approach to these anatomic structures. [61]

True cavitary lung disease, which results from necrosis of granulomatous areas creating airspaces within thick walls or within a fibrotic mass, is rare in sarcoidosis. Sarcoidal cavities must be differentiated from those associated with mycobacterial infection. The radiographic cystic changes that occur in advanced sarcoidosis are typically consistent with saccular bronchiectasis, rather than true cavitations. [57, 61] Saccular or cylindrical bronchiectasis likely results from bronchial wall injury by granulomas, superimposed bronchial infection and radial traction by peribronchial scar tissue. Colonization of the bronchiectatic sacs by Aspergillus sp., may result in the development of an aspergilloma. Patients with aspergillomas complicating sarcoidosis may have life-threatening hemoptysis but, as a result of their advanced lung disease, are usually high-risk surgical candidates. [62]

Intracavitary installation of antifungal agents is an alternative treatment in patients with severe pulmonary dysfunction who are poor operative risks. Percutaneous instillation of amphotericin B guided by CT scans may be effective for the treatment of aspergilloma. [63] In several cases, the intervention has led to resolution of hemoptysis. [63] The response to percutaneous injection of amphotericin B appears to be sustainable for several months. [63]

Israel and associates evaluated the role of surgery in 38 sarcoidosis patients with pulmonary aspergillomas, 10 of whom were considered satisfactory operative candidates. [64] Satisfactory candidates demonstrated a forced vital capacity greater than 50% predicted and a resting PaO2 greater than 80 mmHg. The indication for surgical resection in satisfactory and unsatisfactory candidates was recurrent hemoptysis. Seven satisfactory and 7 unsatisfactory candidates underwent segmental resection, lobectomy or bilobectomy. The authors did not specify the type of procedure that each patient received. Patients were followed postoperatively for an unspecified duration. Among the 7 satisfactory candidates who underwent resection, 1 patient died from empyema immediately after surgery. Three of 7 patients with unsatisfactory pulmonary function died of respiratory failure 1 month, 11 months and 27 months, respectively, after surgery. Twenty-one patients with poor pulmonary function did not have surgery. Four patients died of recurrent hemorrhage 4 months to 3 years after discovery of the aspergilloma. Eleven patients died of respiratory failure and 6 survived at the time of publication (1982) although it is unclear when these patients were diagnosed with their aspergilloma. The principle complications of surgical resection were prolonged air leaks, bronchopleural fistulae and empyema. The authors concluded that surgical resection should generally be avoided in patients with bilateral disease and compromised pulmonary function. The indication for surgery in all patients, especially those with poor pulmonary function, should be recurrent hemoptysis because it may cause exsanguinating hemorrhage, which poses a greater risk to the patient than surgical intervention. [64]

7. Imaging

Computed tomography (CT) is often the imaging method of choice for sarcoidosis of the upper and lower respiratory tract. [40] Braun and associates analyzed the CT findings of 15 patients with sinonasal sarcoidosis. [20] A spectrum of abnormalities were evaluated: nodular lesions of the septum and/or inferior turbinates; mucosal thickening and complete or subtotal opacification of the ethmoidal, maxillary and/or sphenoid sinuses; obstruction of the ostio-meatal units and of the upper part of the nasal cavities; turbinoseptal synechiae; destruction or erosion of the turbinates, nasal bones, septum, ethmoid air cells and sphenoid sinus.

CT scan has a high sensitivity for detecting sarcoidosis of the larynx or trachea. [65] Typically, the CT demonstrates stenosis of the larynx and trachea.

Airways sarcoidosis produces a variety of abnormalities on CT scan of the lungs. Several CT studies performed at near residual volume (end expiration) have demonstrated air-trapping in pulmonary sarcoidosis. [40, 66, 67] Davies and colleagues reported that air-trapping on expiratory CT was present in 95% of 21 sarcoidosis patients and correlated with physiologic obstruction by percentage predicted residual volume (RV)/ total lung capacity (TLC) ($p < 0.05$) and percentage predicted maximal mid-expiratory flow rate between 25% and 75% of the vital capacity (VC) ($p < 0.05$). [41] The CT may also demonstrate focal bronchial lesions, atelectasis, bullous disease, fibrosis/honeycombing, cavitary lung disease, bronchiectasis (saccular or cylindrical) and mycetomas

8. Physiology

The respiratory tract is typically divided into the upper and lower airways at the level of the vocal cords. The physiology of obstruction to the upper airways depends on the location of the obstruction (intrathoracic or extrathoracic) and whether it is fixed or variable within the respiratory cycle. Granulomatous involvement of the larynx results in a fixed upper airway obstruction. When tracheal sarcoidosis results in stenosis, it may cause a fixed upper airway obstruction (figure 4) or a variable extrathoracic or intrathoracic obstruction (figure 4) depending on whether it is located above (extrathoracic) or below (intrathoracic) the thoracic inlet (level of the supra-sternal notch). In a fixed upper airway obstruction, there is flattening of the inspiratory and expiratory limbs of the flow volume loop. A variable extrathoracic obstruction causes flattening of the inspiratory portion of the flow volume loop, while a variable intrathoracic obstruction causes flattening of the expiratory portion of the loop.

Spirometry commonly indicates restrictive ventilatory dysfunction. At least 50% of patients have concurrent obstructive airways disease, evidenced by a reduced ratio of forced expiratory volume in 1 second (FEV1) to forced vital capacity (FVC). [2, 68] Airway hyperreactivity assessed by methacholine challenge test occurs in 5-83% of patients. [47, 68]

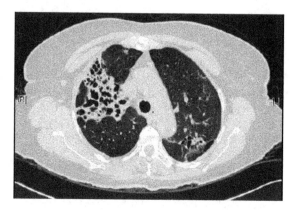

Figure 4. Sarcoidosis patient with "honeycomb lung".

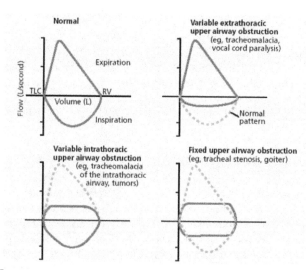

TLC = Total Lung Capacity, RV = Residual Volume
Adapated with permission from Kavuru et al…Essentials of Pulmonary and Critical care Medicine. 5th Edition. Philadel-phia. Lippincott, Williams and Wilkins, 2005.

Figure 5. Flow volume loops demonstrating various types of airways obstruction.

9. Bronchoscopy

The diagnosis of sarcoidosis is confirmed by histologic evidence of non-caseating, epitheliod granulomas. Tissue is obtained from the upper airways by direct nasopharyngoscopy. Transbronchial and/or mucosal biopsies of the lower airways may be obtained by bronchocoscopy, the diagnostic procedure of choice for sarcoidosis.

10. Treatment

There are no controlled studies that examine the variety of therapeutic agents, which are purported to be effective in the treatment of sarcoidosis. There is consensus by experienced physicians that corticosteroids are the most efficacious medication. None of the other therapies share this favorable level of support. Oral corticosteroids are given in the smallest possible dose to limit their adverse effects. Since upper airways obstruction occurs in chronic sarcoidosis, 'steroid-sparing' medications may be administered simultaneously to reduce the corticosteroid dose that would be needed if it is given for many months. Hydroxychloroquine has been used with some success for cutaneous sarcoidosis. [69] Minocycline is also effective for the treatment of skin lesions. [70, 71] Minocycline appears to inhibit metalloproteinases, angiogenesis, apoptosis and in vitro granuloma formation. [68, 72]

The treatment of sinus and nasal sarcoidosis should be tailored to the specific organ system or systems involved and to the extent of disease. [14, 16] Isolated sinonasal disease can be treated by topical corticosteroids and/or intra-lesional steroid injections. [73] Nasal irrigations and emollients may be used to ameliorate nasal crusting. Siltzbach and Teirstein used chloroquine to treat 14 pataients with intrathoracic and cutaneous sarcoidosis. All of the patients showed relative improvement in their cutaneous lesions and most exhibited radiographic improvement of their intrathoracic disease. Johns and colleagues used hydroxychloroquine, a drug with less ocular toxicity, to treat mucosal lesions. [74] Patients taking hydroxychloroquine must have an ophthalmic exam every 6 months. Hassid reported a patient with biopsy-proven sarcoidosis of the paranasal sinuses who was successfully treated with hydroxychloroquine 200 mg orally, twice daily for one month and 200 mg per day for an additional 7 months. [75] Despite these results, the overall response rate for antimalarial drugs is probably less than 50% [76] and the drugs are often reserved for patients with cutaneous or sinonasal sarcoidosis, in whom the response to treatment can be easily observed. [76]

Methotrexate may also be used for the treatment of cutaneous sarcoidosis. In several case reports, skin lesions improved in patients who were treated with methotrexate 10 mg to 15 mg per week. [77] Although azathioprine has been commonly used as a corticosteroid-sparing agent for many forms of sarcoidosis, it has rarely been reported for the treatment of skin sarcoidosis. [7] Tumor necrosis factor-a (TNF-a) antagonists have been reported to be useful in the treatment of sarcoidosis, including cutaneous sarcoidosis. [78] Infliximab appears to be the most efficacious of the biologics. It may be especially useful in the treatment of lupus pernio. [78]

The indication for surgical intervention of sinonasal granulomatous lesions is controversial. While surgery may reduce symptoms, it does not eradicate or prevent recurrence of disease. [14, 17, 79] Neville and associates evaluated 34 patients with sarcoidosis of the upper respiratory tract, [9] 3 of whom, underwent submucous resection. In 2 of 3 patients the resection was complicated by nasal septal perforation. Aubart and colleagues operated on 7 patients. [17] Nasal and sinus involvement recurred in all of them and sinus symptoms worsened in 1 patient after surgery. But two additional studies suggest that endoscopic sinus surgery may have a therapeutic role in patients with nasal obstruction or chronic sinusitis caused by anatomic blockage from sinonasal sarcoidosis. [18, 80] Removal of the obstructing lesion(s) may facilitate improved sinonasal hygiene by permitting endoscopic debridement, nasal irrigation and topical administration of medicines into the sinonasal tract. Surgical intervention should not be used to treat patients with symptoms related to crusting, atrophy or bleeding. While surgery may improve one's quality of life by relieving severe symptoms and may even reduce the need for oral steroids, it is almost never curative.

Laryngeal sarcoidosis may cause life-threatening upper airway obstruction. As a result, early diagnosis and proper management is essential. The treatment of laryngeal sarcoidosis depends on the severity of the symptoms. Asymptomatic patients do not require therapy. [5, 19, 81] But close monitoring is warranted. It may be difficult to assess the efficacy of various treatment modalities because spontaneous remissions of disease punctuate the natural evolution of sarcodosis. [51, 67] Systemic corticosteroids are the mainstay of treatment for laryngeal sarcoidosis, especially for impending laryngeal obstruction. [1, 10] Methotrexate has been used with some success in the treatment of laryngeal sarcoidosis. One patient with granulomatous laryngitis responded to treatment with azathioprine. Intra-lesional steroid injections of the larynx for selected patients with well-circumscribed disease is modestly effective. [5, 21] When the airway is compromised and stridor is present, emergent tracheostomy should be performed. [21] Tracheostomy may also be an appropriate for patients who develop marked adverse effects from systemic corticosteroids. [82] Tracheostomy is often used as a temporizing measure until corticosteroids are able to effectively reduce granulomatous inflammation. Surgical intervention for laryngeal sarcoidosis is effective for patients with well-localized, life threatening lesions. [5] Typically, the goals of surgery are to create an adequate airway, avoid aspiration, avoid tracheostomy and preserve the voice. [5, 83] Low-dose external beam radiation therapy (3000 rads during 6 weeks) has been utilized in selected patients. [5, 84] It is generally reserved for patients in whom intra-lesional steroids or local excision of granulomatous tissue are not feasible and/or in those who are refractory to or cannot tolerate systemic corticosteroids. [5, 82]

Tracheal involvement in sarcoidosis is limited to the description of tracheal dystonia [29] and tracheal stenosis. [29, 30] Brandstetter and colleagues used high-dose systemic corticosteriods to treat a patient with tracheal stenosis. The patient failed to stabilize with the treatment but ultimately underwent successful bronchoscopic tracheal dilatation. [30] Tracheal stents have been used with limited success for tracheobronchial obstruction in pediatric patients. [85]

Patients with bronchostenosis respond poorly to treatment with systemic corticosteroids. [33, 37, 46, 47, 53] Fouty and associates used a flexible fiberoptic bronchoscope and a Fogarty embolectomy catheter to dilate multiple bronchial stenoses under direct vision. [86] The six patients who underwent the procedure were symptomatic and refractory to corticosteroids. All of them obtained subjective symptomatic benefit from the dilatation. Three of the patients required repeated dilatation on a long-term basis. Complications from the procedure were minimal. Collectively, these studies suggest that bronchial dilatation is a safe option for sarcoidosis patients with stenoses who are refractory to systemic corticosteroids.

The majority of patients with sarcoidosis improve with therapy. However, 10-30% of patients develop progressive pulmonary fibrosis, which may result in advanced airways disease such as bronchiectasis, bullae and cavitation. Rarely, patients with bronchiectasis will improve with corticosteroids, antibiotics and/or nonsteroidal anti-inflammatory medications. [87] If patients do respond, it is generally short-lived. Bullectomies performed for bullous sarcoidosis may improve pulmonary function and symptoms. [57, 58] Surgical resection of the cavity and removal of the fungus ball is the mainstay of treatment for aspergilloma(s). [88] The primary indication for resection is recurrent hemoptysis. Bronchial artery embolization is modestly effective in inoperable patients. [89] Taken together, advanced involvement in sarcoidosis is seldom responsive to medical therapy, moderately responsive to surgical therapy depending on the type of underlying disease and has an ominous prognosis. Finally, sarcoidosis patients with fibrotic lung disease and/or airways dysfunction often develop pulmonary hypertension, which often has an unfavorable prognosis.

11. Summary

Sarcoidosis is a chronic granulomatous disease of undetermined etiology that can involve any organ system within the body. Greater than 90% of patients with sarcoidosis have interstitial lung disease. [2] But the upper and lower respiratory tract is also affected. Sarcoidosis is one of a few interstitial lung diseases that involves the entire respiratory tract; beginning at the nose and ending at the terminal bronchioles.

Although many patients are asymptomatic, most complain of dyspnea, cough and/or wheezing. Patients with sarcoidosis of the upper respiratory tract present with a variety of symptoms, which are primarily determined by the anatomic location of the granulomatous inflammation and/or scarring that may result from chronic disease. The diagnosis of upper or lower respiratory tract disease is frequently ascertained by bronchoscopy.

Computed tomography (CT), the imaging method of choice for sarcoidosis of the upper and lower respiratory tract, may demonstrate lesions within the sinonasal tract, larynx and trachea, large and small airways or parenchyma. It may also reveal mediastinal and/or hilar lymphadenopathy.

The physiology of airways obstruction depends on the location of the obstruction (intrathoracic or extrathoracic) and whether it is fixed or variable within the respiratory cycle. Granulomatous involvement of the larynx results in a fixed upper airway obstruction. Tracheal sarcoidosis may cause a fixed upper airway obstruction, or a variable extrathoracic or intrathoracic obstruction, depending on whether the lesion is located above (extrathoracic) or below (intrathoracic) the thoracic inlet (level of the supra-sternal notch).

Patients with pulmonary sarcoidosis may exhibit obstructive, restrictive, restrictive and obstructive, or gas transfer abnormalities. Corticosteroids are the mainstay of therapy for upper respiratory tract disease. However, other immunosuppressive treatments may be effective for the treatment of skin and sinonasal sarcoidosis. Patients with endobronchial or tracheal stenoses who are refractory to steroid therapy may derive some benefit from mechanical dilatation of the airways. [86] Surgical intervention may be required for treatment of bullous sarcoidosis and aspergilloma. [57, 58]

Author details

Adam S. Morgenthau

Address all correspondence to: adam.morgenthau@mssm.edu

The Mount Sinai School of Medicine, Department of Medicine, Division of Pulmonary, Critical Care and Sleep Medicine, New York, NY, USA

Dr. Morgenthau discloses no conflicts of interest.

References

[1] Laohaburanakit, P, & Chan, A. Obstructive sarcoidosis. Clin Rev Allergy Immunol. (2003). Oct;, 25(2), 115-29.

[2] Baughman, R. P, Teirstein, A. S, Judson, M. A, Rossman, M. D, & Yeager, H. Jr., Bresnitz EA, et al. Clinical characteristics of patients in a case control study of sarcoidosis. Am J Respir Crit Care Med. (2001). Nov 15;164(10 Pt 1):1885-9.** A large study that discusses the clinical characteristics of patients with sarcoidosis.

[3] Mccaffrey, T. V, & Mcdonald, T. J. Sarcoidosis of the nose and paranasal sinuses. Laryngoscope. (1983). Oct;, 93(10), 1281-4.

[4] Rosell, A, Garcia-arranz, G, Romero, N, Sendra, J, & Fogue, L. Lupus pernio with involvement of nasal cavity and maxillary sinus. ORL J Otorhinolaryngol Relat Spec. (1998). Jul-Aug;, 60(4), 236-9.

[5] Dean, C. M, Sataloff, R. T, Hawkshaw, M. J, & Pribikin, E. Laryngeal sarcoidosis. J Voice. (2002). Jun;, 16(2), 283-8.

[6] Zeitlin, J. F, Tami, T. A, Baughman, R, & Winget, D. Nasal and sinus manifestations of sarcoidosis. Am J Rhinol. (2000). May-Jun;, 14(3), 157-61.

[7] Marchell, R. M, & Judson, M. A. Cutaneous sarcoidosis. Semin Respir Crit Care Med. (2010). Aug;, 31(4), 442-51.

[8] Maples, C. J, & Counselman, F. L. Lupus pernio. J Emerg Med. (2007). Aug;, 33(2), 187-9.

[9] Neville, E, Mills, R. G, & James, D. G. Sarcoidosis of the upper respiratory tract and its relation to lupus pernio. Ann N Y Acad Sci. (1976). , 278, 416-26.

[10] Polychronopoulos, V. S, & Prakash, U. B. Airway involvement in sarcoidosis. Chest. (2009). Nov;A review article that discusses airway involvement in sarcoidosis., 136(5), 1371-80.

[11] Deshazo, R. D, Brien, O, Justice, M. M, & Pitcock, W. K. J. Diagnostic criteria for sarcoidosis of the sinuses. J Allergy Clin Immunol. (1999). May;103(5 Pt 1):789-95.

[12] Fergie, N, Jones, N. S, & Havlat, M. F. The nasal manifestations of sarcoidosis: a review and report of eight cases. J Laryngol Otol. (1999). Oct;, 113(10), 893-8.

[13] Shipchandler, T. Z, Chung, B. J, & Alam, D. S. Saddle nose deformity reconstruction with a split calvarial bone L-shaped strut. Arch Facial Plast Surg. (2008). Sep-Oct;, 10(5), 305-11.

[14] Gurkov, R, & Berghaus, A. Nasal reconstruction in advanced sinunasal sarcoidosis. Rhinology. (2009). Sep;, 47(3), 327-9.

[15] Reed, J, Deshazo, R. D, Houle, T. T, Stringer, S, Wright, L, & Moak, J. S. rd. Clinical features of sarcoid rhinosinusitis. Am J Med. (2010). Sep;, 123(9), 856-62.

[16] Dessouky, O. Y. Isolated sinonasal sarcoidosis with intracranial extension: case report. Acta Otorhinolaryngol Ital. (2008). Dec;, 28(6), 306-8.

[17] Aubart, F. C, Ouayoun, M, Brauner, M, Attali, P, Kambouchner, M, Valeyre, D, et al. Sinonasal involvement in sarcoidosis: a case-control study of 20 patients. Medicine (Baltimore). (2006). Nov;A study that discusses sinonasal sarcoidosis., 85(6), 365-71.

[18] Long, C. M, Smith, T. L, Loehrl, T. A, Komorowski, R. A, & Toohill, R. J. Sinonasal disease in patients with sarcoidosis. Am J Rhinol. (2001). May-Jun;, 15(3), 211-5.

[19] Devine, K. D. Sarcoidosis and Sarcoidosis of the Larynx. Laryngoscope. (1965). Apr;, 75, 533-69.

[20] Braun, J. J, Gentine, A, & Pauli, G. Sinonasal sarcoidosis: review and report of fifteen cases. Laryngoscope. (2004). Nov;, 114(11), 1960-3.

[21] Baughman, R. P, Lower, E. E, & Tami, T. Upper airway. 4: Sarcoidosis of the upper respiratory tract (SURT). Thorax. (2010). Feb;A review article that discusses upper airways disease in sarcoidosis., 65(2), 181-6.

[22] Coffey, C. S, Vallejo, S. L, Farrar, E. K, Judson, M. A, & Halstead, L. A. Sarcoidosis presenting as bilateral vocal cord paralysis from bilateral compression of the recurrent laryngeal nerves from thoracic adenopathy. J Voice. (2009). Sep;, 23(5), 631-4.

[23] Jaffe, R, Bogomolski-yahalom, V, & Kramer, M. R. Vocal cord paralysis as the presenting symptom of sarcoidosis. Respir Med. (1994). Sep;, 88(8), 633-6.

[24] Teirstein, A. Neuromuscular sarcoidosis. Semin Respir Crit Care Med. (2002). Dec;, 23(6), 505-12.

[25] Tobias, J. K, Santiago, S. M, & Williams, A. J. Sarcoidosis as a cause of left recurrent laryngeal nerve palsy. Arch Otolaryngol Head Neck Surg. (1990). Aug;, 116(8), 971-2.

[26] Fuso, L, Maiolo, C, Tramaglino, L. M, Benedetto, R. T, Russo, A. R, Spadaro, S, et al. Orolaryngeal sarcoidosis presenting as obstructive sleep apnoea. Sarcoidosis Vasc Diffuse Lung Dis. (2001). Mar;, 18(1), 85-90.

[27] Turner, G. A, Lower, E. E, Corser, B. C, Gunther, K. L, & Baughman, R. P. Sleep apnea in sarcoidosis. Sarcoidosis Vasc Diffuse Lung Dis. (1997). Mar;, 14(1), 61-4.

[28] Miller, A, Brown, L. K, & Teirstein, A. S. Stenosis of main bronchi mimicking fixed upper airway obstruction in sarcoidosis. Chest. (1985). Aug;, 88(2), 244-8.

[29] Ellefsen, P. Tracheal dystonia and sarcoidosis. Acta Otolaryngol. (1970). Nov-Dec;, 70(5), 438-42.

[30] Brandstetter, R. D, Messina, M. S, Sprince, N. L, & Grillo, H. C. Tracheal stenosis due to sarcoidosis. Chest. (1981). Nov;80(5):656.

[31] Rockoff, S. D, & Rohatgi, P. K. Unusual manifestations of thoracic sarcoidosis. AJR Am J Roentgenol. (1985). Mar;, 144(3), 513-28.

[32] Corsello, B. F, Lohaus, G. H, & Funahashi, A. Endobronchial mass lesion due to sarcoidosis: complete resolution with corticosteroids. Thorax. (1983). Feb;, 38(2), 157-8.

[33] Hadfield, J. W, Page, R. L, Flower, C. D, & Stark, J. E. Localised airway narrowing in sarcoidosis. Thorax. (1982). Jun;, 37(6), 443-7.

[34] Teo, F, Anantham, D, Feller-kopman, D, & Ernst, A. Bronchoscopic management of sarcoidosis related bronchial stenosis with adjunctive topical mitomycin C. Ann Thorac Surg. (2010). Jun;, 89(6), 2005-7.

[35] Baba, K, Yamaguchi, E, Matsui, S, Niwa, S, Onoe, K, Yagi, T, et al. A case of sarcoidosis with multiple endobronchial mass lesions that disappeared with antibiotics. Sarcoidosis Vasc Diffuse Lung Dis. (2006). Mar;, 23(1), 78-9.

[36] Yamada, G, Aketa, K, Takahashi, H, Satoh, M, & Abe, S. Endobronchial lesions of sarcoidosis. Intern Med. (2005). Aug;, 44(8), 909-10.

[37] Chambellan, A, Turbie, P, Nunes, H, Brauner, M, Battesti, J. P, & Valeyre, D. Endoluminal stenosis of proximal bronchi in sarcoidosis: bronchoscopy, function, and evo-

lution. Chest. (2005). Feb;A study that discusses endobronchial sarcoidosis., 127(2), 472-81.

[38] Olsson, T, Bjornstad-pettersen, H, & Stjernberg, N. L. Bronchostenosis due to sarcoi-dosis: a cause of atelectasis and airway obstruction simulating pulmonary neoplasm and chronic obstructive pulmonary disease. Chest. (1979). Jun;, 75(6), 663-6.

[39] Mendelson, D. S, Norton, K, Cohen, B. A, Brown, L. K, & Rabinowitz, J. G. Bronchial compression: an unusual manifestation of sarcoidosis. J Comput Assist Tomogr. (1983). Oct;, 7(5), 892-4.

[40] Criado, E, Sanchez, M, Ramirez, J, Arguis, P, De Caralt, T. M, Perea, R. J, et al. Pul-monary sarcoidosis: typical and atypical manifestations at high-resolution CT with pathologic correlation. Radiographics. (2010). Oct;, 30(6), 1567-86.

[41] Davies, C. W, Tasker, A. D, Padley, S. P, Davies, R. J, & Gleeson, F. V. Air trapping in sarcoidosis on computed tomography: correlation with lung function. Clin Radiol. (2000). Mar;, 55(3), 217-21.

[42] Fain, S, Schiebler, M. L, Mccormack, D. G, & Parraga, G. Imaging of lung function using hyperpolarized helium-3 magnetic resonance imaging: Review of current and emerging translational methods and applications. J Magn Reson Imaging. (2010). Dec;, 32(6), 1398-408.

[43] Burgel, P. R. The role of small airways in obstructive airway diseases. Eur Respir Rev. (2011). Mar 1;, 20(119), 23-33.

[44] Kamp, D. W. Physiologic evaluation of asthma. Chest. (1992). Jun;101(6 Suppl): 396S-400S.

[45] Kabitz, H. J, Lang, F, Walterspacher, S, Sorichter, S, Muller-quernheim, J, & Wind-isch, W. Impact of impaired inspiratory muscle strength on dyspnea and walking ca-pacity in sarcoidosis. Chest. (2006). Nov;, 130(5), 1496-502.

[46] Pesola, G. R, Kurdi, M, & Olibrice, M. Endobronchial sarcoidosis and hyperreactive airways disease. Chest. (2002). Jun;121(6):2081; author reply

[47] Shorr, A. F, Torrington, K. G, & Hnatiuk, O. W. Endobronchial involvement and air-way hyperreactivity in patients with sarcoidosis. Chest. (2001). Sep;A study that dis-cusses endobronchial disease and airways hyperreactivity in sarcoidosis., 120(3), 881-6.

[48] Viskum, K, & Vestbo, J. Vital prognosis in intrathoracic sarcoidosis with special refer-ence to pulmonary function and radiological stage. Eur Respir J. (1993). Mar;, 6(3), 349-53.

[49] Westney, G. E, Habib, S, & Quarshie, A. Comorbid illnesses and chest radiographic severity in African-American sarcoidosis patients. Lung. (2007). May-Jun;, 185(3), 131-7.

[50] Plusa, T, Chcialowski, A, Piechota, W, & Pirozynski, M. Activity of angiotensin I converting enzyme in sarcoidosis, atopic bronchial asthma and acute bronchitis. Allergol
Immunopathol (Madr). (1990). Jul-Aug;, 18(4), 217-21.

[51] Naccache, J. M, Lavole, A, Nunes, H, Lamberto, C, Letoumelin, P, Brauner, M, et al.
High-resolution computed tomographic imaging of airways in sarcoidosis patients
with airflow obstruction. J Comput Assist Tomogr. (2008). Nov-Dec;, 32(6), 905-12.

[52] Lavergne, F, Clerici, C, Sadoun, D, Brauner, M, Battesti, J. P, & Valeyre, D. Airway
obstruction in bronchial sarcoidosis: outcome with treatment. Chest. (1999). Nov;,
116(5), 1194-9.

[53] Witko, J, Strazzella, W. D, & Safirstein, B. H. Upper lobe collapse due to endobronchial sarcoidosis. AJR Am J Roentgenol. (1990). Apr;, 154(4), 897-8.

[54] Stinson, J. M, & Hargett, D. Prolonged lobar atelectasis in sarcoidosis. J Natl Med Assoc. (1981). , 73(7), 669-71.

[55] Sharma, O. P, & Izumi, T. The importance of airway obstruction in sarcoidosis. Sarcoidosis. (1988). Sep;, 5(2), 119-20.

[56] Rosen, Y. Pathology of sarcoidosis. Semin Respir Crit Care Med. (2007). Feb;A review
article that discusses the granuloma formation and histopathology in sarcoidosis.,
28(1), 36-52.

[57] Judson, M. A, & Strange, C. Bullous sarcoidosis: a report of three cases. Chest. (1998).
Nov;, 114(5), 1474-8.

[58] Jeebun, V, & Forrest, I. A. Sarcoidosis: an underrecognised cause for bullous lung
disease? Eur Respir J. (2009). Oct;, 34(4), 999-1001.

[59] Miller, A. The vanishing lung syndrome associated with pulmonary sarcoidosis. Br J
Dis Chest. (1981). Apr;A review article that discusses the vanishing lung syndrome
associated with sarcoidosis., 75(2), 209-14.

[60] Miller, A, Teirstein, A. S, Jackler, I, Chuang, M, & Siltzbach, L. E. Airway function in
chronic pulmonary sarcoidosis with fibrosis. Am Rev Respir Dis. (1974). Feb;, 109(2),
179-89.

[61] Seaman, D. M, Meyer, C. A, Gilman, M. D, & Mccormack, F. X. Diffuse Cystic Lung
Disease at High-Resolution CT. AJR Am J Roentgenol. (2011). Jun;, 196(6), 1305-11.

[62] Akbari, J. G, Varma, P. K, Neema, P. K, Menon, M. U, & Neelakandhan, K. S. Clinical
profile and surgical outcome for pulmonary aspergilloma: a single center experience.
Ann Thorac Surg. (2005). Sep;, 80(3), 1067-72.

[63] Judson, M. A. Noninvasive Aspergillus pulmonary disease. Semin Respir Crit Care
Med. (2004). Apr;, 25(2), 203-19.

[64] Israel, H. L, Lenchner, G. S, & Atkinson, G. W. Sarcoidosis and aspergilloma. The role of surgery. Chest. (1982). Oct;, 82(4), 430-2.

[65] Glastonbury, C. M. Non-oncologic imaging of the larynx. Otolaryngol Clin North Am. (2008). Feb;vi., 41(1), 139-56.

[66] Hansell, D. M, Milne, D. G, Wilsher, M. L, & Wells, A. U. Pulmonary sarcoidosis: morphologic associations of airflow obstruction at thin-section CT. Radiology. (1998). Dec;, 209(3), 697-704.

[67] Handa, T, Nagai, S, Hirai, T, Chin, K, Kubo, T, Oga, T, et al. Computed tomography analysis of airway dimensions and lung density in patients with sarcoidosis. Respiration. (2009). , 77(3), 273-81.

[68] Iannuzzi, M. C, Rybicki, B. A, & Teirstein, A. S. Sarcoidosis. N Engl J Med. (2007). Nov 22;A clinical review article on sarcoidosis., 357(21), 2153-65.

[69] Jones, E, & Callen, J. P. Hydroxychloroquine is effective therapy for control of cutaneous sarcoidal granulomas. J Am Acad Dermatol. (1990). Sep;23(3 Pt 1):487-9.

[70] Miyazaki, E, Ando, M, Fukami, T, Nureki, S, Eishi, Y, & Kumamoto, T. Minocycline for the treatment of sarcoidosis: is the mechanism of action immunomodulating or antimicrobial effect? Clin Rheumatol. (2008). Sep;, 27(9), 1195-7.

[71] Bachelez, H, Senet, P, Cadranel, J, Kaoukhov, A, & Dubertret, L. The use of tetracyclines for the treatment of sarcoidosis. Arch Dermatol. (2001). Jan;, 137(1), 69-73.

[72] Sapadin, A. N, & Fleischmajer, R. Tetracyclines: nonantibiotic properties and their clinical implications. J Am Acad Dermatol. (2006). Feb;, 54(2), 258-65.

[73] Siltzbach, L. E, & Teirstein, A. S. Chloroquine therapy in 43 patients with intrathoracic and cutaneous sarcoidosis. Acta Med Scand Suppl. (1964). , 425, 302-8.

[74] Johns, C. J, & Michele, T. M. The clinical management of sarcoidosis. A 50-year experience at the Johns Hopkins Hospital. Medicine (Baltimore). (1999). Mar;A review article that discusses the management of sarcoidosis., 78(2), 65-111.

[75] Hassid, S, Choufani, G, Saussez, S, Dubois, M, Salmon, I, & Soupart, A. Sarcoidosis of the paranasal sinuses treated with hydroxychloroquine. Postgrad Med J. (1998). Mar;, 74(869), 172-4.

[76] Baughman, R. P, & Costabel, U. du Bois RM. Treatment of sarcoidosis. Clin Chest Med. (2008). Sep;ix-x.* A review article that discusses the treatment of sarcoidosis., 29(3), 533-48.

[77] Baughman, R. P, & Lower, E. E. Evidence-based therapy for cutaneous sarcoidosis. Clin Dermatol. (2007). May-Jun;, 25(3), 334-40.

[78] Stagaki, E, Mountford, W. K, Lackland, D. T, & Judson, M. A. The treatment of lupus pernio: results of 116 treatment courses in 54 patients. Chest. (2009). Feb;, 135(2), 468-76.

[79] Preminger, B. A, Hiltzik, D. H, Segal, J, & Morrison, N. G. An operative approach to the treatment of refractory cutaneous nasal sarcoid: a case report and review of the literature. Ann Plast Surg. (2009). Dec;, 63(6), 685-7.

[80] Kay, D. J, & Har-el, G. The role of endoscopic sinus surgery in chronic sinonasal sarcoidosis. Am J Rhinol. (2001). Jul-Aug;, 15(4), 249-54.

[81] Benjamin, B, Dalton, C, & Croxson, G. Laryngoscopic diagnosis of laryngeal sarcoid. Ann Otol Rhinol Laryngol. (1995). Jul;, 104(7), 529-31.

[82] Levey, M. Extensive sarcoidosis involving the upper respiratory tract. Int Surg. (1979). Apr;, 64(3), 73-7.

[83] Gallivan, G. J, & Landis, J. N. Sarcoidosis of the larynx: preserving and restoring airway and professional voice. J Voice. (1993). Mar;, 7(1), 81-94.

[84] Fogel, T. D, Weissberg, J. B, Dobular, K, & Kirchner, J. A. Radiotherapy in sarcoidosis of the larynx: case report and review of the literature. Laryngoscope. (1984). Sep;, 94(9), 1223-5.

[85] Anton-pacheco, J. L, Cabezali, D, Tejedor, R, Lopez, M, Luna, C, Comas, J. V, et al. The role of airway stenting in pediatric tracheobronchial obstruction. Eur J Cardiothorac Surg. (2008). Jun;, 33(6), 1069-75.

[86] Fouty, B. W, Pomeranz, M, Thigpen, T. P, & Martin, R. J. Dilatation of bronchial stenoses due to sarcoidosis using a flexible fiberoptic bronchoscope. Chest. (1994). Sep;, 106(3), 677-80.

[87] ten Hacken NHWijkstra PJ, Kerstjens HA. Treatment of bronchiectasis in adults. BMJ. (2007). Nov 24;, 335(7629), 1089-93.

[88] Panjabi, C, Sahay, S, & Shah, A. Aspergilloma formation in cavitary sarcoidosis. J Bras Pneumol. (2009). May;, 35(5), 480-3.

[89] Corr, P. Management of severe hemoptysis from pulmonary aspergilloma using endovascular embolization. Cardiovasc Intervent Radiol. (2006). Sep-Oct;, 29(5), 807-10.

Chapter 6

Clinical Manifestations of Sarcoidosis

Luis Jara-Palomares, Candela Caballero-Eraso,
Cesar Gutiérrez, Alvaro Donate and
Jose Antonio Rodríguez-Portal

Additional information is available at the end of the chapter

1. Introduction

Sarcoidosis is a systemic granulomatous disease of unknown etiology that is characterized from the point of view of pathology of the presence of noncaseating granulomas in affected organs. Typically affects young adults and is often present initially with one or more of the following conditions: 1) bilateral hilar lymphadenopathy, 2) pulmonary reticular pattern, 3) Involvement of the skin, joints and / or eyes.

In this chapter we are going to review and update the clinical features and sign of sarcoidosis.

2. Airway involvement

Patients with pulmonary sarcoidosis may have impaired upper and/or lower airway, and could be impossible or difficult to detect with routine imaging, but are recognized by alternative diagnostic tests (eg, bronchoscopy) [1]. Endobronchial disease exists in approximately 40% of patients with stage I disease, and approximately 70% of patients with stage II or III. Airway stenosis clinically significant is rare but can be unwieldy when severe [2, 3]. Table 1 summarize the airway involvement in sarcoidosis.

In the fibrotic stage of the disease can be observed thinning of the mucosa, pallor, and scarring can lead to a decrease in the light of the airways and the stenosis [4-6].

Type of involvement	Comments
Mucosal erythema and edema	Nonspecific finding*
Granular mucosa	Nonspecific*
Cobblestone mucosa	More common in lobar and segmental bronchi*
Mucosal plaques (yellowish)	Also occurs in other disorders*
Mucosal nodules (waxy yellow)	Characteristic feature*; may occlude bronchi
Bronchial stenosis	Lobar and segmental bronchi affected more frequently than central airways; mucosal biopsy may or may not show granulomas
Airway distortion	More likely in advanced parenchymal disease
Bronchiectasis	Traction bronchiectasis associated with advanced parenchymal disease; usually asymptomatic
Bronchiolitis	Uncommon; CT scan may suggest diagnosis*
Extrinsic compression	Uncommon; may occur with significant thoracic lymphadenopathy
Airway hyperreactivity	Occurs in up to 20% of sarcoid patients; endobronchial involvement increases the risk
Airflow limitation (FEV1/FVC ratio < 80)	Occurs in 60% of sarcoid patients; seen in any stage
Hemoptysis	Uncommon from airway involvement
Obstructive sleep apnea	Due to laryngeal involvement; more common in patients with lupus pernio
Supraglottic structures	Oral, nasal, and pharyngeal mucosal changes as noted above, hoarseness, dysphagia, laryngeal paralysis, and airway obstruction

*A biopsy required to document the presence of a noncaseous granuloma; in other types of involvement, a biopsy specimen may or may not demonstrate noncaseous granulomas.

Modified from Ref. 1

Table 1. Airway involvement in sarcoidosis

2.1. Supraglottic airways

Nasal passages, oropharynx, supraglottic structures, and the larynx develop sarcoid granulomas in approximately 6% of patients with sarcoidosis [7-10]. Debería sospecharse en todos los pacientes con sarcoidosis sistémica y síntomas de vía aérea superior [4, 5, 8, 11-12]. Sarcoid lesions can occur in nasal and oral mucosa, occasionally with ulceration; anosmia improves after steroid therapy [13]. A nasal examination may reveal granulomatous mass, yellow-white mucosal papules, and adhesions and crusting of septal and turbinate mucosa. Nodular sarcoidosis of supraglottic and glottic structures can lead to dyspnea, stridor, dysphonia, irritating cough with pharyngolaryngeal discomfort, dysphagia, retronasal obstruction, and/or hyponasal speech. Rhinopharyngolaryngeal endoscopy may reveal reddish or yellow granulomatous lesions (2-4 mm in diameter) [14]. Laryngoscopy may show epiglottic thickening and granularity, granulomatous mass and infiltrative sarcoid nodules of epiglottis, aryepiglottic folds, and false cords. These may cause respiratory distress, requiring tracheostomy [15]. Flow-volume curves and laryngeal examination are helpful in the diagnosis and management [16]. Obstructing polypoid sarcoid lesions have been managed with laryngoscopic resection, tracheostomy, or local injection of a corticosteroid [17].

Obstructive sleep apnea, which occurs in about 5% of the general population, seems to occur with increased frequency in patients with sarcoidosis, especially in patients with lupus pernio [18]. Sarcoidosis of the upper airways has been suggested as one of the possible mechanisms for sleep apnea in patients with sarcoidosis and lupus pernio, although the overwhelming majority of obstructive sleep apnea in sarcoidosis is most probably related to obesity from corticosteroids. Sarcoidosis of the supraglottic airways in children is rare [19].

2.2. Larynx

Laryngeal sarcoidosis often occurs as an isolated phenomenon and is usually attributed to asthma [20]. Occasionally, laryngeal sarcoid can lead to progressive life-threatening airway obstruction [15]. Laryngeal sarcoidosis is uncommon [21]. The incidence of laryngeal sarcoidosis is estimated to be about 1.2%. Laryngeal sarcoidosis could be treated with systemic and intralesional injections of a corticosteroid, surgical intervention, carbon dioxide laser ablation, and external beam radiation [22, 23].

Paralysis of the left vocal cord and hoarseness can occur from compression of the left recurrent laryngeal nerve by enlarged lymph nodes [24, 25]. Systemic corticosteroid therapy has resulted in resolution of the hoarseness [24].

2.3. Central airways

The trachea and main bronchi are less frequently affected than the lobar, segmental, subsegmental, and distal airways. Sarcoid granulomas of trachea, main carina, and major bronchi by themselves seldom produce significant obstructive symptoms or airway dysfunction [26, 27]. Cough is the main symptom. Symptoms, clinical examination, flow-volume curves, and bronchoscopy help in assessing the severity of the central airway stenosis [28].

Mainstem bronchial stenoses as well as segmental stenosis have been described in patients with sarcoidosis [29]. Disabling inspiratory and expiratory airflow limitation mimicking fixed upper airway obstruction has been reported [27]. Bronchoscopy may demonstrate other changes as: mucosal erythema, edema, friability, granularity, fine cobblestoning, and sarcoid nodules. The characteristic yellow waxy nodules typical of sarcoidosis are less likely to occur in the trachea and main bronchi, but when seen in these areas, they tend to be sparsely distributed.

Extrinsic compression of the central airways by the enlarged mediastinal and hilar lymph nodes is uncommon. Right middle lobe syndrome caused by extrinsic compression and intraluminal sarcoidosis has been described [30].

2.4. Distal airways

Sarcoidosis could affect lobar, segmental, subsegmental, and more distal bronchi as well as bronchioles, which is manifested as mucosal inflammation, endobronchial granulomas, stenosis, extrinsic compression, distortion, bronchiectasis, bronchiolitis, airway hyperreactivity, and streaky hemoptysis.

These can lead to airway dysfunction and respiratory symptoms. Sarcoid granulomas tend to develop along the bronchovascular bundle or in the vicinity of the airways. All of these changes are more likely to affect the airways in upper and mid-lung regions.

The various types of airway abnormalities encountered in patients with sarcoidosis are described in the following paragraphs.

a. Endobronchial Granulomas

The definitive diagnosis of endobronchial granulomata requires a biopsy of the airway mucosa because a normal-appearing airway mucosa does not exclude the presence of granulomas [31]. The mucosal abnormalities can be diffuse or patchy. These findings are nonspecific and may be seen in other disorders. Therefore, biopsies of the mucosa and submucosa are essential for making a histologic diagnosis. Segmental and lobar bronchial lumen can be compromised by extrinsic compression by an enlarged adjacent lymph node. Endobronchial characteristics of sarcoid granulomas are well documented [32]. The classic endobronchial sarcoidosis is characterized by mucosal islands of waxy yellow mucosal nodules, measuring 2 to 4 mm in diameter. These nodules appear dull gray or waxy yellow. The mucosal lesions tend to be diffuse but more profuse in the lobar and segmental bronchi. Bronchial luminal occlusion by sarcoid granulomas can mimic an obstructing malignant mass. Endobronchial granulomas produce cough, wheezing, and dyspnea. The mucosal nodules seldom ulcerate or bleed.

b. Bronchial Stenosis

Bronchial stenosis is reported to occur in up to 14% of patients with sarcoidosis [33]. Bronchoscopy is helpful in evaluating the location, types, and severity of bronchial stenosis. The stenoses can be solitary or multiple, lobar or segmental bronchial stenoses, with or without atelectasis, and they may occur at any stage of respiratory sarcoidosis [33-35]. Extensive and multiple stenotic lesions of larger bronchi may cause or contribute to pulmonary symptoms.

c. Bronchiolitis

Bronchiolar involvement from sarcoidosis can also occur in early sarcoidosis without pulmonary parenchymal involvement [36, 37]. Bronchiolitis obliterans organizing pneumonia, bronchiolar narrowing and occlusion, and sarcoidosis coexisting with asthma have been described [38, 39]. Airtrapping is a common feature in sarcoidosis and correlates with evidence of small airways disease on pulmonary function testing.

d. Airway Distortion

Airway distortion is common in later stages of sarcoidosis and is caused by granulomatous changes in and around the airways and the secondary traction bronchiectasis associated with pulmonary parenchymal fibrosis [40, 41].

e. Bronchiectasis

Traction bronchiectasis becomes evident as the parenchymal disease progresses [40]. Traction bronchiectasis has been reported in up to 40% of patients with fibrotic stages of sarcoid [41]. Localized bronchiectasis of the right middle lobe caused by obstructing sarcoid granuloma has been described [42]. Traction bronchiectasis and bronchial distortion, as described earlier, seldom cause bronchiectatic symptoms [43].

f.   Hemoptysis

Hemoptysis in patients with sarcoidosis is usually the result of a complication such as the development of an aspergilloma in advanced fibrotic and cavitary sarcoid [44-46]. Large pulmonary cystic lesions occur in advanced stages of sarcoidosis, and these could potentially become infected with *Aspergillus* and aspergilloma could develop. Fatal massive hemoptysis has been described in such patients [46]. Traction bronchiectasis is observed in patients with advanced sarcoidosis and endobronchial sarcoidosis rarely causes hemoptysis.

g.   Airway Hyperreactivity

Airway hyperreactivity has been reported in up to 20% of patients with sarcoidosis, and, as a result, cough and wheezing may prompt patients to seek medical help [47, 48]. The airway hyperreactivity is also responsible for the cough, wheezing, and dyspnea and is independent of the airway involvement. Airway hyperreactivity in patients with sarcoidosis remains a difficult entity to define because of the airway involvement by sarcoidosis. The smaller baseline diameter of the diseased airway can potentially increase airway resistance and lead to a false-positive bronchoprovocation test result.

2.5. Bronchoscopy

Bronchoscopy plays a significant role in the diagnosis and management of airway sarcoidosis. The role of the technique in the retrieval of immune effector cells and infectious organisms by analyzing bronchoalveolar lavage (BAL) fluid, biopsy specimens of pulmonary parenchymal sarcoid, and needle aspiration/biopsy samples of enlarged lymph nodes in the mediastinum and hilar regions is well known [49]. These bronchoscopic techniques have an important role in the diagnosis of infectious diseases in sarcoid patients in whom complications such as aspergilloma and other infections develop. Bronchoscopy also helps in excluding disorders that may resemble sarcoidosis.

Bronchoscopic abnormalities have been observed in up to 60% of patients with sarcoidosis [48]. These include "retinalization" of mucosa from increased mucosal vascularity, mucosal coarseness, pallor, flat yellow mucosal plaques, wartlike excrescences, "bleb-like" formations, irregular mucosal thickening, ulceration, and atrophic mucosa. The three common findings were bronchial mucosal hyperemia or edema, distortion of the bronchial anatomy, and bronchial narrowing. The classic endobronchial sarcoidosis is mucosal islands of waxy yellow mucosal nodules, 2 to 4 mm in diameter. Bronchoscopy may reveal endobronchial occlusion by sarcoid granulomas in the submucosa or an endobronchial polyp caused by sarcoid granulomas [35].

Bronchoscopic biopsy of endobronchial lesions confirms the diagnosis of endobronchial sarcoidosis in up to 70% patients with the disease [48, 50, 51]. Patients with abnormal-appearing airways are much more likely to have positive results, with a diagnostic yield of 75% [48]. Even when the airway mucosa appears normal, mucosal biopsy specimens may demonstrate mucosal or submucosal noncaseous granulomas in up to 50% of patients with sarcoidosis [48]. In typical cases, the identification of noncaseous granulomas on frozen section analysis may render lung biopsy unnecessary.

3. Lung disease

Sarcoidosis occurs in patients aged between 10-40 years in 70-90% of cases. In about half the cases the disease is detected incidentally by alterations in the chest radiograph. The organ most frequently affected is the lung. The most common symptoms are cough, dyspnea and chest pain. In patients in the eighth decade of life is more common than systemic symptoms such as fatigue and anorexia, although dyspnea is often present at the same time [52].

A pulmonary auscultation crackles or roncus uncommon to hear, but wheezing may be present.

3.1. Pulmonary imaging

Pulmonary involvement occurs in 90% of patients with sarcoidosis [10]. The typical chest radiograph shows bilateral hilar lymphadenopathy. This finding, however, may be absent, or if present may occur in combination with opacities in the parenchyma. Parenchymal opacities may be interstitial, alveolar or both. Pleural involvement is uncommon (<5%), but may occur as lymphocytic exudate in the pleural effusion, chylothorax, hemothorax, or pneumothorax [54-56].

a.   Chest x-ray:

Stage of lung involvement is established based on chest radiography. Although the chest radiograph provides an anatomical guide of lung disease can not measure disease activity or functional damage assessment. The sarcoid nodule is defined as pulmonary nodules, bilateral and multiple in the chest radiograph, which may mimic metastatic disease. When viewed through the computerized tomography (CT) revealed a nodular consolidation with well defined borders [56]. Radiological stages are (Figure 1):

• Stage I: is defined as the presence of bilateral hilar lymphadenopathy, which are often accompanied with an increase in right paratracheal adenopathy. 50% of patients initially present as bilateral hilar lymphadenopathy. In 75% of cases, hilar lymphadenopathy return within the first through third year, while 10% will persist for 10 years or more.

• Stage II: Defined as bilateral hilar lymphadenopathy and reticular opacities (the latter occurs more often in the upper lobes). These findings are initially in 25% of patients. In two thirds of these cases the lesions regress spontaneously, while the rest can be progression of the disease or remain unchanged over time. Normally the stage II patients have mild or moderate. The most common symptoms are usually: cough, dyspnea, fever, and/or fatigue.

• Stage III: This is defined as reticular opacities without hilar lymphadenopathy. Reticular opacities are distributed predominantly in the upper lobes.

- Stage IV: Is characterized by reticular opacities with evidence of volume loss, chiefly distributed in the upper lobes. Can also be observed: adenopathic clusters with marked traction bronchiectasis, or extensive calcification, cavitation or cyst formation [57].

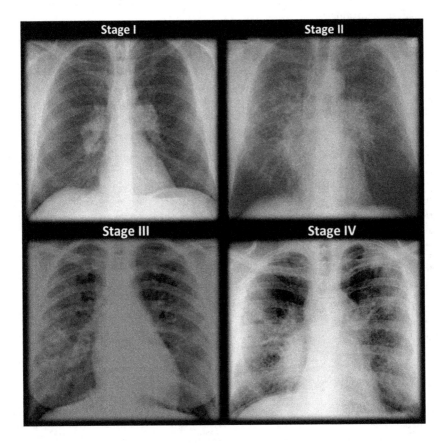

Figure 1. Staging of sarcoidosis on basis of chest radiographs

b. Computerized Axial Tomography (CT) scan:

Sarcoidosis patient can show a variety of abnormalities [58, 59]: Hilar and mediastinal lymphadenopathy, beaded or irregular thickening of the bronchovascular bundles, nodules along bronchi, vessels, and subpleural regions, bronchial wall thickening, ground glass opacification, parenchymal masses or consolidation, parenchymal bands, cysts, traction bronchiectasis, fibrosis with distortion of the lung architecture.

High-resolution CT has proved superior to conventional CT for assessing subtle parenchymal details and discriminating between inflammation and fibrosis in patients with pulmonary sarcoidosis [58, 60]. The thin-section collimation (1- to 1.5- mm section thickness) and high-spatial-frequency reconstruction algorithms that are used to generate high-resolution CT images allow improved detection of nodular and reticular opacities, thickened interlobular septa, and faint ground-glass opacities, making the technique especially useful for identifying and managing sarcoidosis.

High-resolution CT may be particularly helpful for distinguishing active inflammation from irreversible fibrosis in selected patients with stage 2 or 3 sarcoidosis. Nodules, ground-glass opacities, and alveolar opacities are suggestive of granulomatous inflammation that may be reversed with therapy [61]. By contrast, honeycomb-like cysts, bullae, broad and coarse septal bands, architectural distortion, volume loss, and traction bronchiectasis are indicative of irreversible fibrosis [62]. High-resolution CT may be useful also for verifying specific diagnoses in patients with atypical clinical manifestations or unusual radiographic features [63].

In the appropriate clinical context, the observation of typical imaging features of sarcoidosis (eg, bilateral hilar lymph node enlargement with a perilymphatic micronodular pattern) and the anatomic distribution of those abnormalities (eg, upper lobe predominance) may point to a highly specific diagnosis. However, atypical manifestations may necessitate a broader differential diagnosis that includes tuberculosis and other granulomatous infections, silicosis, malignancies, and pneumoconiosis.

We are going to explain some typical patterns of sarcoidosis. Criado et al. [64] published and extensive review about typical and typical patterns of sarcoidosis. Table 2 shows typical and atypical features of pulmonary sarcoidosis at high-resolution CT.

Typical features	Atypical features
Lymphadenopathy: hilar, mediastinal (right paratracheal), bilateral, symmetric, and well defined	Lymphadenopathy: unilateral, isolated, anterior and posterior mediastinal
Nodules: micronodules (2–4 mm in diameter; well defined, bilateral); macronodules (≥5 mm in diameter, coalescing)	Airspace consolidation: masslike opacities, conglomerate masses, solitary pulmonary nodules, confluent alveolar opacities (alveolar sarcoid pattern)
Lymphangitic spread: peribronchovascular, subpleural, interlobular septal	Linear opacities: interlobular septal thickening, intralobular linear opacities
Fibrotic changes: reticular opacities, architectural distortion, traction bronchiectasis, bronchio-lectasis, volume loss	Fibrocystic changes: cysts, bullae, blebs, emphysema, honeycomb-like opacities with upper- and middle-zone predominance
Bilateral perihilar opacities	Ground-glass opacities
Predominant upper- and middle-zone locations of parenchymal abnormalities	Miliary opacities
	Airway involvement: mosaic attenuation pattern, tracheobronchial abnormalities, atelectasis
	Pleural disease: effusion, chylothorax, hemothorax, pneumothorax, pleural thickening, calcification
	Mycetoma, aspergilloma

Table 2. Typical and Atypical Features of Pulmonary Sarcoidosis at High-Resolution CT. Modified from ref. 64.

• Typical Patterns of Lymphadenopathy

The most common pattern is well-defined, bilateral, symmetric hilar and right paratracheal lymph node enlargement. Bilateral hilar lymph node enlargement, alone or in combination with mediastinal lymph node enlargement, occurs in an estimated 95% of patients affected with sarcoidosis [65, 66]. Middle mediastinal nodes (at the left paratracheal level, subcarinal level, and level of the aortopulmonary window), prevascular nodes, or both are involved in approximately 50% of patients [60].

Bilateral hilar lymph node enlargement may be a feature of infection (particularly fungal or mycobacterial infection) or malignancy (eg, lymphoma). However, in the absence of specific symptoms or signs, sarcoidosis is the most common cause of bilateral lymph node enlargement. Histologic confirmation is not required for a diagnosis of sarcoidosis in these patients. However, a biopsy should be performed if the chest radiographic findings worsen or specific signs and symptoms develop [67].

• Typical Parenchymal Manifestations

1.   Micronodules with a Perilymphatic Distribution

A perilymphatic distribution of micronodular lesions is the most common parenchymal disease pattern seen in patients with pulmonary sarcoidosis (75%–90% of cases). High-resolution CT shows sharply defined, small (2–4 mm in diameter), rounded nodules, usually with a bilateral and symmetric distribution, predominantly but not invariably in the upper and middle zones. The nodules are found most often in the subpleural peribronchovascular interstitium and less often in the interlobular septa. Although sarcoid granulomas arise as micronodular lesions, they may coalesce over time, forming larger lesions (macronodules) [56, 58, 63].

Sarcoid granulomas frequently cause nodular or irregular thickening of the peribronchovascular interstitium. Extensive peribronchovascular nodularity on high-resolution CT images is strongly suggestive of sarcoidosis. However, interstitial thickening is not extensive in most patients with sarcoidosis.

2.   Fibrotic Changes

In most patients, sarcoid granulomas resolve with time. However, in an estimated 20% of patients, fibrosis becomes more prominent over time, producing CT and radiographic findings of linear opacities, traction bronchiectasis, and architectural distortion (displacement of fissures and bronchovascular bundles). Fibrosis is seen predominantly in the upper and middle zones, in a patchy distribution [41].

Extensive interstitial fibrosis can cause pulmonary arterial hypertension and resultant right heart failure. Imaging findings that may be predictive of such an event include a prominent main pulmonary artery, enlarged right and left pulmonary arteries, right ventricular enlargement, and attenuation of peripheral vessels.

3.   Bilateral Perihilar Opacities

Confluent nodular opacities that appear on high-resolution CT images as bilateral areas of lung consolidation with irregular edges and blurred margins, radiating from the hilum toward the periphery, are often seen with or without air bronchograms. These areas of consolidation are less homogeneous peripherally and are usually accompanied by micronodules [41, 60].

c.   Positron emission tomography (PET):

A PET fluorine-18-fluorodeoxyglucose (18F-FDG) can help identify occult lesions and potentially reversible granulomatous disease [69, 70]. This test does not differentiate sarcoidosis from malignant lesions, as 18F-FDG PET can be positive in both processes. However, in a small study of 24 sarcoidosis and 17 lung cancer, the combination of 18F-FDG and 18F-FMT (L-[3-18F]-methyltyrosine) PET scanning was able to differentiate sarcoidosis cancer. Sarcoid lesions were positive in 18 F-FDG PET but negative on 18 F-FMT PET, and both were positive for cancer patients [71]. More studies are needed to confirm these findings. Besides the latter tracer may not be available in all centers.

d.   Radiotracer scanning - Gallium-67 lung scanning:

Is a noninvasive test for staging the "alveolitis" found in interstitial lung diseases. This compound located the site of inflammation of the lung [72-74]. The role of gallium-67 scanning in the diagnosis and management of sarcoidosis is currently controversial [75]. It has been suggested that there is a direct relationship between a visual index of gallium-67 uptake in the lung and the number of inflammatory cells (particularly macrophages) obtained from bronchoalveolar lavage in patients with sarcoidosis (and idiopathic pulmonary fibrosis). As a result the uptake of gallium-67 may be useful to determine the degree of alveolar inflammation, which will focus more lower alveolar macrophages and neutrophils [72-74].

Unfortunately there has not been adequate study to make any correlation of the gallium-67 level with the stage of swelling or how the level of radionuclide uptake may correspond to the stage of disease. Furthermore, studies in normal subjects demonstrate that there may be a small but significant uptake of gallium-67 in alveolar macrophages obtained by bronchoalveolar lavage despite negative imaging test [76].

As a result, actually is not recommended for routine evaluation with gallium-67 lung scanning in these patients because of the difficulty of interpretation, since it is not specific, and that a negative test does not exclude the disease.

Other types of radiotracer-based scanning may help in future diagnosis and clinical management of patients with sarcoidosis [77, 78]. As an example, one study of 22 patients with sarcoidosis scans performed after administration of technetium-labeled Depreotide, which binds to somatostatin receptors [77]. The scan was positive in 18 patients (81%) and in 4 of whom was negative had a normal chest radiograph. The features of this test are still unknown, and clinical use is experimental.

3.2. Pulmonary function test

Characteristically, pulmonary function tests show a restrictive pattern with reduced diffusing capacity for carbon monoxide. Yet we must bear in mind that pulmonary function tests may be normal [79]. Endobronchial sarcoidosis may show involvement of airflow obstruction and respiratory pattern.

The greatest value of pulmonary function tests is to verify the course of the disease individually by sequential measurements. Mean it will not detect pulmonary sarcoidosis or provide a reliable estimate of the extent of parenchymal disease. In addition, the clinician can not predict the natural course of lung disease or response to treatment based solely on these tests.

3.3. Bronchoalveolar Lavage (BAL)

BAL can be used as an adjuvant as to support the diagnosis of sarcoidosis, showing a reduced number of CD8 cells, an elevated CD4/CD8 ratio and an increase in activated T cells, CD4, immunoglobulins, and IgG-secreting cells [80-83]. BAL may also be useful to exclude infections as an alternative diagnosis.

Lymphocytosis in BAL is neither sensitive nor specific for the diagnosis of sarcoidosis. In addition, this test can be misinterpreted [80].

The D-dimer in BAL also supports the diagnosis of sarcoidosis. An observational study found that 8 of the 10 patients with sarcoidosis had detectable D-dimer in the BAL (defined as D-dimer> 78ng) Compared to none of 18 healthy controls [82]. Among patients with sarcoidosis are more likely to have a higher D-dimer black patients than whites [83].

3.4. Histopathology

The morphological feature of sarcoidosis is the noncaseating granuloma of the lung, which is most often found in the alveolar septa, the walls of the bronchi and pulmonary arteries and veins. Sarcoid granuloma formation probably is preceded by alveolitis which involves more than the interstitium and alveolar spaces is characterized by the accumulation of inflammatory cells, including monocytes, macrophages and lymphocytes [84, 85].

The sarcoid granuloma is a chronic inflammatory reaction and focal accumulation formed by epithelial cells, monocytes, lymphocytes, macrophages and fibroblasts. Multinucleated giant cells are frequently found between epithelial cells in the follicle of the granuloma and often have cytoplasmic inclusions such as asteroid bodies, Schaumann bodies and birefringent crystalline particles (calcium oxalate and other calcium salts) [86]. Most sarcoid granulomas gradually resolved and leave little or no residual manifestation of prior inflammation.

3.5. Allocation pulmonary vs. extrapulmonary

Health status is a subjective parameter that is being used more frequently to assess health interventions. Questionnaires have been developed, both generic and disease-specific, to assess health status. Differences in patients reported outcomes between sarcoidosis patients with isolated pulmonary involvement and those with extrapulmonary manifestations have not been well described. In this way, Gvozdenovic et al. [68] develop a study to assess the differences of the severity of fatigue and dyspnea symptoms, activities of daily living and health status between the patients with isolated pulmonary and those with pulmonary plus extrapulmonary sarcoidosis. This study concluded that patients with pulmonary and extrapulmonary sarcoidosis are more fatigued, have more dyspnea, are more limited in their everyday physical activities, and have lower health status in comparison with those with isolated pulmonary involvement. They proposed several mechanisms to explain these differences, although remained conjectural and are potential fruitful areas for future research.

4. Pulmonary hypertension complicating sarcoidosis

Pulmonary hypertension (PH) is defined as the presence of a mean pulmonary artery pressure (mPAP) $\geq$ 25 mm Hg [87]. Although in most cases sarcoidosis is a disease with good prognosis, the presence of PH is a serious complication that occurs in cases with severe pulmonary involvement, although there have been cases of PH in any stages of the disease. An early diagnosis that may consider different treatment options is critical to improve the prognosis of these patients.

The prevalence of pulmonary hypertension (SAPH) asociated to sarcoidosis is unknown. Prospective and retrospective studies describe prevalence from 5 to 28% [88] (see Table 3). This variability is mainly due to the use of different diagnostic methods, non-homogeneous patient populations and stages of the disease included in those studies. It has been described that in patients with mild lung disease in which PH is defined as that PAP $\geq$ 40 mm Hg measured by transthoracic echocardiography (TTE), the prevalence is 5.7% [89].

Author/reference	Population	Number	Method	Prevalence (%)
Handa (89)	Prospective study of unselected patients	212	TTE	5.7
Baughmann (88)	Subjects with dyspnea out of proportion	53	RHC	47
Sulica (98)	Retrospective study of TTE	106	TTE	51

Table 3. Ascertained prevalence of Sarcoidosis-associated pulmonary hypertension in several populations

A retrospective study of 53 patients with sarcoidosis and persistent dyspnea showed that in 47% of them had a mPAP $\geq$ 25 mm Hg. Only 69% of these cases had stage 3-4 of sarcoidosis [90].

4.1. Pathophysiology

According to Dana Point classification [91] of pulmonary hypertension, the group 3 includes cases of PH due to lung disease or hypoxia (including interstitial lung disease). The group 5 includes the cases where PH has not a clarified mechanism; group 5 also includes sarcoidosis because the pathogenesis of SAPH is associated with complex mechanisms.

a. Destruction of the distal capillary bed

Most patients with sarcoidosis and PH are in advanced stages, presenting a significant alteration of lung parenchyma with destruction of the capillary bed and leading of hypoxemia. However, there are cases of SAPH with minimal lung disorder (Stages 0-1) and hemodynamic measurements detected in the right heart catheterization (RHC) are not always correlated directly with lung function or PaO2 [92]. When comparing cases of idiopathic pulmonary fibrosis and sarcoidosis there are differences in mPAP of 9 mm Hg for an equivalent functional alteration, so this mechanism does not explain the development of PH in all the patients.

b. Increased vasoreactivity

Few years ago was found that production of endothelin 1 (ET-1) in the lung of patients with sarcoidosis is increased [93]. The ET-1 is a potent vasoconstrictor with mitogenic and inflammatory activity and one of the therapeutic targets for the treatment of PH, using receptor antagonists of ET-1. The synthesis and release of nitric oxide (NO) by endothelial cells causes vasodilatation, the decreased of NO production has been associated with PH. Has been suggested that the decrease of NO, found in some studies of patient with sarcoidosis, may participate in the development of SAPH and that could have therapeutic implications [94].

c. Extrinsic compression of pulmonary vessels

There is extrinsic compression of major pulmonary arteries by adenopathies up to 21.4% of patients with SAPH and pulmonary fibrosis [95]. This alteration is often seen in cases with mediastinal and bilateral hillar adenopathies. Compression of the pulmonary vasculature can also be found in cases of mediastinal fibrosis.

d. Vasculopathy

Granulomatous involvement of the pulmonary vessel occurs in 69-100% of the cases studied by lung biopsy specimens. Exits occlusive or destructive granulomas or the patient may develop a perivascular fibrosis. These findings are more frequent in small veins [96].

e. Post-capillary pulmonary hypertension

We mustn`t forget that myocardial involvement in sarcoidosis occurs in up to 5% of cases and cause ventricular systolic or diastolic failure which contribute to the development of PH [97]. However, the symptomatic myocardial abnormality is lower than that found in necropsy studies. We can conclude that the mechanisms involved in the development of PH in sarcoidosis are multiple, involving various anatomical structures and with different therapeutic implications.

4.2. Clinical presentation

The diagnosis of PH in sarcoidosis is difficult because the most common symptom is dyspnea, and many times, this symptom is attributed to the presence of parenchymal involvement. The PH should be suspected in patients with sarcoidosis and dyspnea, hypoxemia, or clinical evidence of the presence of right heart failure, particularly, if these symptoms have not a proportional relationship to the degree of parenchymal involvement. Symptoms of right heart failure are independent predictors of increased pressure in the right cavities. However, these symptoms have low sensitivity, and are only manifested in 21% of patients with confirmed PH. The symptoms are: progressive dyspnea, cough, chest pain, palpitations or syncope [98]. Table 4 shows the distribution of the symptoms.

Sudden death caused by compression of large pulmonary arteries, occlusion of the pulmonary veins by a sarcoid involvement intravascular or combination of SAPH and portal hypertension is infrequent.

Symptoms	Frequency %
Dyspnea on exertion	85
Cough	36
Chest pain	10
Palpitations	10
Asymptomatic	8

Table 4. Presenting symptoms in Sarcoidosis-associated pulmonary hypertension

4.3. Diagnosis

Patients with SAPH usually present with restrictive dysfunction on pulmonary function tests, and decrease in carbón monoxide diffusion capacity (DLCO) out of proportion to the decrease in total lung capacity (TLC). Forced vital capacity (FVC), forced expiratory volumen in 1 second (FEV1) and DLCO have been reported to be significantly lower in patients with Sarcoidosis and PH when compared with patients without PH [99].La hipoxemia esta frecuentemente presente en los pacientes con SAPH siendo este grupo uno de los que con probabilidad va a requerir oxigeno suplementario y por otra parte recorren menos metros en el 6-minute walking test cuando se comparan con pacientes que tienen Sarcoidosis en el mismo estadio radiológico pero sin PH [99].

Transthoracic echocardiography (TTE) represents a noninvasive screening method to evaluate the presence of PH in sarcoidosis. It is helpful to describe other potential cardiac abnormalities, such as left heart disease, presence of shunts or pericardial effusion, and to evaluate the right heart anatomically and functionally. Echocardiography may be used to estimate the right ventricular systolic pressure (RVSP) if a tricuspid regurgitation jet is present. Echocardiographically estimated RVSP had inadequate positive and negative predictive value in diagnosing PH in advanced lung disease, so it's a screening test that cannot supplant right heart cathetetization (RHC) for the SAPH diagnosis.

RHC is the diagnostic gold standard for SAPH. TTE was unable to detect RVSP in 30% of the patients and 24% of the patients with elevated PAP had a pulmonary capillary wedge pressure (PCWP) in excess of 20 mm Hg, underscoring the importance of left ventricular disease in the pathogenesis of PH in some Sarcoidosis patients. RHC should be performed in all cases in which SAPH is suspected or when echocardiography is suggestive of right heart pathology.

5. Cardiac sarcoidosis

5.1. Epidemiology

The presence of cardiac sarcoidosis is influenced by race. Over 25% of Japanese sarcoidosis patients present cardiac disease, only 5% of patients in the United States and Europe are affected at this level. Although clinical evidence of myocardial involvement is present in 5% of patients, there are autopsy studies that indicate that sublinical cardiac disease is present in 20-30% of cases.

5.2. Clinical manifestations

Cardiac Sarcoidosis can be an incidental finding, has a benign course or being a life-threatening disorder. Clinicians should suspect this disease in young or middle-aged patients with cardiac symptoms and in any patients with a history of sarcoidosis who develop arrhythmias, conduction disturbances or other cardiac symptoms.

Clinical manifestations depend on the location and extent of granulomatous infiltration, being the most common cause of cardiac involvement secondary to infiltration of the myocardium. Usually, cardiac disease appears with any other organ involvement (lung, skin…). The most frequent manifestations of cardiac sarcoidosis are heart failure and arrhythmias, produced in both cases,by the infiltration of the myocardium.

5.3. Cardiac arrhythmias

The most common are ventricular arrhythmias, caused by infiltration of granulomas in the ventricular myocardium causing a focus for abnormal automaticity, or a disruption of ventricular activation and recover [100]. In patients with cardiac sarcoidosis, ventricular arrhythimias and sudden death, due to ventricular tachycardia, are common causes of death. Ventricular tachycardia is one of the most common manifestations of cardiac involvement, being the 24-h ambulatory monitoring the best way to detect them. Supraventricular arrhythmias are infrequent.

5.4. Conduction abnormalities

Caused by the granulomatous infiltration at the atrioventricular node or bundle of His leading to a first degree heart block. Initially, patients are usually asymptomatic but they can progress to complete heart block [101].This can be detected by routine electrocardiography.

5.5. Heart failure

Caused by extensive granulomatous infiltration of the myocardium. May cause impairment of systolic or diastolic function. Diagnostic is difficult and many patients with heart failure due to sarcoidosis disease are diagnostic of idiopathic dilated cardiomyopathy.

5.6. Other clinical manifestations

a. *Valvular dysfunction:* The most frequent is the involvement of the mitral valve caused by diastolic dysfunction and left ventricular dilatation or granulomatous involvement of the papillary muscle [102]. Less common is the tricuspid valve dysfunction.

b. Aorta aneurysm: Although are infrequent, has been described descending thoracic and abdominal aorta aneurysm [103].

c. Cor pulmonale: May occur secondary to pulmonary fibrosis.

6. Gastrointestinal and liver sarcoidosis

6.1. Liver disease

Occurs in 13% of patients with systemic sarcoidosis [104]. Isolated liver involvement is infrequent. In most cases there are no symptoms but can appear hepatosplenomegaly, elevated liver enzymes, cholestasis or portal hypertension. In addition, 60% of patients with liver disease have fever and / or concomitant arthralgia [104].

Although in most cases the granulomas in the liver are small and are located in the portal space, symptoms consistent with chronic cholestasis [105] portal hypertension or Bud-Chiari syndrome can appear [106] Intrahepatic cholestasis can resemble primary biliary cirrhosis or sclerosing cholangitis.

Usually liver function is normal, but the most common abnormality is an elevation of alkaline phosphatase level.

6.2. Gastrointestinal involvement

Affects less than 1% of patients with sarcoidosis, being the stomach the most affected organ of the digestive tract. The symptoms of patients with gastric involvement are inespecific: epigastric pain, heartburn, abdominal discomfort, nausea or vomiting, diarrhea and significant weight loss.

Involvement of the intestine is very infrequent and can occasionally coexist with Crohn's disease [107].

7. Neurosarcoidosis

Neurosarcoidosis is the neurologic manifestation of sarcoidosis, a system granulomatous disease. The most affected organ is the lung, but it can also affect eyes, liver and nervous system. It affects the 5-15% of patients with sarcoidosis. It can be manifested by a wide variety of symptoms: peripheral neuropathy, central symptoms, loss of memory and behavior changes. Psiquiatric manifestations include, but not exclusively, psychosis and delirium, with

20% prevalence in patients with neurosarcoidosis or 1% in those affected with sarcoidosis. The prevalence of neurosarcoidosis is similar to schizophrenia, between 0,50-1,46% of general population. Thus, a study shows that 2 of each 268 patients with a first schizophrenia episode, they had neurosarcoidosis.

Neurologic complications occur in approximately 5 percent of patients with sarcoidosis [108-112]. Neurosarcoidosis is a diagnostic consideration in patients with known sarcoidosis who develop neurologic complaints and in patients presenting de novo with a constellation of findings consistent with the disease [113, 114]. About 50 percent of patients with neurosarcoidosis present with neurologic difficulties at the time of the diagnosis. One-third of those with neurosarcoidosis has or develops more than one neurologic manifestation of their disease.

7.1. Clinical presentation

Any portion of the central or peripheral nervous system can be affected by sarcoidosis. Neuropsychiatric: seizures, amnesia, psychosis and disorientation. Cranial mononeuropathy. Peripheral facial nerve palsy develops in 25 to 50 percent of patients with neurosarcoidosis [111, 114, 115]. The facial nerve palsy can be unilateral or bilateral (simultaneous or sequential) and recurrent. Optic neuropathy and cranial nerve VIII dysfunction can lead to intermittent or progressive visual, auditory, or vestibular dysfunction. Neuroendocrine dysfunction typically occurs with hypothalamic inflammation, resulting in polyuria or disturbances in thirst, sleep, appetite, temperature, or libido. Hypothalamic or pituitary lesions may also cause thyroid, gonadal, or adrenal abnormalities [115, 117]. Polyuria can result from one or more factors in patients with sarcoidosis. Direct hypothalamic involvement can lead to central diabetes insipidus or primary polydipsia, while hyperkalemia (due to production of calcitriol by activated macrophages) can cause nephrogenic diabetes insipidus [117]. Thus, all patients with sarcoidosis and polyuria require a water restriction test to establish the correct diagnosis. Granulomatous inflammation in a perivascular distribution can involve the brain and produce partial or generalized seizures, or a restricted or generalized encephalopathy/vasculopathy [114, 115]. Patients can present with cognitive or behavioral problems and/or focal neurologic deficits referable to the anatomic area involved. In rare cases, this manifests as a focal cerebral infarction [118]. A myelopathy or radiculopathy can occur if granulomatous inflammation affects the spinal cord [114, 115, 119, 120]. The lesions are typically perivascular, they can be extra medullary or intramedullary, and can involve the caudal equine. Communicating or no communicating hydrocephalus may develop acutely or subacutely. Asymptomatic ventricular enlargement may be incidentally detected by imaging studies. Sudden death can rarely result from acute obstruction to CSF flow. Meningeal involvement can take the form of either acute aseptic meningitis or chronic meningitis. Meningeal mass lesions also can develop. Peripheral neuropathic presentations include a mononeuropathy, mononeuritis multiplex, and generalized sensory, small fiber sensory, sensorimotor, autonomic and motor polyneuropathies [122]. The symptoms can be acute, subacute, or chronic; electromyography usually reveals an axonal neuropathy. In addition, an acute generalized demyelinating motor neuropathy similar to the Guillain-Barré syndrome also has been described [123]. Carpal tunnel syndrome appears to be more common among patients with sarcoidosis than the general population [124-126].

Muscle involvement includes asymptomatic microscopic nodules, isolated palpable nodules, an acute or chronic proximal myopathy, and muscle atrophy [127].

In some series of patients affected with intracranial hypertension syndrome, whose manifestation is headache, the diagnosis is neurosarcoidosis. It is uncommon, however, it must be include in differential diagnosis [109].

Patients presenting with neurosarcoidosis may have no systemic features of the disease. In one case series, non-neurologic symptoms were present in less than one-fourth of patients and were most commonly anterior uveitis, cough and dyspnea, renal impairment, rash, and polyarthritis [114].

7.2. Diagnosis

Neurosarcoidosis is a diagnostic consideration in patients with known sarcoidosis who develop neurologic findings, although an intercurrent infection or malignancy must be excluded. Patients who develop a neurologic illness consistent with neurosarcoidosis but are not known to have sarcoidosis present a diagnostic challenge. Table 5 summarizes findings in patients with Neurosarcoidosis.

Findings in patients with Neurosarcoidosis	Frequency (%)
Findings in Chest Rx	24-68%
Cranial mononeuropathy	25-50%
MRI meningeal enhancement	40%
Psychiatric symptoms	20%
Findings in Cerebrospinal fluid	**Frequency (%)**
Elevated total protein	66%
Pleocytosis	50%
Elevated openning pressure	10%

Table 5. Findings in patients with Neurosarcoidosis

a.   Clinical evaluation:

If neurosarcoidosis is suspected, the patient should be evaluated for evidence of extra neural disease because obtaining nerve tissue for diagnostic evaluation is often difficult. Corticosteroids can eliminate evidence of systemic inflammation, and the diagnostic evaluation should be pursued in a rapid fashion while withholding immunosuppressive therapy unless severe illness mandates its use.

The search for extra neural sarcoidosis should include a thorough evaluation of the skin, lymph nodes, and lungs. Other tests that may be useful are:

1.   Ophthalmologic examination

2.   Endoscopic nasal and sinus examination. A chest x-ray or computed tomographic scan of the chest to look for hilar adenopathy or parenchymal changes consistent with pulmonary sarcoidosis. Positive findings suggestive of sarcoidosis on chest imaging have been reported in 24 to 68 percent of individuals who present with neurologic sarcoidosis [114, 115].

3.   Serum angiotensin converting enzyme (ACE) assay, which may be helpful if elevated; however, an elevated serum ACE is not specific for sarcoidosis, and the ACE concentration may not necessarily be elevated if the patient has isolated neurosarcoidosis

4.   In occasional cases, a magnetic resonance, gallium, or fluorodeoxyglucose positron emission tomographic scan, may highlight otherwise occult areas of inflammation that might be amenable to biopsy

b.   Neurodiagnostic testing:

Neurologic evaluation should proceed if no extra neural tissue is available for biopsy. Unfortunately, no neurodiagnostic tests are pathognomonic for neurosarcoidosis. However, neurodiagnostic tests help define the extent of disease and eliminate other diagnostic considerations, particularly infection and malignancy. Furthermore, a presumptive diagnosis of neurosarcoidosis is often made on the basis of MRI and lumbar puncture results in the appropriate clinical setting [128].

c.   Neuroimaging:

The imaging procedure of choice for CNS disease is contrast-enhanced MRI [115, 116, 129]. Meningeal or parenchymal enhancement suggests active inflammation with disruption of the blood brain barrier, and parenchymal or meningeal masses and hydrocephalus are easily identified. Involvement of the optic nerve or other cranial nerves can be documented, and spinal cord and cauda equine inflammation is well seen on targeted images. Multiple parenchymal nodules may actually represent inflammation extending along the Virchow-Robin spaces deep into the brain or spinal cord. In one series of 29 patients with neurosarcoidosis, approximately 40 percent demonstrated meningeal enhancement and/or multiple white matter lesions on MRI [128].

d.   Lumbar puncture:

Cerebrospinal fluid (CSF) abnormalities occur frequently in patients with CNS sarcoidosis [114, 115]: The CSF opening pressure is elevated in approximately 10 percent of patients, and the total protein is increased in two-thirds of patients, typically up to 250 mg/dL. A pleocytosis is present in approximately 50 percent of patients. Glucose can be normal or low, as can be seen in CNS infections or carcinomatous meningitis. A predominantly mononuclear cell pleocytosis is common. The IgG index can be elevated, and oligoclonal bands may be present.

The CSF ACE concentration is occasionally elevated, but reliable normal values are lacking and CSF ACE may also be increased with infection or carcinomatous meningitis.

Caution should be applied in performing a LP in patients with neurosarcoidosis if there is evidence of increased intracranial pressure. A funduscopic examination to exclude papilledema and an MRI to exclude ventricular enlargement, cerebral edema, and a mass lesion should precede LP [130].

e.   Other tests:

Other diagnostic tests, such as electroencephalography, evoked potentials, and angiography, are occasionally indicated to exclude other conditions. Nerve conduction studies (NCS) and electromyography (EMG) can help localize neuromuscular lesions, depending on the clinical syndrome.

Although false-positive reactions to the Kveim-Siltzbach test are reported to be rare; the test has limited utility [114]. The test is not standardized; it is not universally available; and there are concerns regarding the transmission of HIV and hepatitis.

f.   Biopsy:

If the diagnosis remains in doubt, meningeal, brain, or spinal cord biopsy is occasionally indicated. Extra neural tissue biopsy from other clinically affected organs is generally preferable when possible, as it is less risky; skin, lymph node, and lung (trans bronchial) biopsies can be of high yield [114, 115]. Muscle and peripheral nerve biopsy, including an epidermal biopsy with quantitative nerve terminal analysis to document small fiber sensory neuropathy, can all be easily performed for the appropriate syndrome.

8. Cutaneous manifestations of sarcoidosis

Cutaneous lesions of sarcoidosis may present with variety of morphologies [131]. Although not life-threatening, the unsightly skin lesions of sarcoidosis can be emotionally devastating [132]. Given the wide variability of clinical manifestations, it is one of the "great imitators," making it necessary to consider clinical, epidemiological, radiographic, laboratory, and histopathological criteria to make the diagnosis [133]

Skin involvement is common (occurring in 25 to 35 % of patients with sarcoidosis). Cutaneous manifestation of sarcoidosis could be one of the two following: specific lesions, which demonstrate granuloma on biopsy; and nonspecific lesions that do not have granulomas but are inflammatory reactions [134].

Specific lesions are estimated to occur in 9 to 15 percent of patients with sarcoidosis. Although their histopathologic features are similar, the clinical manifestations of specific lesions vary widely [135]. Papules, nodules, plaques, and infiltrated scars are among the most common presentations; other manifestations also occur.

8.1. Specific eruptions

a.   Papular sarcoidosis

Papular sarcoidosis is a common specific cutaneous manifestation of sarcoidosis. Papular sarcoidosis most frequently occurs on the face, with predilection for the eyelids and nasolabial folds. Upon resolution, faintly discolored, occasionally atrophic macules may remain at previous sites of involvement [135, 136].

b. Nodular sarcoidosis

Nodular sarcoidosis is a relatively common form of cutaneous sarcoidosis that results from large collections of sarcoidal granulomas in the dermis or subcutaneous tissue [135]. Nodules tend to be between 1 and 2 cm in diameter and may be single or multiple. On the nose, nodular sarcoidosis can resemble rhinophyma [135, 137]-

c. Maculopapular sarcoidosis

Characteristically, lesions are asymptomatic or pruritic, and consist of slightly infiltrated, slightly hyperpigmented patches studded with slightly raised papules that are often around 1 mm in diameter [136]. Facial skin, especially the periorifial or eyelid area, is the most common site of involvement.

d. Plaque sarcoidosis

Presents with oval or annular, indurated, discrete plaques that are flesh – colored, erythematous, or brown. Frequent site of involvement include the shoulders and arms, back, and buttocks [131].

e. Lupus pernio

Lupus pernio is characterized by violaceous or erythematous indured papules, plaques, or nodules that are primarily distributed on the central face [138]. The alar rim of the nose is often affected. Lupus pernio is more common in women than in men and is associated with chronic disease and extrapulmonary involvement [138, 139]. Without treatment, the lesions progressively increase in thickness, size, and induration, eventually resulting in considerable cosmetic disfigurement.

The presence of lupus pernio appears to be associated with an increased risk for extra cutaneous disease, particularly sarcoidosis involving the respiratory tract [140]. When severe, granulomatous inflammation of the upper respiratory tract can result in airway obstruction [141].

8.2. Non-Specific eruptions

a. Erythema nodosum

Erythema nodosum develops in up to 25 percent of patients with sarcoidosis and is clinically and histologically identical to erythema nodosum secondary to other causes. García Porrúa et al in Spanish study of 106 biopsy proven cases of erythema nodosum, 20 percent of patients had sarcoidosis [142]. Arthritis, lower extremity edema, and low grave fever are the most common systemic symptoms associated with erythema nodosum.

The clinical feature of subcutaneous sarcoidosis can resemble erythema nodosum. Biopsy is useful for distinguishing between these disorders. Biopsy specimens of erythema nodosum lesions show nonspecific septal panniculitis, which neither confirms nor negates the diagnosis of sarcoidosis [143].

b. Löfgren's syndrome

Löfgren's syndrome is an acute presentation of sarcoidosis characterized by the triad of hilar adenopathy, erythema nodosum, and polyarthralgia or arthritis, with or without parenchymal infiltrates or fever [132, 144]. The presence of bilateral hilar adenopathy and erythema nodosum is usually, but no always, caused by acute sarcoidosis. More recently, the definition has been expanded to include patients with hilar adenopathy and periarticular inflammation with or without erythema nodosum [145].

8.3. Management of cutaneous sarcoidosis

a. First line agents:

Formal studies of local therapies for cutaneous sarcoidosis are limited, and the widespread use of topical and intralesional corticosteroids for this disease primarily are based upon clinical experience.

Topical corticosteroids: Superpotent topical corticosteroids are widely used for the treatment of cutaneous sarcoidosis: Clobetasol, halobetasol.

Intralesional Corticosteroids: Generally accepted that intralesional injection of corticosteroids can lead to flattening or resolution of cutaneous lesions: Triamcinolone

b. Seconds line agents

Systematic glucocorticoids (prednisone 20 to 40 mg/day)

Antimalarials: Hydroxychoroquine and chloroquine.

Methotrexate (10 to 25mg/week)

c. Refractory disease:

Patients who fail to respond to conventional first – and second – line therapies may benefit from treatment with infliximab or thalidomide.

9. Sarcoid arthropathy

Arthritis is the most common musculoskeletal manifestation in sarcoidosis [146]. Approximately 25 percent of patients with sarcoidosis have an associated arthropathy [147]. Real incidence is unclear since the diagnosis may be difficult when a patient presents with articular complaints alone; in this setting, the presence of sarcoidosis is established only after more commonly involved organs, such as the eye or lung, become affected [148].

9.1. Acute arthritis

Acute sarcoid arthritis may present in isolation or as part of Lofgren's syndrome (association of arthritis, erythema nodosum and bilateral hilar lymphadenopathy). Joint effusion is discrete [149]. Rheumatoid factor and ANA may be positive, as in the general sarcoidosis [146]. The acute polyarthritis most commonly involves ankles (>90 percent), often bilaterally, followed by other larger joints of lower extremity and may be mistaken for a reactive arthritis. The arthritis is mostly oligoarticular (87%), and involvement is typically symmetrical (76%). Glennas et al, in a prospective study of 189 patients presenting with symptoms suggestive of reactive arthritis, 17 (9%) were eventually diagnosed with acute sarcoid arthritis. Ten had Löfgren's syndrome, and 17 had bilateral ankle involvement [150].

Löfgren's syndrome: The triad of hilar adenopathy, acute polyarthritis and erythema nodosum characterizes Löfgren's syndrome. Löfgren's syndrome is usually self-limiting. Erythema nodosum typically disappears in a few months [144]. Approximately one third of patients have persistent arthritis; rarely, the arthritis symptoms are recurrent. Hilar adenopathy tends to resolve over time up to 90 percent of patients. Erythema nodosum is more often seen in female compared with male patients presenting with Löfgren's syndrome [142].

Sarcoid arthritis can resemble rheumatic fever when the polyarthritis is migratory. It may resemble patients with juvenile idiopathic arthritis in young children presenting with both uveitis and arthritis [151].

9.2. Chronic arthritis

Patients presenting with chronic arthritis are typically older than patients with acute arthritis or Löfgren's syndrome [144]. The ankle, knees, hands, wrist, metacarpophalangeal and proximal interphalangeal joint are the joints most frequently involved; rarely, the sacroiliac and temporomandibular joints may also be affected [144]. Chronic arthritis is frequently associated with parenchymal lung disease and other extrapulmonary manifestations [144].

The correlation between extremely high serum of angiotensin converting enzyme levels and extrathoracic sarcoidosis, including chronic arthritis, probably reflects the high total body load of granulomas.

9.3. Diagnosis

Diagnosis of sarcoid arthropathy is based upon suggestive clinical, imaging, synovial fluid, and, in selected cases, synovial tissue biopsy. Classic Löfgren's syndrome can be diagnosed based upon clinical features alone [132].

9.4. Treatment

Sarcoid arthritis should be treated with nonsteroidal antiinflammatory agents. Corticosteroids and other immunosuppressive drugs as colchicine and hydroxychloroquine should be reserved for refractory cases. Biological therapies such as the anti-TNFa and the anti-CD20 were showed to be effective in some case reports of severe and refractory disease [152].

10. Ocular manifestations in sarcoidosis

The eye or adnexa are affected in 25 to 80% of the sarcoidosis patients. The disease can involve the orbit, lacrimal gland, anterior and posterior segments of the eye [153].

The disease can involve the orbit, lacrimal gland, anterior and posterior segments of the eye. Anterior uveitis is the most common manifestation, occurring in 65% of patients with ophthalmologic involvement [132]. Inflammation can affect the uveal tract leading to glaucoma, cataracts, and blindness. Typical sarcoid uveitis presents with bilateral mutton-fat keratic precipitates, cells, flare, iris nodules, anterior and posterior synechia, and increased ocular pressure. Posterior involvement includes vitreitis, vasculitis, choroidal lesions, and optic neuropathy. Long-term complications are common, and cystoid macular edema is the most important and sight-threatening consequence [153]. Acute uveitis presents with eye redness, cloudy vision, photophobia, and watering or can present asymptomatically (with a "quiet eye").

The gold standard for the diagnosis of sarcoidosis should be obtained with histologic examination. However, an international workshop has recently established diagnostic criteria of "intraocular sarcoidosis" (sarcoidosis uveitis) on the basis of a combination of suggestive ophthalmological findings and laboratory tests, when biopsy is not performed or is negative. More recent techniques such as PET-scan and endoscopic ultrasound-guided fine-needle biopsy of intrathoracic nodes should be assessed in future prospective studies [154].

Chronic anterior uveitis, with insidious symptoms leading to glaucoma and vision loss, is more common than acute anterior uveitis. In about 10 to 15% of patients with uveitis, both the anterior and posterior segments are involved.

Lacrimal gland enlargement can cause dry eyes. Conjunctival follicles, dacryoscystitis, keratoconjunctivitis sicca, and retinal vasculitis also occur. Optic neuritis is an ophthalmologic emergency that requires immediate systemic therapy as it can result in a rapid permanent loss of vision.

Papillitis, papilledema, and neovascularization are seen under funduscopic examination leading to optic atrophy. Other less common manifestations include periphlebitis retinae, retinal hemorrhage, retinitis proliferans, band keratopathy, proptosis, and exophthalmos [155, 156].

Routine evaluation for eye involvement should include a slit-lamp examination and funduscopic examination to evaluate the anterior and posterior uveal tract, respectively [132]. Fluorescence angiography may also be considered if a posterior uveitis is suspected [156].

Oral corticosteroids are the mainstay of treatment of sarcoidosis. Systemic cytotoxic agents like methotrexate, azathioprine, and chlorambucil may be used in refractory cases. The visual prognosis of sarcoidosis is usually good [153].

Patients should be warned that skin atrophy could occur if steroids come into contact with skin surfaces. Intraocular corticosteroid injections can provide the patient with longer control of symptoms. Systemic steroids can be used if uveitis does not resolve with topical therapy or for cases where vision loss is possible. Alternative agents include tacrolimus, methotrexate, and photodynamic therapy [157].

Minocycline may be an option for patients with comorbidities that make steroids a less appealing option [158].

Interferon-alpha is commonly used to treat hepatitis C viral infection and has been reported to induce sarcoidosis and more recently ocular sarcoidosis with granulomatous panuveitis with choroidal granulomas.

In these cases topical steroids were used to treat ocular uveitis with systemic steroids for systemic findings.

Author details

Luis Jara-Palomares, Candela Caballero-Eraso, Cesar Gutiérrez, Alvaro Donate and Jose Antonio Rodríguez-Portal

*Address all correspondence to: luisoneumo@hotmail.com

Pneumologist, Medical-Surgical Unit of Respiratory Diseases. University Hospital Virgen del Rocio. Seville, Spain

References

[1] Polychronopoulos VS, Prakash UB. Airway involvement in sarcoidosis. Chest 2009; 136:1371.

[2] James JC, Simpson CB. Treatment of laryngeal sarcoidosis with CO2 laser and mito-mycin-C. Otolaryngol Head Neck Surg 2004; 130:262.

[3] Fouty BW, Pomeranz M, Thigpen TP, Martin RJ. Dilatation of bronchial stenoses due to sarcoidosis using a flexible fiberoptic bronchoscope. Chest 1994; 106:677.

[4] Baughman RP, Lower EE, Tami T. Upper airway. 4: Sarcoidosis of the upper respira-tory tract (SURT). Thorax 2010; 65:181.

[5] Reed J, deShazo RD, Houle TT, et al. Clinical features of sarcoid rhinosinusitis. Am J Med 2010; 123:856.

[6] Aubart FC, Ouayoun M, Brauner M, et al. Sinonasal involvement in sarcoidosis: a case-control study of 20 patients. Medicine (Baltimore) 2006; 85:365.

[7] Hunninghake GW, Costabel U, Ando M, et al. ATS/ERS/WASOG statement on sar-coidosis: American Thoracic Society/European Respiratory Society/World Associa-

tion of Sarcoidosis and other Granulomatous Disorders. Sarcoidosis Vasc Diffuse Lung Dis 1999; 16:149–173

[8] Rottoli P, Bargagli E, Chidichimo C, et al. Sarcoidosis with upper respiratory tract involvement. Respir Med 2006; 100:253–257

[9] Rizzato G, Palmieri G, Agrati AM, et al. The organ-specific extrapulmonary presentation of sarcoidosis: a frequent occurrence but a challenge to an early diagnosis; a 3-year-long prospective observational study. Sarcoidosis Vasc Diffuse Lung Dis 2004; 21:119–126

[10] Baughman RP, Teirstein AS, Judson MA, et al. Clinical characteristics of patients in a case control study of sarcoidosis. Am J Respir Crit Care Med 2001; 164:1885–1889

[11] Fouty BW, Pomeranz M, Thigpen TP, Martin RJ. Dilatation of bronchial stenoses due to sarcoidosis using a flexible fiberoptic bronchoscope. Chest 1994; 106:677.

[12] Long CM, Smith TL, Loehrl TA, et al. Sinonasal disease in patients with sarcoidosis. Am J Rhinol 2001; 15:211

[13] Black JI. Sarcoidosis of the nose. J Laryngol Otol 1966; 80:1065–1068

[14] Braun JJ, Imperiale A, Schultz P, et al. Pharyngolaryngeal sarcoidosis: report of 12 cases. Otolaryngol Head Neck Surg 2008; 139:463–465

[15] Davis C, Girzadas DV Jr. Laryngeal sarcoidosis causing acute upper airway obstruction. Am J Emerg Med 2008; 26:e111–e113

[16] Becker GL, Tenholder MF, Hunt KK. Obligate mouth breathing during exercise: nasal and laryngeal sarcoidosis. Chest 1990; 98:756–757

[17] Carasso B. Sarcoidosis of the larynx causing airway obstruction. Chest 1974; 65:693–695

[18] Turner GA, Lower EE, Corser BC, et al. Sleep apnea in sarcoidosis. Sarcoidosis Vasc Diffuse Lung Dis 1997; 14: 61–64

[19] Roger G, Gallas D, Tashjian G, et al. Sarcoidosis of the upper respiratory tract in children. Int J Pediatr Otorhinolaryngol 1994; 30:233–240

[20] Bower JS, Belen JE, Weg JG, et al. Manifestations and treatment of laryngeal sarcoidosis. Am Rev Respir Dis 1980; 122:325–332

[21] Israel HL, Sones M. Sarcoidosis: clinical observation on one hundred sixty cases. AMA Arch Intern Med 1958; 102:766–776

[22] Gerencer RZ, Keohane JD Jr, Russell L. Laryngeal sarcoidosis with airway obstruction. J Otolaryngol 1998; 27:90–93.

[23] Fogel TD, Weissberg JB, Dobular K, et al. Radiotherapy in sarcoidosis of the larynx: case report and review of the literature. Laryngoscope 1984; 94:1223–1225

[24] Chijimatsu Y, Tajima J, Washizaki M, et al. Hoarseness as an initial manifestation of sarcoidosis. Chest 1980; 78:779–781

[25] Jaffe R, Bogomolski-Yahalom V, Kramer MR. Vocal cord paralysis as the presenting symptom of sarcoidosis. Respir Med 1994; 88:633–636.

[26] Brandstetter RD, Messina MS, Sprince NL, et al. Tracheal stenosis due to sarcoidosis. Chest 1981; 80:656

[27] Miller A, Brown LK, Teirstein AS. Stenosis of main bronchi mimicking fixed upper airway obstruction in sarcoidosis. Chest 1985; 88:244–248

[28] Harrison BD, Shaylor JM, Stokes TC, et al. Airflow limitation in sarcoidosis: a study of pulmonary function in 107 patients with newly diagnosed disease. Respir Med 1991; 85:59–64

[29] Murray ME, Stokes TC. Endobronchial sarcoidosis presenting as severe upper airways narrowing with normal chest radiograph. Respir Med 1991; 85:425–426

[30] Mendelson DS, Norton K, Cohen BA, et al. Bronchial compression: an unusual manifestation of sarcoidosis. J Comput Assist Tomogr 1983; 7:892–894

[31] Armstrong JR, Radke JR, Kvale PA, et al. Endoscopic findings in sarcoidosis: characteristics and correlations with radiographic staging and bronchial mucosal biopsy yield. Ann Otol Rhinol Laryngol 1981; 90:339–343

[32] Yamada G, Aketa K, Takahashi H, et al. Endobronchial lesions of sarcoidosis. Intern Med 2005; 44:909–910

[33] Olsson T, Bjornstad-Pettersen H, Stjernberg NL. Bronchostenosis due to sarcoidosis: a cause of atelectasis and airway obstruction simulating pulmonary neoplasm and chronic obstructive pulmonary disease. Chest 1979; 75:663–666

[34] Westcott JL, Noehren TH. Bronchial stenosis in chronic sarcoidosis. Chest 1973; 63:893–897

[35] Corsello BF, Lohaus GH, Funahashi A. Endobronchial mass lesion due to sarcoidosis: complete resolution with corticosteroids. Thorax 1983; 38:157–158

[36] Chapman A, Rgyropoulou PK, Patakas DA, Louridas GE. Airway function in stage I and stage II pulmonary sarcoidosis. Respiration 1984; 46:17–25

[37] Dutton RE, Renzi PM, Lopez-Majano V, et al. Airway function in sarcoidosis: smokers versus nonsmokers. Respiration 1982; 43:164–173

[38] Rodriguez E, Lopez D, Buges J, et al. Sarcoidosis-associated bronchiolitis obliterans organizing pneumonia. Arch Intern Med 2001; 161:2148–2149

[39] Carbonelli C, Roggeri A, Cavazza A, et al. Relapsing bronchiolitis obliterans organising pneumonia and chronic sarcoidosis in an atopic asthmatic patient. Monaldi Arch Chest Dis 2008; 69:39–42

[40] Akira M, Kozuka T, Inoue Y, et al. Long-term follow-up CT scan evaluation in patients with pulmonary sarcoidosis. Chest 2005; 127:185–191.

[41] Abehsera M, Valeyre D, Grenier P, et al. Sarcoidosis with pulmonary fibrosis: CT patterns and correlation with pulmonary function. AJR Am J Roentgenol 2000; 174:1751–1757

[42] Rockoff SD, Rohatgi PK. Unusual manifestations of thoracic sarcoidosis. AJR Am J Roentgenol 1985; 144:513–528

[43] Lewis MM, Mortelliti MP, Yeager H Jr, et al. Clinical bronchiectasis complicating pulmonary sarcoidosis: case series of seven patients. Sarcoidosis Vasc Diffuse Lung Dis 2002; 19:154–159

[44] Rubinstein I, Baum GL, Hiss Y, et al. Hemoptysis in sarcoidosis. Eur J Respir Dis 1985; 66:302–305

[45] Rubinstein I, Solomon A, Baum GL, et al. Pulmonary sarcoidosis presenting with unusual roentgenographic manifestations. Eur J Respir Dis 1985; 67:335–340

[46] Wollschlager C, Khan F. Aspergillomas complicating sarcoidosis: a prospective study in 100 patients. Chest 1984; 86:585–588

[47] Marcias S, Ledda MA, Perra R, et al. Aspecific bronchial hyperreactivity in pulmonary sarcoidosis. Sarcoidosis 1994; 11:118–122

[48] Shorr AF, Torrington KG, Hnatiuk OW. Endobronchial involvement and airway hyperreactivity in patients with sarcoidosis. Chest 2001; 120:881–886

[49] Chapman JT, Mehta AC. Bronchoscopy in sarcoidosis: diagnostic and therapeutic interventions. Curr Opin Pulm Med 2003; 9:402–407

[50] Mihailovic -Vucinic V, Jovanovic D. Pulmonary sarcoidosis. Clin Chest Med 2008; 29:459–473

[51] Judson MA. The diagnosis of sarcoidosis. Clin Chest Med 2008; 29:415–427 fsd

[52] Chevalet P, Clément R, Rodat O, et al. Sarcoidosis diagnosed in elderly subjects: retrospective study of 30 cases. Chest 2004; 126:1423.

[53] Soskel NT, Sharma OP. Pleural involvement in sarcoidosis. Curr Opin Pulm Med 2000; 6:455.

[54] Navaneethan SD, Venkatesh S, Shrivastava R, et al. Recurrent pleural and pericardial effusions due to sarcoidosis. PLoS Med 2005; 2:e63.

[55] Huggins JT, Doelken P, Sahn SA, et al. Pleural effusions in a series of 181 outpatients with sarcoidosis. Chest 2006; 129:1599.

[56] Koyama T, Ueda H, Togashi K, et al. Radiologic manifestations of sarcoidosis in various organs. Radiographics 2004; 24:87.

[57] Hours S, Nunes H, Kambouchner M, et al. Pulmonary cavitary sarcoidosis: clinico-radiologic characteristics and natural history of a rare form of sarcoidosis. Medicine (Baltimore) 2008; 87:142.

[58] Müller NL, Kullnig P, Miller RR. The CT findings of pulmonary sarcoidosis: analysis of 25 patients. AJR Am J Roentgenol 1989; 152:1179-1182.

[59] Müller NL, Mawson JB, Mathieson JR, et al. Sarcoidosis: correlation of extent of disease at CT with clinical, functional, and radiographic findings. Radiology 1989; 171:613.

[60] Brauner MW, Grenier P, Mompoint D, Lenoir S, de Crémoux H. Pulmonary sarcoidosis: evaluation with high-resolution CT. Radiology 1989;172(2): 467–471.

[61] Müller NL, Miller RR. Ground-glass attenuation, nodules, alveolitis, and sarcoid granulomas. Radiology 1993;189(1):31–32.

[62] Baughman RP, Winget DB, Bowen EH, Lower EE. Predicting respiratory failure in sarcoidosis patients. Sarcoidosis Vasc Diffuse Lung Dis 1997;14(2): 154–158.

[63] Hamper UM, Fishman EK, Khouri NF, Johns CJ, Wang KP, Siegelman SS. Typical and atypical CT manifestations of pulmonary sarcoidosis. J Comput Assist Tomogr 1986;10(6):928–936.

[64] Criado E, Sánchez M, Ramírez J, Arguis P, de Caralt TM, Perea RJ, Xaubet A. Pulmonary sarcoidosis: typical and atypical manifestations at high-resolution CT with pathologic correlation. Radiographics. 2010 Oct;30(6):1567-86. Review.

[65] Henke CE, Henke G, Elveback LR, Beard CM, Ballard DJ, Kurland LT. The epidemiology of sarcoidosis in Rochester, Minnesota: a population-based study of incidence and survival. Am J Epidemiol 1986;123(5):840–845.

[66] Lynch JP 3rd, Kazerooni EA, Gay SE. Pulmonary sarcoidosis. Clin Chest Med 1997;18(4):755–785.

[67] Winterbauer RH, Belic N, Moores KD. Clinical interpretation of bilateral hilar adenopathy. Ann Intern Med 1973;78(1):65–71.

[68] Gvozdenovic BS, Mihailovic-Vucinic V, Ilic-Dudvarski A, Zugic V, Judson MA. Differences in symptom severity and health status impairment between patients with pulmonary and pulmonary plus extrapulmonary sarcoidosis. Respir Med. 2008 Nov; 102(11):1636-42.

[69] Teirstein AS, Machac J, Almeida O, et al. Results of 188 whole-body fluorodeoxyglucose positron emission tomography scans in 137 patients with sarcoidosis. Chest 2007; 132:1949.

[70] de Prost N, Kerrou K, Sibony M, et al. Fluorine-18 fluorodeoxyglucose with positron emission tomography revealed bone marrow involvement in sarcoidosis patients with anaemia. Respiration 2010; 79:25.

[71] Kaira K, Oriuchi N, Otani Y, et al. Diagnostic usefulness of fluorine-18-alpha-methyl-tyrosine positron emission tomography in combination with 18F-fluorodeoxyglucose in sarcoidosis patients. Chest 2007; 131:1019.

[72] Line BR, Hunninghake GW, Keogh BA, et al. Gallium-67 scanning to stage the alveolitis of sarcoidosis: correlation with clinical studies, pulmonary function studies, and bronchoalveolar lavage. Am Rev Respir Dis 1981; 123:440.

[73] Schoenberger CI, Line BR, Keogh BA, et al. Lung inflammation in sarcoidosis: comparison of serum angiotensin-converting enzyme levels with bronchoalveolar lavage and gallium-67 scanning assessment of the T lymphocyte alveolitis. Thorax 1982; 37:19.

[74] Beaumont D, Herry JY, Sapene M, et al. Gallium-67 in the evaluation of sarcoidosis: correlations with serum angiotensin-converting enzyme and bronchoalveolar lavage. Thorax 1982; 37:11.

[75] Baughman RP, Shipley R, Eisentrout CE. Predictive value of gallium scan, angiotensin-converting enzyme level, and bronchoalveolar lavage in two-year follow-up of pulmonary sarcoidosis. Lung 1987; 165:371.

[76] Braude AC, Chamberlain DW, Rebuck AS. Pulmonary disposition of gallium-67 in humans: concise communication. J Nucl Med 1982; 23:574.

[77] Shorr AF, Helman DL, Lettieri CJ, et al. Depreotide scanning in sarcoidosis: a pilot study. Chest 2004; 126:1337.

[78] Lebtahi R, Crestani B, Belmatoug N, et al. Somatostatin receptor scintigraphy and gallium scintigraphy in patients with sarcoidosis. J Nucl Med 2001; 42:21.

[79] Dunn TL, Watters LC, Hendrix C, et al. Gas exchange at a given degree of volume restriction is different in sarcoidosis and idiopathic pulmonary fibrosis. Am J Med 1988; 85:221.

[80] Winterbauer RH, Lammert J, Selland M, et al. Bronchoalveolar lavage cell populations in the diagnosis of sarcoidosis. Chest 1993; 104:352.

[81] Lin YH, Haslam PL, Turner-Warwick M. Chronic pulmonary sarcoidosis: relationship between lung lavage cell counts, chest radiograph, and results of standard lung function tests. Thorax 1985; 40:501.

[82] Perez RL, Duncan A, Hunter RL, Staton GW Jr. Elevated D dimer in the lungs and blood of patients with sarcoidosis. Chest 1993; 103:1100.

[83] Perez RL, Kimani AP, King TE Jr, et al. Bronchoalveolar lavage fluid D dimer levels are higher and more prevalent in black patients with pulmonary sarcoidosis. Respiration 2007; 74:297.

[84] Keogh BA, Hunninghake GW, Line BR, Crystal RG. The alveolitis of pulmonary sar-
      coidosis. Evaluation of natural history and alveolitis-dependent changes in lung
      function. Am Rev Respir Dis 1983; 128:256.

[85] Takemura T, Hiraga Y, Oomichi M, et al. Ultrastructural features of alveolitis in sar-
      coidosis. Am J Respir Crit Care Med 1995; 152:360.

[86] Myers JL, Tazelaar HD. Challenges in pulmonary fibrosis: 6--Problematic granulom-
      atous lung disease. Thorax 2008; 63:78.

[87] Badesh DB, Champion HC, Sanchez MA et al. Diagnosis and assesment of pulmona-
      ry arterial hypertension. J Am Coll Cardiol 2009; 54(1. Suppl): S55-S66.

[88] Baughman RP, Engel PJ, Meyer CA, Barret AB, Lower EE. Pulmonary hypertension
      in Sarcoidosis. Sarcoidosis Vasc Diffuse Lung Dis 2006; 23: 108-16.

[89] Handa T, Nagai S, Miki S et al. Incidence of pulmonary hypertension and its clinical
      relevance in patients with Sarcoidosis . Chest 2006; 129: 1246

[90] Días-Guzmán E, Farver C, Parambil J, Culver DA. Pulmonary hypertension caused
      by Sarcoidosis. Clin Chest Med 2008; 29 (3): 549-71.

[91] Simonneau G, Robbins JM, Beghetti M et al. Update clinical classification of pulmo-
      nary hypertension. J Am Coll Cardiol 2009; 54: S43-S54

[92] Baughman RP, Engel PJ, Meyer CA, Berret AB, Lower EE. Survival in Sarcoidosis as-
      sociated pulmonary hypertension: the importance of hemodinamyc evaluation.
      Chest 2010;138(5): 1078-85.

[93] Giaid A, Yanagisawa M, Langleben D et al. Expression of endotelin 1 in the lungs of
      patients with pulmonary hypertension. N Eng J Med 1993; 328:1732-39.

[94] Preston IR, Klinger JR, Landzberg MJ, Houtchens J, Nelson D, Hill NS. Vasorespon-
      siveness of Sarcoidosis-associated pulmonary hypertension. Chest 2001; 120:866-72.

[95] Nunes H, Humbert M, Capron F et al. Pulmonary hypertension associated with Sar-
      coidosis: mechanisms, haemodynamics and prognosis. Thorax 2006; 61: 68-74.

[96] Palmero V, Sulica R. Sarcoidosis-associated pulmonary hypertension: assessment
      and management. Semin Respir Crit Care Med 2010; 31: 494-500

[97] Nunes H, Freynet O, Naggara N et al. Cardiac Sarcoidosis. Semin Respir Crit Care
      Med 2010; 31: 428-41.

[98] Sulica R, Teirstein AS, Kakarla S, Nemani N, Behnegar A, Padilla ML. Distinctive
      clinical, radiographic, and functional characteristics of patients with Sarcoidosis-as-
      sociated pulmonary hypertension. Chest 2005;128:1483-89.

[99] Shlobin OA, Nathan D. Management of end-stage Sarcoidosis: pulmonary hyperten-
      sion and lung transplantation . Eur Respi J 2012; 39: 1520-33.

[100] Sekiguchi M, Numao Y, Imai M, et al. Clinical and histopathological profile of sarcoidosis of the heart and acute idiopathic myocarditis. Concepts through a study employing endomyocardial biopsy. I. Sarcoidosis. Jpn Circ J 1980; 44:249

[101] Yoshida Y, Morimoto S, Hiramitsu S, et al. Incidence of cardiac sarcoidosis in Japanese patients with high-degree atrioventricular block. Am Heart J 1997; 134:382.

[102] Sato Y, Matsumoto N, Kunimasa T, et al. Multiple involvements of cardiac sarcoidosis in both left and right ventricles and papillary muscles detected by delayed-enhanced magnetic resonance imaging. Int J Cardiol 2008; 130:288.

[103] Numata S, Kanda K, Hatta T, et al. Sarcoidosis with double saccular abdominal aortic aneurysms. J Vasc Surg 2005; 41:1065.

[104] Mueller S, Boehme MW, Hofmann WJ, Stremmel W. Extrapulmonary sarcoidosis primarily diagnosed in the liver. Scand J Gastroenterol 2000; 35: 1003-1008

[105] Dupas B, Gournay J, Frampas E, Leaute F, Le Borgne J. Anicteric cholestasis: imaging and diagnostic strategy. J Radiol 2006; 87: 441-459

[106] Nataline MR, Goyette RE, Owensby LC, Rubin RN. The Budd-Chiari syndrome in sarcoidosis. JAMA 1978; 239: 2657-2657

[107] Fries W, Grassi SA, Leone L, et al. Association between inflammatory bowel disease and sarcoidosis. Report of two cases and review of the literature. Scand J Gastroenterol 1995; 30:1221.

[108] Burns TM. Neurosarcoidosis. Arch Neurol 2003; 60:1166.

[109] Vargas DL, Stern BJ. Neurosarcoidosis: diagnosis and management. Semin Respir Crit Care Med 2010; 31(4): 419-27.

[110] Titilic M, Bradic-Hammoud M, Miric L, Punda A. Clinical manifestations of neurosarcoidosis. Bratisl Lek Listy 2009; 110(9):576-9.

[111] Stern BJ, Krumholz A, Johns C, et al. Sarcoidosis and its neurological manifestations. Arch Neurol 1985; 42:909.

[112] Joseph FG, Scolding NJ. Sarcoidosis of the nervous system. Pract Neurol 2007; 7:234.

[113] Scott TF. Neurosarcoidosis: progress and clinical aspects. Neurology 1993; 43:8.

[114] Joseph FG, Scolding NJ. Neurosarcoidosis: a study of 30 new cases. J Neurol Neurosurg Psychiatry 2009; 80:297.

[115] Pawate S, Moses H, Sriram S. Presentations and outcomes of neurosarcoidosis: a study of 54 cases. QJM 2009; 102:449.

[116] Bihan H, Christozova V, Dumas JL, et al. Sarcoidosis: clinical, hormonal, and magnetic resonance imaging (MRI) manifestations of hypothalamic-pituitary disease in 9 patients and review of the literature. Medicine (Baltimore) 2007; 86:259.

[117] Stuart CA, Neelon FA, Lebovitz HE. Disordered control of thirst in hypothalamic-pituitary sarcoidosis. N Engl J Med 1980; 303:1078.

[118] Navi BB, DeAngelis LM. Sarcoidosis presenting as brainstem ischemic stroke. Neurology 2009; 72:1021.

[119] Junger SS, Stern BJ, Levine SR, et al. Intramedullary spinal sarcoidosis: clinical and magnetic resonance imaging characteristics. Neurology 1993; 43:333.

[120] Reda HM, Taylor SW, Klein CJ, Boes CJ. A case of sensory ataxia as the presenting manifestation of neurosarcoidosis. Muscle Nerve 2011; 43:900.

[121] Brouwer MC, de Gans J, Willemse RB, van de Beek D. Neurological picture. Sarcoidosis presenting with hydrocephalus. J Neurol Neurosurg Psychiatry 2009; 80:550.

[122] Zuniga G, Ropper AH, Frank J. Sarcoid peripheral neuropathy. Neurology 1991; 41:1558.

[123] Saifee TA, Reilly MM, Ako E, et al. Sarcoidosis presenting as acute inflammatory demyelinating polyradiculoneuropathy. Muscle Nerve 2011; 43:296.

[124] Niemer GW, Bolster MB, Buxbaum L, Judson MA. Carpal tunnel syndrome in sarcoidosis. Sarcoidosis Vasc Diffuse Lung Dis 2001; 18:296.

[125] Nakatani-Enomoto S, Aizawa H, Koyama S, et al. Transient swelling of peripheral nerves in a case of neurosarcoidosis. Intern Med 2004; 43:1078.

[126] Shambaugh GE, Cirksena WJ, Newcomer KL. Carpal tunnel syndrome as manifestation of sarcoidosis. Arch Intern Med 1964; 114:830.

[127] Ando DG, Lynch JP 3rd, Fantone JC 3rd. Sarcoid myopathy with elevated creatine phosphokinase. Am Rev Respir Dis 1985; 131:298.

[128] Zajicek JP, Scolding NJ, Foster O, et al. Central nervous system sarcoidosis--diagnosis and management. QJM 1999; 92:103.

[129] Sherman JL, Stern BJ. Sarcoidosis of the CNS: comparison of unenhanced and enhanced MR images. AJNR Am J Neuroradiol 1990; 11:915.

[130] Scott TF. Cerebral herniation after lumbar puncture in sarcoid meningitis. Clin Neurol Neurosurg 2000; 102:26.

[131] Lodha S, Sanchez M, Prystowsky S. Sarcoidosis of the skin: a review for the pulmonologist. Chest 2009; 136:583.

[132] Iannuzzi MC, Rybicki BA. Sarcoidosis. N Engl J Med 2007; 357: 2153-65

[133] Fernandez Fait E, MacDonnel J. Cutaneous sarcoidosis: differential diagnosis. Clin Dermatol. 2007 May-Jun; 25(3):276-87.

[134] Holmes J, Lazarus A. Sarcoidosis extrathoracic manifestations. Disease a month. Vol 55 (11). Elsevier. Nov 1, 2009

[135] Yanardag H, Pamuk ON, Karayel T. Cutaneous involvement in sarcoidosis: analysis of the features in 170 patients. Respir Med 2003; 97: 978.

[136] Elgart ML, Cutaneous sarcoidosis: definitions and types of lesions. Clin Dermatol 1986; 4:35.

[137] Ben Jennet S, Benmously R, Chaabane S, et al. Cutaneous sarcoidosis through a hospital series of 28 cases. Tunis Med 2008; 86: 447

[138] Dumitrescu SM, Schwartz RA, Baredes S, et al. Mutilating facial sarcoidosis. Dermatology 1999; 199:265.

[139] Young RJ, Gilson RT, Yanase D. Cutaneous sarcoidosis. Int J Dermatol 2001; 40:249.

[140] Yanardag H, Pamuk ON, Pamuk GE. Lupus pernio in sarcoidosis: clinical features and treatment outcomes of 14 patients. J Clin Rheumatolol 2003; 9: 72-6

[141] Cardoso JC, Cravo M, Reis JP, Tellechea O. Cutaneous sarcoidosis: a histophatological study. J Eur Acad Dermatol Venereol 2009; 23:678.

[142] García Porrúa C, Gonzalez–Gay MA, Vázquez–Caruncho M, et al. Erythema nodosum: etiologic and predictive factors in a defined population. Arthritis Rheum 2000; 100:183.

[143] Okamoto H, Mizuno K, Imamura S, et al. Erythema nodosum like eruption in sarcoidosis. Clin Exp Dermatol 1994; 19:507.

[144] Grunewald J, Eklund A. Sex-specific manifestations of Löfgren´s syndrome. Am J Respir Crit Care Med 2007; 175:40.

[145] Grunewald J, Eklund A. Löfgren´s syndrome: human leukocyte antigen strongly influences the disease course. Am J Respir Crit care Med 2009; 179: 307.

[146] Valverde García J, García Gómez C. Sarcoidosis. Medicine 2009, 10 (33): 2192-8

[147] Abril A, Cohen MD. Rheumatologic manifestations of sarcoidosis. Curr Opin Rheumatol 2004; 16:51.

[148] Siltzbach LE, Duberstaein JL. Arthritis in sarcoidosis. Clin Orthop Relat Res 1968; 57:31.

[149] Visser H, Vos K, Zanelli E, et al. Sarcoid arthritis: clinical characteristics, diagnostic aspects, and risk factors. Ann Rheum Dis 2001; 61:499.

[150] Glennas A, Kvien TK, Melby K, et al. Acute sarcoid arthritis: occurrence. Seasonal onset, clinical features and outcome. Br J Rheumatol 1995; 34:45

[151] Shetty AK, Gedalia A. Sarcoidosis: a pediatric prospective. Clin Pediatr 1998; 37:707.

[152] Awada H, Abi–Karam G, Fayad F. Musculoskeletal and other extrapulmonary disorders in sarcoidosis. Best Pract Res Clin Rheumatol 2003; 17: 971.

[153] Bonfioli AA, Orefice F. Sarcoidosis. Sem Ophthalmol. 2005 Jul – Sep; 20 (3): 177-82

[154] Varron L, Abad S, Kodjikian L, Seve P. Sarcoid uveitis: Diagnostic and therapeutic update. Rev Med Interne. 2011 Feb; 32(2): 86 – 92. Epub 2010 Oct 20.

[155] American Thoracic Society: Statement on sarcoidosis. Am J Respir Crit Care Med 1999;160:736-55.

[156] Judson M. Extrapulmonary sarcoidosis. Semin Respir Crit Care Med 2007;28: 83-101

[157] White ES, Lynch JP. Current and emerging strategies for the management of sarcoidosis. Exp Opin Pharmacother 2007;8:1293-311.

[158] Park DJJ, Woog JJ, Pulido JS, et al. Minocycline for the treatment of ocular and ocular adnexal sarcoidosis. Arch Ophthalmol 2007;125:705-9.

Chapter 7

Physiological Manifestation in Pulmonary Sarcoidosis

Kentaro Watanabe

Additional information is available at the end of the chapter

1. Introduction

Sarcoidosis is a granulomatous disease involving multiple organs with unknown cause. More than 90% of patients with sarcoidosis have lung disease [1–3]. However, respiratory function in patients with sarcoidosis often remains normal, even when pulmonary parenchymal involvement is extensive. Not only the lung parenchyma but also the lung airways are involved, which sometimes makes it difficult to evaluate the relationship between functional impairment and morphological/imaging patterns.

Respiratory function impairment in sarcoidosis has not been considered to be a major concern in either clinical or basic research. However, the marked restrictive ventilatory impairment in sarcoidosis with end-stage pulmonary fibrosis is a serious problem in clinical practice.

Obstructive disease is another manifestation of respiratory function impairment in sarcoidosis that is sometimes associated with the end-stage fibrosis of sarcoidosis, with marked reduction of vital capacity and total lung capacity. However, obstructive ventilatory impairment also appears without restrictive disease of sarcoidosis, especially in the early stage of sarcoidosis [4–6].

This chapter will review the functional impairment in patients with pulmonary sarcoidosis, especially restrictive and obstructive ventilatory impairments, taking the histological background into consideration.

2. Restrictive impairment

Restrictive impairment is mainly caused by extensive fibrosis secondary to sarcoid granulomas or by interstitial pneumonia coexistent with pulmonary sarcoidosis.

Histologically, sarcoidosis manifests itself as multiple nodules of nonnecrotizing granulomas consisting of epithelioid histiocytes and multinucleated giant cells with mononuclear inflammatory cells at the periphery of the nodules. Granulomas are usually situated in the interstitium (Figures 1, 2), and sometimes in the air spaces (Figure 3) [7–9], thus forming space-occupying lesions. Granulomas are typically scattered along the lymphatic routes. Peribronchial and perivascular tissues are richly supplied by lymphatics, where granulomas grow larger (Figures 1, 2). The imaging pattern is, therefore, quite characteristic; that is, opacities are situated along the bronchovascular bundles. High-resolution computed tomography (HRCT) describes well multiple nodules located along airways and pulmonary vasculatures and on the pleura, including the interlobar pleura (Figure 4). Sarcoid granulomas may spontaneously regress or become fibrotic (Figure 5).

It is reasonable to hypothesize that restrictive impairment in sarcoidosis depends on the extent of parenchymal involvement of the granulomas, even if they later become fibrotic [10]. Generally, respiratory function worsens with more advanced disease stages, but the radiographic stage does not correlate well with the severity of respiratory function impairment [11].

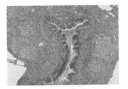

Figure 1. Low-magnification view of pulmonary sarcoidosis in a biopsy specimen. Nodular lesions are situated along the bronchovascular bundles. (Courtesy of Dr. Thomas V. Colby, Mayo Clinic, Arizona, USA.)

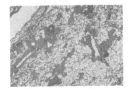

Figure 2. High-magnification view of the specimen shown in Figure 1. Nonnecrotizing epithelioid granulomas surround a bronchiole. (Courtesy of Dr. Thomas V. Colby, Mayo Clinic, Arizona, USA.)

A mild interstitial mononuclear cell infiltration is said to occur occasionally in pulmonary sarcoidosis, but in practice this is rarely seen [12]. However, some investigators have paid attention to coexistent interstitial pneumonia in patients with sarcoidosis. Interstitial pneumonia or secondary fibrosis in end-stage sarcoidosis may play a more important role in the restrictive impairment of sarcoidosis. Rosen et al. examined interstitial pneumonia in patients with sarcoidosis [13]. They found that the incidence of interstitial pneumonia decreases as the density of parenchymal granulomas increases, and that interstitial pneumonia is significantly more prevalent in patients with sarcoidosis of stage I than stages 2 or 3. They concluded that sarcoid granulomas are preceded by lymphocytic infiltration or that interstitial pneumonia typically occurs in the early stage of sarcoidosis.

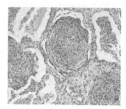

Figure 3. An epithelioid cell granuloma located in the peripheral airway. Another granuloma is embedded in the interstitium in the right lower quadrant (69-year-old woman).

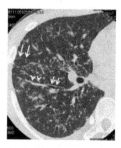

Figure 4. Chest CT scan of a 28-year-old man with pulmonary sarcoidosis. Small nodules are found along the bronchial wall (short arrows) and pulmonary artery (arrowheads). Nodules are also found on the pleural surface, including the interlobar pleura (long arrows).

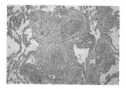

Figure 5. Nonnecrotizing epithelioid granulomas with giant cells are surrounded by concentric layers of fibrotic bundles.

Here, we present a 49-year-old woman with a nine-year history of progressive pulmonary sarcoidosis with stages from early cellular interstitial pneumonia to late fibrotic interstitial pneumonia. She underwent transbronchial lung biopsy at 40 years of age, when she noticed dyspnea and cough. Chest radiograph revealed bilateral diffuse ground-glass shadows and CT revealed ground-glass opacities along the bronchovascular bundles. The imaging features appeared like nonspecific interstitial pneumonia (Figures 6a and b). A transbronchial lung biopsy specimen collected at that time showed cellular interstitial pneumonia and focal aggregates of epithelioid cells with giant cells, which is compatible with sarcoidosis (Figures 6c and d). But for the sarcoid granulomas, the histological features would be similar to those of cellular pattern of nonspecific interstitial pneumonia, a subset of idiopathic interstitial pneumonias [14]. The ground-glass opacities on chest CT were attributable to the infiltration of mononuclear cells in the alveolar septa. At that stage, restrictive impairment and gas exchange impairment were prominent (Table 1). The pathophysiological mechanisms under-lying the functional impairment described in Figures 6c and 6d are probably similar to those of the cellular interstitial pneumonias described above. In contrast to the decrease in DLco, DLco/VA was normal. The decrease in DLco observed in the patient can be mainly attributed to diffusion impairment caused by thickened alveolar septa.

At the later stage, the ground-glass opacities disappeared and traction bronchiectasis became the main imaging finding (Figures 6e and 6f), although outer-zone-dominant honeycombing at both lung bases, which is the hallmark of usual interstitial pneumonia (UIP), was absent. Restrictive impairment progressed during the 8.6 years of follow-up, but the annual decrease in FVC was gradual (Table 2 and Figure 6g).

To summarize the disease of this woman, ground-glass opacities at the initial stage were replaced by traction bronchiectasis in the course of 8.6 years of follow-up. It is probable that cellular interstitial pneumonia associated with pulmonary sarcoidosis progressed to fibrosing interstitial pneumonia with gradual decrease in FVC. However, the pulmonary fibrosis in this case did not look like idiopathic pulmonary fibrosis (IPF).

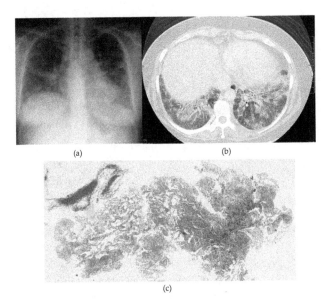

(a)   (b)

(c)

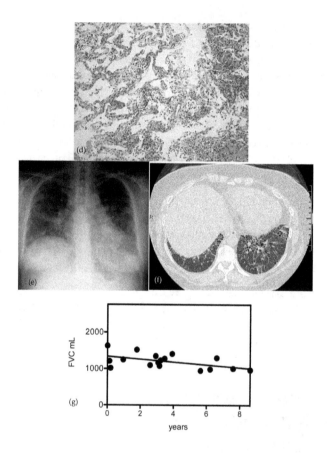

Figure 6. Chest radiograph (a) of a woman with sarcoidosis showing diffuse ground-glass opacities in the bilateral lung fields. Chest CT (b) of the same woman showing ground-glass opacities mainly along the bronchovascular bundles. (c) A transbronchial lung biopsy specimen obtained from the same woman. Alveolar septa are thickened. Granulomas are sparsely found. (d) A high-magnification view of Figure 6c. Alveolar septa are thickened with mononuclear cell infiltration. Small foci of epithelioid granulomas are found on the right side of the specimen. Thickened alveolar septa may be the barrier to gas exchange. Chest radiograph (e) and CT (f) of the woman with sarcoidosis, which were taken 7.1 years after the first CT (Figure b). Ground-glass opacities disappeared, but many bronchi were densely concentrated in the left lung base, forming traction bronchiectasis. (g) Yearly decline of FVC in the course of the 8.6 years of follow-up of advanced pulmonary sarcoidosis. The annual decline of FVC calculated using linear regression was 38 mL (2.9% of the initial FVC at year 0), which is far milder than that observed in IPF. The top of the vertical axis shows the 100% level for FVC as predicted for the patient at year 0.

Restrictive impairment and gas exchange impairment are serious presentations in advanced sarcoidosis, as is the case in IPF. However, honeycomb-like cysts, which are the imaging hallmark of IPF/UIP, are atypical radiographic manifestations in sarcoidosis [11]. Moreover, the most important diagnostic feature in sarcoidosis is the prognosis or the slope of the deterioration of respiratory functions, as seen in Figure 6g. Nardi et al. reported that the 10-year survival of patients with stage IV sarcoidosis was 84.1%, which is far better than that of IPF [15].

FVC mL (% pred)	1210 mL (44%)
FEV₁ mL (% pred)	870 mL (36%)
FEV/FVC %	71%
TLC mL (% pred)	2510 mL (68%)
FRC mL (% pred)	1160mL (53%)
RV mL (% pred)	810mL (70%)
DLco mL/min/mmHg (% pred)	11.3 (54%)
DLco/VA mL/min/mmHg/L (%pred)	5.49 (103%)

FVC: forced vital capacity; FEV1: forced expiratory volume in 1 second; TLC: total lung capacity; FRC: functional reserve capacity; RV: reserve volumeDLco: diffusing capacity of carbon monoxide; DLco/V$_A$: diffusing capacity of carbon monoxide/alveolar volume

Table 1. Respiratory function data for a 40-year-old woman with sarcoidosis

FVC mL (% pred)	970 mL (38%)
FEV₁ mL (% pred)	800 mL (37%)
FEV/FVC %	82%

Table 2. Spirometry 8.6 years after the first measurement (Table 1)

In contrast to patients with sarcoidosis associated with interstitial pneumonia, functional impairment in patients with sarcoidosis without interstitial pneumonia may be less extensive, if present. We frequently encounter patients with sarcoidosis who have extensive imaging findings, but almost normal respiratory function. Such differences in functional impairment raise the possibility that interstitial pneumonia could be independently coexistent with pulmonary sarcoidosis [16], although the histological findings in which sarcoid granulomas are embedded in cellular interstitial pneumonia, as shown in Figures 6c and d, suggest that interstitial pneumonia is one of the fundamental histological manifestations of sarcoidosis.

Shigemitsu et al. reviewed the microscopic slides of explanted lungs to examine chronic interstitial pneumonia (interstitial infiltration by lymphocytes and/or plasma cells) in seven patients with end-stage sarcoidosis who ultimately underwent lung transplantation [17]. In their report, four of the seven patients had diffuse interstitial pneumonia, which was atypical of end-stage sarcoidosis, and two of these four patients had a pattern that was indistinguishable from the UIP pattern, with fibroblastic foci. Furthermore, these four patients had undergone lung transplantation with a shorter time to transplant than the remaining three patients without interstitial pneumonia. These results raise the possibility that there is a subset of patients with sarcoidosis that progresses to pulmonary fibrosis resembling IPF/UIP with poorer prognosis [18].

Stage IV sarcoidosis might encompass two subsets of end-stage sarcoidosis, as described above: sarcoid granuloma-derived secondary fibrosis and fibrosing interstitial pneumonia, which is not secondary but coexistent, although it may be rare.

3. Obstructive impairment

1. Obstructive impairment as a minor component of functional impairment?

Although sarcoidosis involving thoracic lymph nodes and pulmonary parenchyma is familiar to most pulmonologists, airway involvement is often overlooked [19]. Airway dysfunction is an important component of the disease, but is often ignored when the interstitial disease is dominant.

As sarcoidosis commonly affects the pulmonary parenchyma, one could often misunderstand that airways are less commonly involved and restrictive impairment occurs more frequently than does obstructive impairment. However, airway involvement, as judged based on clinical features, physiological testing, imaging techniques, bronchoscopy, and airway mucosal biopsy, has been observed in two-thirds of patients with sarcoidosis [19]. According to a case–control etiologic study of sarcoidosis consisting of 736 patients [3], the majority of patients (477/736) had normal FVC defined as > 80% of FVC, in contrast to a smaller percentage of normal FEV1/FVC% defined as > 80% of FEV1/FVC% (340/736). As described above, clinicians should notice that airflow obstruction is more frequently encountered than is restrictive impairment and is the commonest physiological abnormality in patients with sarcoidosis in clinical practice.

Airway sarcoidosis occurring over the entire length of the respiratory tract – from the upper airway to the lower airway, including the respiratory bronchioles – causes a broad spectrum of airway dysfunction or obstructive ventilatory impairment [20]. In addition, airway sarcoidosis causing obstructive impairment and lung parenchymal sarcoidosis causing restrictive impairment could modify their physiological manifestations mutually.

As airway obstruction in sarcoidosis is reported to be associated with increased morbidity and increased mortality risk [21, 22], obstructive impairment, as well as restrictive impairment, should be checked carefully in the routine follow-up.

2. Upper-airway sarcoidosis

In this section, the trachea is conveniently included in the upper airway. The nose, sinuses, oropharynx, supraglottic structures, larynx, and trachea are less frequently affected with sarcoidosis than is the lower airway [1, 2, 19, 20, 23]. The presenting symptoms of laryngeal sarcoidosis are dysphagia, hoarseness, dyspnea, stridor, and cough [20, 23]. Hoarseness can occur from the granulomatous lymphadenopathy in the mediastinum compressing recurrent nerve or from polyneuropathy by granulomatous inflammation of the vagus nerve [24–26]. Sometimes, these may cause respiratory distress, requiring tracheostomy.

Obstructive sleep apnea syndrome occurs with increased frequency in patients with laryngeal sarcoidosis. Turner et al. reported that 14 of 83 consecutive patients with sarcoidosis (17%) had sleep apnea, which was significantly more frequent than that observed in the general population [27]. It may be secondary to laryngeal sarcoidosis, or may result from obesity associated with the long-term administration of corticosteroids.

Tracheal stenosis and dystonia are the primary manifestations of tracheal sarcoidosis, although tracheal involvement is rare compared with sarcoidosis of lobar or segmental bronchi. Cough is the main symptom.

The flow-volume curve is quite characteristic. Sarcoid lesions located in the upper airway cause flattening of the inspiratory and/or expiratory loops of the flow-volume curve, although this is not specific to sarcoidosis. In general, fixed airway stenosis caused by upper-airway sarcoidosis, regardless of whether it is extrathoracic or intrathoracic, induces flattening of both the inspiratory and expiratory loops. Variable extrathoracic or intrathoracic stenosis induces flattening of the inspiratory and expiratory loops of the flow-volume curve, respectively [28, 29] (Figures 7a–d).

3.   Lower-airway sarcoidosis

As described above, the lower airways are also affected, similarly to the lung parenchyma. As granulomatous lesions also occur in the bronchial mucosa and submucosa [30], endoscopic examination frequently identifies these submucosal lesions. Endoscopic examination also identifies indirect findings derived from peribronchial lesions, such as extrinsic bronchial compression by enlarged lymph nodes. The morphological characteristics of airway involvement include bronchial stenosis, mucosal nodularity, hypervascularity, and mucosal edema (Figures 8a–d) [19, 20, 23, 31–33]. Some investigators have emphasized the mucosal vessels that run perpendicular to cartilaginous rings as an early manifestation of sarcoidosis (Figure 8c) [31, 32, 34].

Bronchial mucosal biopsy confirms the histological diagnosis (Figure 9). These lesions can lead to respiratory symptoms and signs, such as cough and wheezes in auscultation, which are often misdiagnosed as asthma.

Lower-airway involvement in sarcoidosis may lead to airflow limitation (Figure 10, Table 3). However, bronchial mucosal findings in fiberoptic bronchoscopy are not always correlated with the severity of airflow limitation, because airflow limitation is due not only to proximal airway lesions but also to distal airway lesions that are not visible using conventional fiberoptic bronchoscopy. According to the report of Stjernberg et al., an obstructive spirometry pattern was found in only three patients among 21 patients with bronchial sarcoidosis that was confirmed by bronchoscopy [5].

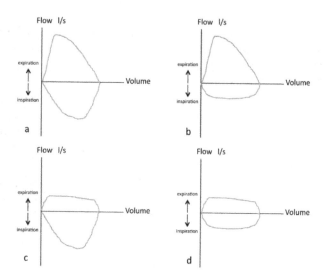

Figure 7. a) Normal flow-volume curve, b) Variable extrathoracic stenosis, c)Variable intrathoracic stenosis, d)Fixed extrathoracic or intrathoracic stenosis.

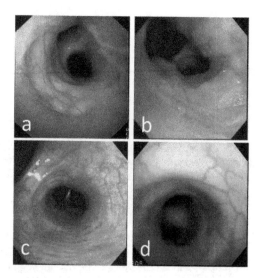

Figure 8. Endoscopic findings of bronchial sarcoidosis. a) Flattened and pale-colored plaques arising from the bronchial mucosa, forming a "cobblestone appearance" (right main bronchus, 38-year-old woman), b) Bronchial lumen is crowded by pale-colored multiple nodules (left upper lobe bronchus, 61-year-old woman), c) Mucosal hypervascularity with vessels running perpendicular to cartilaginous rings (left lingular bronchus, 38-year-old man), d) Network formation of mucosal vessels in the left main bronchus, and mucosal edema of the left second carina (29-year-old man).

Airflow obstruction is reported in 4–63% of patients with sarcoidosis, depending on the spirometry criteria used by different authors [3, 5, 6, 10, 22, 35–40]. Sharma et al. reported that airway obstruction defined as less than 75% of FEV1/FVC was found in 63% of black American nonsmoking patients with sarcoidosis [37]. Airflow obstruction defined as less than 70% of FEV1/FVC, the criterion for COPD, occurs in 9–14% of patients with sarcoidosis [3, 39]. We demonstrated that 21% of patients with sarcoidosis (12/56) had airflow obstruction, which was defined as less than 70% of FEV1/FVC, obtained at least once in repeated spirometry during the entire follow-up period [41].

Airflow obstruction is often associated with an advanced stage of sarcoidosis or decreased VC and FVC [39], but occurs without any relationship to radiographic stage or restrictive impairment [6, 37]. Small airway dysfunction is common in early sarcoidosis without restrictive defects [4–6]. The previous investigations described above tell us that airflow obstruction occurs in all stages of sarcoidosis and should always be looked for in patients with sarcoidosis who have respiratory symptoms [38].

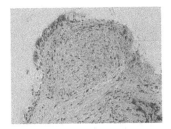

Figure 9. An epithelioid cell granuloma obtained using bronchial mucosal biopsy.

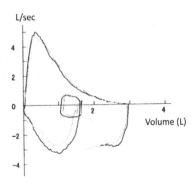

Figure 10. Flow-volume curve of a 61-year-old woman with bronchial sarcoidosis. Her mucosal finding under bronchoscopy is shown in Figure 10b. She never smoked and the expiratory flow is reduced, with a downward convex, as observed bronchial asthma. However, FEV1 did not significantly improve after the inhalation of a β-2 agonist (thick line: basal flow-volume curve; thin line: flow-volume curve after inhalation of salbutamol).

FVC mL (% pred)	3150 mL (120%)
FEV₁ mL (% pred)	1990 mL (94%)
FEV/FVC %	63%
TLC mL (% pred)	4540 mL (115%)
FRC mL (% pred)	2710 mL (105%)
RV mL (% pred)	1240 mL (81%)
DLco mL/min/mmHg (% pred)	21.3 (137%)
DLco/VA mL/min/mmHg/L (%pred)	5.63 (121%)

FVC: forced vital capacity; FEV1: forced expiratory volunme in 1 second; TLC: total lung capacity; FRC: functional reserve capacity; RV: reserve volume; DLco: diffusing capacity of carbon monoxide; DLco/V$_A$: diffusing capacity of carbon monoxide/alveolar volume

Table 3. Respiratory function data for a 61-year-old woman with sarcoidosis

As described above, airflow obstruction is frequently encountered in sarcoidosis. Lavergne et al. demonstrated that airway obstruction by sarcoid granulomas in the bronchial mucosa that were histologically confirmed via endobronchial biopsy was partially or completely reversed by steroid treatment, with improved pulmonary symptoms [21]. However, airflow obstruction in sarcoidosis is often refractory to inhaled steroid or bronchodilator therapy in clinical practice [20, 23, 38, 39, 41]. This presentation is not likely to be caused by coexistent asthma or COPD, because of its poor response to inhaled steroids and/or β-agonists. At what level of the airways does airflow obstruction occur?

Airways with endobronchial lesions that are visible on fiberoptic bronchoscopy are not the only airways that are responsible for airflow obstruction. Small airways or the lung parenchyma may also be involved in airflow obstruction. In general, the extent of decreased attenuation with a mosaic pattern is related to small airway disease, whereas a reticular pattern is considered to be a typical pattern of pulmonary fibrosis on CT. Air trapping, which presents as decreased attenuation exaggerated at expiratory CT, is a common feature of sarcoidosis, and there have been reports examining the correlation between air trapping and airflow obstruction [42, 43]. However, Hansell et al. reported that airflow obstruction is more closely related to a reticular pattern than to the extent of decreased attenuation on expiratory CT [44]. It is possible that progression to fibrosis of granulomatous inflammation adjacent to the small airways is critically associated with airflow obstruction.

4. Treatment of obstructive impairment

As described above, obstructive impairment appears at an early stage of sarcoidosis and also with advancing radiographic stage. The efficacy of treatment may depend on the anatomical sites of sarcoid granulomas, associated fibrosis, and severity of the symptoms.

Upper-airway or tracheal sarcoidosis with airway stenosis needs systemic corticosteroids. In some cases, methotrexate or cytotoxic drugs, such as azathiopurine, may be added. Laryngeal sarcoidosis may cause life-threatening upper-airway obstruction. Surgical intervention is indicated for patients with well-localized, life-threatening lesions. When stridor is present, emergent tracheostomy may be needed [20, 45].

As the symptoms of bronchial sarcoidosis are, if present, cough and wheezing, and spirometry shows reduced rate of FEV1/FVC, which is misdiagnosed as asthma, inhaled β2-agonists and/ or corticosteroids are often administered. However, we have often experienced unfavorable results in such cases, especially when parenchymal lesions are associated with the condition.

As described above, Lavergne et al. [21] examined the effect of systemic steroid therapy for patients who had histologically proven bronchial sarcoidosis with airflow obstruction (< 70% of FEV1/FVC), but their radiographic stages were 1 to 3. They obtained a favorable result after administration of 0.6 mg/kg of oral corticosteroids initially, and concluded that airflow obstruction by bronchial sarcoidosis without fibrosis-related airway obstruction is treatable.

5. Airway hyperreactivity

The prevalence of airway hyperreactivity, as demonstrated by a positive methacholine or histamine challenge test, is significantly higher in patients with sarcoidosis compared with normal controls [46–49]. It is unclear whether airway hyperreactivity is a physiological manifestation of endobronchial sarcoidosis or is due to concomitant asthma [20]. However, Wilsher et al. examined the prevalence of asthma in patients with sarcoidosis and demonstrated that it was the same as that observed in the normal population [50]. Airway hyperreactivity in sarcoidosis and asthma can be distinguished by the response to inhaled corticosteroids and β2-agonists. Airway hyperreactivity associated with asthma is improved by these agents, whereas airway hyperreactivity caused by sarcoidosis requires oral corticosteroids [20, 47, 48].

6. Pulmonary hypertension

Pulmonary hypertension (PH) occurs in 1–28% of patients with sarcoidosis [51–53]. PH is a serious complication in advanced stage VI sarcoidosis and has a poor prognosis. PH is largely attributed to the destruction of the capillary bed by pulmonary fibrosis. As the severity of PH does not always correlate with parenchymal changes, other factors may contribute to the development of PH, such as specific vasculopathy, local increased vasoreactivity, mechanical compression of pulmonary vessels, and portopulmonary hypertension.

According to the Dana Point Classification of 2008 [54], PH in sarcoidosis falls under category 3 (PH owing to lung disease and/or hypoxia) or 5 (PH with unclear multifactorial mechanisms) [53].

There is no specific therapy for PH associated with sarcoidosis. The management of sarcoidosis with PH mainly relies on supportive therapy (supplemental O_2 and diuretics, as needed) [52]. Lung transplantation is now an important therapeutic option for these patients [53].

Patients with "out of proportion" pulmonary hypertension (characterized by dyspnea insufficiently explained by lung mechanical disturbances and mean pulmonary artery pressure $\geq$ 40–45 mmHg at rest) should be referred to expert centers and enrolled in clinical trials of pulmonary artery hypertension-specific drugs [55]. Endothelin receptor antagonists, phosphodiesterase type 5 inhibitors, and intravenous epoprosterol, etc., have been tried, and some patients experienced a beneficial effect. However, large-scale prospective clinical trials are needed before these therapies can be universally adopted.

Author details

Kentaro Watanabe

Address all correspondence to: watanabe@fukuoka-u.ac.jp

Department of Respiratory Medicine, Fukuoka University School of Medicine, Fukuoka, Japan

References

[1] Hunninghake GW, Costabel U, Ando M, et al. ATS/ERS/WASOG Statement on Sarcoidosis. Sarcoidosis Vasc Diffuse Lung Dis 1999; 16: 149-173.

[2] Hunninghake GW, Costabel U, Ando M, et al. Statement on Sarcoidosis. Am J Respir Crit Care Med 1999; 160: 736-755.

[3] Baughman RP, Teirstein AS, Judson MA, et al. Clinical characteristics in a case control study of sarcoidosis. Am J Respir Crit Care Med 2001; 164(10 Pt 1): 1885-1889.

[4] Dines D and Stubbs SE. Obstructive disease of the airways associated with stage I sarcoidosis. Mayo Clin Proc 1978; 53: 788-791.

[5] Stjernberg N and Thunell M. Pulmonary function in patients with endobronchial sarcoidosis. Acta Med Scand 1984; 215:121-126.

[6] Argyropoulou PK, Patakas DA, Louridas GE. Airway function in stage I and stage II pulmonary sarcoidosis. Respiration 1984; 46: 17-25.

[7] Shigematsu N, Emori K, Matsuba K, et al. Clinicopathologic characteristics of pulmonary acinar sarcoidosis. Chest 1978; 73: 186-188.

[8] Harada T, Nabeshima K, Matsumoto T, et al. Histological findings of the computed tomography halo in pulmonary sarcoidosis. Eur Respir J 2009; 34: 281-283.

[9] Katzenstein AA. Katzenstein and Askin's Surgical pathology of non-neoplastic lung disease, 4th ed. Philadelphia: Elsevier Saunders; 2006, p196-206.

[10] Bergin CJ, Bell DY, Coblentz CL, et al. Sarcoidosis: Correlation of pulmonary paren-chymal pattern at CT with results of pulmonary function tests. Radiology 1989; 171: 619-624.

[11] Criado E, Sanchez M, Ramirez J, et al. Pulmonary sarcoidosis: Typical and atypical manifestations at high-resolution CT with pathologic correlation. Radiographics 2010; 30: 1567-1586.

[12] Leslie KO and Wick MR., editors. Practical pulmonary pathology. A diagnostic ap-proach, 2nd ed. Philadelphia: Elsevier Saunders; 2011, p250-252.

[13] Rosen Y, Athanassiades TJ, Moon S, et al. Nongranulomatous interstitial pneumoni-tis in sarcoidosis. Relationship to development of epithelioid granulomas. Chest 1978; 74: 122-125.

[14] American Thoracic Society/European Respiratory Society international multidiscipli-nary consensus classification of the idiopathic interstitial pneumonias. Am J Respir Crit Care Med 2002; 165: 277-304.

[15] Nardi A, Brillet P-Y, Letoumelin P, et al. Stage IV sarcoidosis: comparison of survival with the general population and causes of death. Eur Respir J 2011; 38: 1368-1373.

[16] Matsui Y, Akagawa S, Masuda K, et al. Nine cases of pulmonary sarcoidosis predom-inantly affecting the lower lung fields. Nihon Kokyuki Gakkai Zasshi 2010; 48:883-891.

[17] Shigemitsu H, Oblad JM, Sharma OP, et al., Chronic interstitial pneumonitis in end-stage sarcoidosis. Eur Respir J 2010; 35: 695-697.

[18] Shigemitsu H, Arata A. Sarcoidosis and interstitial pulmonary fibrosis; two distinct disorders or two ends of the same spectrum. Curr Opin Pulm Med 2011; 17: 303-307.

[19] Polychronopoulos VS, Prakash UBS. Airway involvement in sarcoidosis. Chest 2009; 136: 1371-1380.

[20] Morgenthau AS, Teirstein AS. Sarcoidosis of the upper and lower airways. Expert Rev Respir Med 2011; 5: 823-833.

[21] Lavergne F, Clerici C, Sadoun D, et al. Airway obstruction in bronchial sarcoidosis. Outcome with treatment. Chest 1999; 116:1194-1199.

[22] Viskum K, Vestbo J. Vital prognosis in intrathoracic sarcoidosis with special refer-ence to pulmonary function and radiological stage. Eur Respir J 1993; 6: 349-353.

[23] Baughman RP, Lower EE, Gibson K. Pulmonary manifestation of sarcoidosis. Presse Med 2012; 41: e289-e302.

[24] Chijimatsu Y, Tajima J, Washizaki M, et al. Hoarseness as an initial manifestation of sarcoidosis. Chest 1980; 78:779-781.

[25] Jaffe R, Bogomolski-Yahalom V, Kramer MR. Vocal cord aralysis as the presenting symptom of sarcoidosis. Respir Med 1994; 88: 633-636.

[26] Hughes P, McGavin C. Recurrent laryngeal palsy and mediastinal lymphadenopathy. Respir Med 1995; 89 :584-585.

[27] Turner GA, Lower EE, Corser BC, et al. Sleep apnea in sarcoidosis. Sarcoidosis Vasc Diffuse Lung Dis 1997; 14: 61-64.

[28] Miller RD, Hyatt RE. Evaluation of obstructing lesions of the trachea and larynx by flow-volume loops. Am Rev Respir Dis 1973; 108: 475-481.

[29] Kryger M, Bode F, Antic R, et al. Diagnosis of obstruction of the upper and central airways. Am J Med 1976; 61: 85-93.

[30] Chambellan A, Turbie P, Nunes H, et al. Endoluminal stenosis of proximal bronchi in sarcoidosis. Bronchoscopy, function, and evolution. Chest 2005; 127: 472-481.

[31] Friedman OH, Blaugrund SM, Siltzbach LE. Biopsy of the bronchial wall as an aid in diagnosis of sarcoidosis. JAMA 1963; 183: 120-124.

[32] Armstrong JR, Radke JR, Kvale PA, et al. Endoscopic findings in sarcoidosis. Characteristics and correlations with radiographic staging and bronchial mucosal biopsy yield. Ann Otol Rhinol Iaryngol 1981; 90: 339-343.

[33] Chapman JT, Mehta AC. Bronchoscopy in sarcodosis: diagnostic and therapeutic interventions. Curr Opin Pulm Med 2003; 9: 402-407.

[34] Huzly A. Atlas der Bronchoscopie. Stuttgart: Georg Thieme Verlag; 1960.

[35] Loddenkemper R, Kloppenborg A, Schoenfeld N, et al. Clinical findings in 715 patients with newly detected pulmonary sarcoidosis – Results of a cooperative study in former West Germany and Switzerland. Sarcoidosis Vasc Diffuse Lung Dis 1998; 15: 178-182.

[36] Levinson RS, Metzger LF, Stanley NN, et al. Airway function in sarcoidosis. Am J Med 1977; 62: 51-59.

[37] Sharma OP, Johnson R. Airway obstruction in sarcoidosis. A study of 123 nonsmoking black American patients with sarcoidosis. Chest 1988; 94: 343-346.

[38] Harrison BD, Shaylor JM, Stokes TC, et al. Airflow limitation in sarcoidosis – a study of pulmonary function in 107 patients with newly diagnosed disease. Respir Med 1991; 85: 59-64.

[39] Handa T, Nagai S, Fushimi Y, et al. Clinical and radiographic indices associated with airflow limitation in patients with sarcoidosis. Chest 2006; 130: 1851-1856.

[40] Naccache J-M, Laveole A, Nunes H, et al. High-resolution computed tomographic imaging of airways in sarcoidosis patients with airflow obstruction. J Comput Assist Tomogr 2008; 32: 905-912.

[41] Hirano R, Matsumoto T, Kodama M, et al. Obstructive impairment in sarcoidosis. Jpn J Sarcoidosis other Granulomatous Disorders 2011; 31(suppl.): 39.

[42] Davies CW, Tasker AD, Padley SP, et al. Air trapping in sarcoidosis on computed tomography: correlation with lung function. Clin Radiol 2000; 55: 217-221.

[43] Fazzi P, Sbragia P, Solfanelli S, et al. Functional significance of the decreased attenuation sign on expiratory CT in pulmonary sarcoidosis. Report of four cases. Chest 2001; 119: 1270-1274.

[44] Hansell DM, Milne DG, Wilsher ML, et al. Pulmonary sarcoidosis: Morphologic associations of airflow obstruction at thin-section CT. Radiology 1998; 209:697-704.

[45] Baughman RP, Lower EE, Tami T. Upper airway. 4: Sarcoidosis of the upper respiratory tract (SURT). Thorax 2010; 65: 181-186.

[46] Bechtel JJ, Starr T 3rd, Dantzker DR, et al. Airway hyperreactivity in patients with sarcoidosis. Am Rev Respir Dis 1981; 124: 759-761.

[47] Shorr AF, Torrington KG, Hnatiuk OW. Endobronchial involvement and airway hyperreactivity in patients with sarcoidosis. Chest 2001; 120: 881-886.

[48] Laohaburanakit P, Chan A. Obstructive sarcoidosis. Clin Rev Allergy Immunol 2003; 25: 115-129.

[49] Young LM, Good N, Milne D, et al. The prevalence and predictors of airway hyperresponsiveness in sarcoidosis. Respirology 2012; 17: 653-659.

[50] Wilsher M, Hopkins R, Zeng I, et al. Prevalence of asthma and atopy in sarcoidosis. Respirology 2012; 17: 285-290.

[51] Handa T, Nagai S, Miki S, et al. Incidence of pulmonary hypertension and its clinical relevance in patients with sarcoidosis. Chest 2006; 129: 1246-1252.

[52] Nunes H, Uzunhan Y, Frevnet O. Pulmonary hypertension complicating sarcoidosis. Presse Med 2012; 41(6 Pt 2) : e303-e316.

[53] Shlobin OA, Nathan D. Management of end-stage sarcoidosis: pulmonary hypertension and lung transplantation. Eur Respir J 2012; 39: 1520-1533.

[54] Simonneau G, Robbins IM, Beghetti M, et al. Updated clinical classification of pulmonary hypertension. J AM Col Cardiol 2009; 54(suppl.): S43-S54.

[55] Galie N, Hoeper MM, Humbert M, et al. Guidelines for the diagnosis and treatment of pulmonary hypertension. Eur Heart J 2009; 30: 2493-2537.

Chapter 8

Neurosarcoidosis

Mohankumar Kurukumbi, Preema Mehta,
Isha Misra and Jayam-Trouth Annapurni

Additional information is available at the end of the chapter

1. Introduction

Sarcoidosis is an inflammatory granulomatous disease that can affect multiple organ systems, most commonly the lungs. It can also affect other organs, such as the nervous system and heart. Although the exact etiology of sarcoidosis is unknown, it involves the development of noncaseating granulomas in various organs. Noncaseating epithelioid granulomas are the pathological hallmarks of sarcoidosis and symbolize the inflammatory sign of the disease. granulomas are structured masses of activated macrophages and their derivatives (i.e., epitheloid and giant cells). Neurosarcoidosis is a manifestation of sarcoidosis specifically in the nervous system. It is caused by inflammation and abnormal cell deposits in the central and/ or peripheral nervous system, including the brain, spinal cord, or peripheral nerves. In this chapter, we intend to give a brief overview of the common neurologic manifestations of sarcoidosis, as well as diagnosis and management of these symptoms. We will also discuss management of steroid resistant neurosarcoidosis and atypical cases, as well as the overall prognosis of the disease.

2. Epidemiology

Cases of sarcoidosis have been reported worldwide, with a prevalence of approximately 10-80 cases per 100,000 in North America and Europe. Within the United States, African Americans have a greater lifetime risk of developing sarcoidosis than Caucasians (2.4% vs. 0.85%). Worldwide, females have a slightly greater risk of developing this disease. The incidence of sarcoidosis can be described as having a bimodal pattern, with most cases occurring between the ages of 20-40 years old and a second commonly affected group being females who are over the age of 50 [1].

About 5-16% of patients with sarcoidosis have neurologic involvement. The most frequent neurologic abnormality includes cranial and peripheral neuropathy, followed by mononeuropathy, myopathy, psychiatric disorders, cerebellar ataxia, hydrocephalus and papilledema. Neurosarcoidosis is also more prevalent in people of African descent and uncommon in people of Chinese descent and Southeast Asians. It is estimated that isolated neurosarcoidosis, without clinical evidence of systemic sarcoidosis, occurs in less than 1% of sarcoidosis patients [2].

3. History

Sarcoidosis was first clinically described in 1878 by a dermatologist Dr. Johnathan Hutchinson, who called the disease 'Mortimer's Malady', in reference to his patient's name [3]. He wanted to prove it by a biopsy but the patient refused. Then in 1889, Dr. Ernest Besnier described a similar case which he called lupus pernio due to the "chillblain-like swelling" of the nose and the lupus-vulgaris appearance of the fingers. Besnier also did not have histologic findings. It was not until 1892, Tenneson showed a second case of lupus pernio accompanied by histological studies showing lesions which contained epithelioid cells and giant cells. This was the first description of a sarcoid granuloma. Cesar Boeck, in 1899, called it 'Multiple Benign Sarcoid of Skin' which later gave birth to the term 'sarcoidosis'. A few years later, central nervous system (CNS) involvement by sarcoidosis was recognized in 1905 by Winkler [3].

4. Etiology and pathogenesis

Currently, the etiology of sarcoidosis is unknown. There have been hypotheses made including infectious agents, occupational/environmental factors, genetic factors and autoimmune disorders. There has not been a specific pathogen or pathogenic agent linked to the disease. One thought is that the inflammatory response in sarcoidosis, which is characterized by large numbers of activated macrophages and T lymphocytes bearing the CD4-helper phenotype, along with cytokine production is most consistent with a Th1-type immune response commonly triggered by antigens [4]. Also, seeing the trends of blacks and family clusters having increased numbers of the disease, there is a possibility that it is genetic. Many patients with sarcoidosis have the HLA-Factor B 8 (on chromosome 6) and DR 3. Another theory includes inhalation of an antigen that causes granulomatous inflammation in mediastinal lymph nodes and then extends to the lungs and other tissues.[5] Environmental factors involve infections, such as *Mycobacterium tuberculosis* and *Propionibacterium acnes* or *P. granulosum* and non-infectious environmental exposures, such as pesticides and insecticides, pine pollen, silica or talc, metal dusts, and man-made mineral fibers. Exposure to these factors can cause diseases that are histologically and clinically indistinguishable from sarcoidosis [4].

Neurosarcoidosis and multiple sclerosis can present with similar symptoms, such as optic neuritis. It is important to be able to differentiate the two, due to different responses to management and therapy. Since sarcoidosis is often a multisystem disease, solitary nervous-system sarcoidosis is difficult to diagnose, which may delay treatment. The neurological symptoms make it a serious and commonly devastating complication of sarcoidosis [6].

5. Clinical manifestations of neurosarcoidosis

Neurosarcoidosis is seen in approximately 5% of sarcoidosis patients. Of these patients, some may have neurological findings on initial presentation, while others present de novo with neurological signs and symptoms that are consistent with a diagnosis of sarcoidosis [7]. Onset of neurosarcoidosis is most common in the fourth or fifth decades, and typically occurs after patients have had systemic symptoms for some time.

5.1. Cranial nerve findings

Cranial mononeuropathies frequently occur in neurosarcoidosis. In 2009, Joseph and Scolding conducted a study of 30 new cases of sarcoidosis, and reported cranial neuropathies in 80% of the patients [8]. The 7th cranial nerve is often affected. In fact, peripheral facial nerve palsy has been noted in up to 50% of patients with neurosarcoidosis. Oftentimes, Bell palsy is found to be the first manifestation of sarcoidosis and may resolve prior to development of additional symptoms. While facial neuropathies may arise due to basilar meningitis, some cases can be attributed to granulomatous inflammation of the extracranial part of the nerve [9].

Recent studies have found optic neuropathy to be a more common manifestation than previously thought. Patients can present with myriad complaints, ranging from blurry vision and papilledema to retro-bulbar pain and pupillary abnormalities. Palsies of the 8th cranial nerve also occur, leading to auditory and vestibular problems. Extra-ocular movements can become impaired due to involvement of the 3rd, 4th, and 6th cranial nerves. Olfactory involvement is rare, but has been reported in some cases, leading to anosmia and impaired taste.

5.2. Neuroendocrine manifestation

Neuroendocrine dysfunction is often seen in neurosarcoidosis patients, causing them to present with polyuria, changes in thirst, sleep, appetite, temperature, or libido. The hypothalamus and pituitary gland are also often affected, leading to thyroid, gonadal, and adrenal- related symptoms. This usually occurs as a result of subependymal granulomatous infiltration of the 3rd ventricle [9]. Other common symptoms include impaired taste and smell, slurred speech, weakness of trapezius and sternocleidomastoid muscles, and tongue deviation and atrophy. Additionally, carpal tunnel syndrome appears to occur more often in sarcoidosis patients, than in the general population. Occasionally, patients may present with the rare Heerfordt syndrome, characterized by fever, uveitis, parotid gland swelling, and facial nerve palsy [10].

5.3. Other CNS findings

In addition to the hypothalamus and pituitary gland, central nervous system involvement can affect the cerebral cortex, cerebellum, and occasionally the spinal cord. This can occur due to granulomatous inflammation in a perivascular pattern. Granulomas in various parts of the brain parenchyma have even been known to mimic brain tumors such as gliomas, meningiomas, and schwannomas.

Meningeal symptoms have been reported in a substantial number of patients; and can cause many of the aforementioned symptoms. Examination of the cerebrospinal fluid typically shows a mononuclear infiltrate and elevated protein. Cognitive and behavioral problems, along with focal neurologic deficits can occur. If the spinal cord is affected, myelopathies and radiculopathies can occur, and the cauda equina may be affected. Communicating and non-communicating hydrocephalus have been seen in these patients, and sudden death can also occur due to an acute obstruction of CSF flow. Seizures may also occur due to a variety of causes. They are seen as an initial finding in 10% of patients. Sudden death can also occur with involvement of the brainstem leading to central hypoventilation [9].

5.4. Peripheral neuropathy and myopathy

Patients can present with various types of peripheral neuropathies, including, but not limited to mononeuropathy, sensory polyneuropathy, and acute and chronic inflammatory polyneuropathy. Nerve biopsy typically shows noncaseating granulomas, but necrotizing vasculitis may also be seen. Muscle involvement is commonly seen, and is typically secondary to granulomas in the perimysium; however, only a very small number of patients are actually symptomatic. Onset of myopathy usually occurs later in the course of the disease, after involvement of other organ systems has already been noted. Patients may present with acute myopathy, in a similar manner to polymyositis, or may have more chronic symptoms with associated muscle wasting [9].

5.5. Atypical presentations

Sarcoidosis has been shown to affect many parts of both the central and peripheral nervous systems, and patients present with a wide variety of neurological symptoms. Often this can cause difficulties in making a diagnosis, as the reported symptoms are diverse and can mimic several other disease processes, such as Guillain-Barre Syndrome, Multiple Sclerosis, and even psychiatric diagnoses. In April 2012, Spiegel et al noted psychiatric manifestations, such as delirium and psychosis, in about 20% of neurosarcoidosis patients, which is equivalent to approximately 1% of all patients with sarcoidosis. Although this is a rare occurrence, these patients can experience striking auditory and visual hallucinations and delusions [11].

Patients have also reportedly presented with hypersomnolence and hyperphagia consistent with Kleine-Levine-Critchley syndrome [12]. In sum, as neurosarcoidosis can present in many ways, clinicians should maintain a high index of suspicion for the disease, especially in those patients who are not known to have sarcoidosis prior to presenting with neurological manifestations. The disease can be very severe and often life-threatening.

6. Diagnosis

Neurosarcoidosis has no pathognomonic sign, therefore it is a diagnosis of exclusion. This presents a great challenge, especially when the patient does not previously have a confirmed diagnosis of systemic sarcoidosis. The differential diagnosis encompasses a diverse number of pathologies such as Bell's palsy due to Lyme disease, optic neuropathy due to MS, tuberculosis, carcinomatous or lymphomatous meningitis causing multiple cranial nerve palsies. Additional pathologies include metastatic lesions, encephalopathy via syphilis or CNS vasculitis, peripheral neuropathy, or parenchymal lesions such as astrocytomas. Therefore, it is important to think of all the possibilities and rule them out [8].

If neurosarcoidosis is suspected, the patient should be evaluated for evidence of extraneural disease due to the difficulty of obtaining nerve tissue for evaluation. It is imperative to check the skin, lymph nodes and lungs. Other tests that may be useful include ophthalmologic examination, endoscopic nasal and sinus examinations. Radiological tests include neuroimaging (discussed later) and chest x-ray or CT scan to search for hilar adenopathy or parenchymal changes consistent with pulmonary sarcoidosis, serum angiotensin converting enzyme (ACE) assays (nonspecific) and lumbar puncture to analyze CSF. CSF findings may show an increased opening pressure, protein up to 250mg/dL, mononuclear pleocytosis, IgG elevation, oligoclonal bands, glucose normal or low; and CSF ACE is possibly elevated. CSF ACE levels have a relative low sensitivity. Although most studies do not mention immunoglobulins levels in CSF, there is evidence that elevation of immunoglobulin IgG with a high CSF to serum IgG index may be common in CNS sarcoidosis [13]. CSF eosinophilia has also been reported as a consequence of neurosarcoidosis, [14] but may also be present in other infections, inflammatory, and neoplastic conditions, including lepto-meningeal spread of gliomas [15]. Of note, always be cautious of doing a LP in a patient that possibly has increase intracranial pressure. If this is suspected, check for papilledema by using a fundoscope and MRI imaging preceding the LP [8]. Routine laboratory tests may show hyperglobulinemia, hypercalcemia or elevation of alkaline phosphatase [16]. Hypercalcemia occurs in approximately 13-20% of cases due to high levels of 1,25-dihydroxy-vitamin D causing hyperabsorption of calcium [17,18].

Sarcoid lesions in the CNS do not differ from those encountered in other organs. Most cases of CNS sarcoidosis diagnosed by histology have shown variable degrees of meningoencephalomyelitic infiltration, either localized or widespread. This results in focal or disseminated meningeal nodules or plaques, and affecting particularly the basal meninges. Although sarcoid lesions can occur almost anywhere in the central nervous structures, most often they are located perivascularly, with varying degrees of associated gliosis and fibroblast proliferation [3].

One may need to use other tests such as EEG, evoked potentials, and angiography to exclude other causes. Another test, the Kveim-Siltzbach, is not standardized and is not available universally. However, it can show positive granuloma results 4-6 weeks after injecting part of a spleen from a patient with known sarcoidosis into the skin. According to a study by C K Liam and A Menon, the Kveim-Siltzbach test can show false negative results when done in

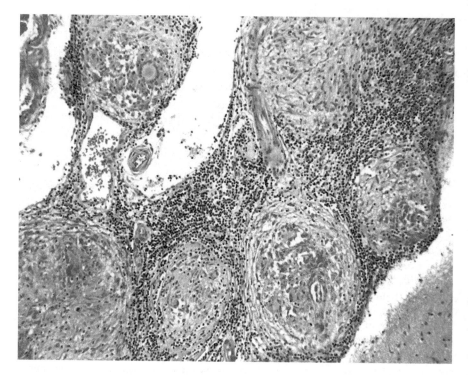

Figure 1. Noncaseating granuloma in parietal lobe showing the granuloma surrounded by epithelioid cells and nodular inflammatory infiltrates (hematoxylin and eosin, 10x). [35]

conjunction with corticosteroid use possibly due immunosuppressive effects. There is also concern that HIV and hepatitis transmission could occur through this technique [8].

As a last resort, a biopsy is done of the meninges, brain, or spinal cord. Biopsies from extra-neural tissue are recommended as it is less risky, but if it is highly suspected and a person with known sarcoidosis with neurologic involvement is deteriorating despite therapy, the neural tissue can be sampled [19]. Most common sites include the meninges and mass lesions.

7. Neuroimaging

Neurosarcoidosis does not have a specific finding on imaging that can assure the diagnosis. However, neuroimaging along with neurologic evaluation, CSF analysis, biopsy and others can aid in making the diagnosis. Oftentimes, it is a brain contrast-enhanced MRI and CSF analysis that gives the presumptive diagnosis. Contrast MRI allows one to visualize meningeal or parenchymal involvement of active inflammation with disruption of the blood brain barrier as well as masses and hydrocephalus.

As mentioned previously, cranial nerve palsies are the most common presentation in neurosarcoidosis, which can be seen on MRI with inflammation along with spinal cord involvement as well [20]. There have been studies done in which enhanced CT was shown to be normal, but the enhanced MRI was abnormal, implying greater sensitivity of MRI for detection neurosarcoidosis lesions [21].

In neurosarcoidosis, leptomeningeal disease is a common pattern of involvement, which may be localized or widespread. Less commonly, granulomatous masses can be found within the cerebral parenchyma. There have been cases showing patients with cranial nerve palsies demonstrating clear evidence of focal meningeal disease on gadolinium-DTPA enhanced MRI brain scans. Neurosarcoidosis is difficult to diagnose when patients have no evidence of granulomatous disease outside the nervous system because of the difficulty of obtaining tissue for histological examination. Therefore, primarily neurological evaluation, neuroimaging and lumbar puncture are done. However, diffuse meningeal infiltration particularly in the skull base region is frequently found at necropsy. Two cases presented by Khaw et al showed Gadolinium-DTPA enhanced MRI's in patients with cranial nerve palsies; one with solely cranial nerve palsies and the other along with gynecologic manifestations. In both of these cases, the meninges were affected by the disease and patients presented with multiple lower cranial nerve palsies, which was not picked up by CT or non-contrast MRI [22].

According to Pawate et al, a study done on 54 cases of neurosarcoidosis, the majority (23%) were found to have intraparenchymal T2 hyperintense lesions on brain MRI. 19% were found to have meningeal involvement seen with gadolinium enhanced MRI. Few of these cases showed intracranial masses, normal brain or solely spinal cord involvement on MRI [23].

When the CNS is involved, brain enhanced MRI and CSF studies are sensitive in the detection of CNS inflammation, however they lack specificity. This continues to make diagnosing neurosarcoidosis a clinical challenge.

8. Management of neurosarcoidosis

While sarcoidosis is a progressive autoimmune disease and there is currently no cure, symptomatic treatment is available. Corticosteroids have become the treatment of choice for neurosarcoidosis. The dosage and duration of therapy varies based upon the type and severity of the symptoms. For instance, patients who present with peripheral facial nerve palsy or meningeal symptoms are given about 0.5mg/kg/day of prednisone for two weeks. On the other hand, a patient with myopathy is given the same dosage for four weeks, and a patient with a mass lesion or symptomatic hydrocephalus is given two to three times this amount for four weeks. Very severe cases of neurosarcoidosis benefit from IV methylprednisone 20mg/kg/day for three days, followed by 1-1.5mg/kg/day of prednisone for two to four weeks [24].

The exact mechanism by which corticosteroids have benefited patients with neurosarcoidosis is unclear, but is generally believed to be secondary to its anti-inflammatory and immunomodulatory effects. Corticosteroids are known to prevent leukocytes from gaining access to sites

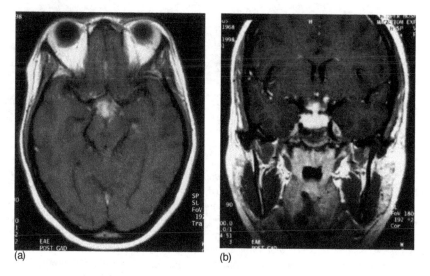

Figure 2. Neurosarcoidosis involving the pituitary-hypothalamic axis. T-1 gadolinium-enhanced Axial (a) and coronal (b) views shows an area of abnormal enhancement involving the sellar, suprasellar regions and the interpeduncular cistern. The diagnosis was confirmed by a biopsy [3].

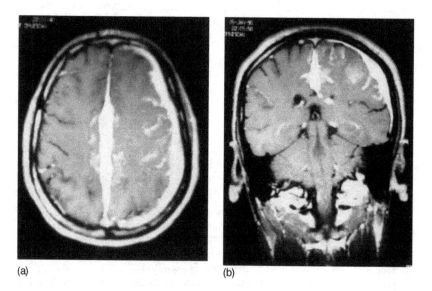

Figure 3. Meningeal neurosarcoidosis. Axial (a) and coronal (b) MRI T-1 weighted images post infusion of gadolinium DTPA in a patient with systemic sarcoidosis show thickening and enhancement of the dura surrounding the left hemisphere [3].

of inflammation, interfere with their function along with that of endothelial cells and fibroblasts, and suppress production of various humoral factors [25]. It is always important to keep in mind, however, that as with all medications, corticosteroids are not without side effects. Common side effects of corticosteroids include cognitive and personality changes, weight gain with central obesity, development of striae, diabetes mellitus, cataracts and predisposition to various infections. Cardiovascular effects are also known to occur, such as hypertension, dyslipidemia, and increased risk of myocardial infarction and stroke. Patients receiving long term corticosteroid therapy are at risk for osteoporotic fractures, especially in the setting of other general risk factors such as being over age 60 or having osteoporosis prior to corticosteroid treatment. Additionally, avascular necrosis, especially of the hip, has been known to occur in a number of patients [1]. Therefore, it is important to carefully monitor the dosage, and to always use the lowest possible effective dose. If treatment with corticosteroids is to be discontinued, it is essential to decrease the dose gradually. Abrupt discontinuation of corticosteroid therapy can cause adrenal insufficiency.

8.1. Alternative therapies for refractory neurosarcoidosis

Several therapies have been proposed for those patients in whom corticosteroid treatment is unsuccessful, or in those who have contraindications to treatment. Many of these studies have shown methotrexate to be an effective treatment. Methotrexate has been successful in two-thirds of sarcoidosis patients regardless of the organ systems that are affected. In one study, EE Lower et al observed 554 sarcoidosis patients, of which 71 had neurosarcoidosis. They found that treatment with methotrexate and cyclophosphamide was associated with higher response rates than treatment with corticosteroids only [26].

In 2007, TF Scott et al used aggressive therapy with corticosteroids and alternative immunosuppressants in 48 patients. Over half of these cases had favorable outcomes [27]. Later, in 2011, G Androdias et al observed a small group of patients with neurosarcoidosis, and found evidence suggesting that Mycophenolate mofetil was effective in treatment of CNS symptoms. The agent was also found to have a steroid sparing effect and was better tolerated than several other immunosuppressive agents [28]. Additional studies have shown anti-TNF agents such as infliximab to be effective; and cytokine modulators such as thalidomide and pentoxifylline have also been used in a limited number of cases [29].

8.2. Other treatments

Surgical resection of CNS mass lesions is usually not recommended, unless the mass persists or continues to enlarge despite appropriate immunomodulatory therapy. If the patient presents with symptomatic hydrocephalus, a ventriculoperitoneal shunt can be placed. It is important to continue immunosuppressive treatment following placement of the shunt as inflammation can lead to obstruction. Cranial or spinal irradiation is suggested in refractory cases if no response is seen with corticosteroids and at least two other agents [30]. Additionally, symptom-specific treatment may be needed, such as hormone replacement therapy for hypopituitarism, and antipsychotics for patients with psychosis.

9. Prognosis of neurosarcoidosis

While many patients with neurosarcoidosis have a monophasic illness, relapsing-remitting and progressive disease patterns are also seen. RA Luke et al followed 25 patients with neurosarcoidosis for a minimum of 5 years or until death. 68% of the patients were found to have the monophasic pattern and 32% had a relapsing pattern [31]. The authors also noted that relapses were more common in patients with cerebral symptoms and in those presenting with hydrocephalus. Furthermore, relapses occurred more frequently in those who were taking smaller doses of corticosteroids (10mg or less).

Although the long term outcomes in neurosarcoidosis patients have not yet been clearly defined in studies, some general conclusions can be made. Patients with peripheral facial nerve palsy often show improvement within 2-4 weeks. Some patients with optic neuropathy show improvement, while others with a more progressive disease pattern can become blind. In 1999, G.A. Christoforidis et al conducted a retrospective study of 461 patients with sarcoidosis, confirmed on biopsy. These researchers reported that patients with optic nerve involvement often did not respond as well to corticosteroid treatment as those with other CNS manifestations did. The researchers suggest that because the other cranial nerves are surrounded by Schwann cells, they can regenerate more easily than the optic nerve, whose myelin sheath is produced by oligodendrocytes [32].

Symptoms such as peripheral neuropathy and myopathy also tend to follow a more chronic and progressive pattern. Aseptic meningitis usually improves within a few weeks, yet CSF abnormalities (asymptomatic chronic pleocytosis) can persist for some time after. Mass lesions often persist for some time, but can also resolve on occasion. Additionally, patients with encephalopathy often exhibit a progressive pattern. Typically immunomodulatory medications are not helpful in patients with endocrinopathies, and these patients need to be treated with hormonal replacement therapy. Also, a series of 68 patients were followed by JP Zajicek et al in 1998, who noted spinal cord involvement in 28% of the patients [33]. The authors concluded that spinal cord disease had a poorer prognosis, as a significant percentage of these patients were found to have deteriorated at follow-up. Patients with seizures have historically been shown to have a poorer prognosis, but more recent studies have disproved this [8].

In general, as the outcome in patients with neurosarcoidosis depends on the severity and types of neurological symptoms, it is difficult to make a conclusive statement regarding the prognosis of the disease. Reportedly, about 10% of patients with neurosarcoidosis die of the disease, typically secondary to CNS parenchymal involvement, hydrocephalus, or other severe symptoms; or due to immune-compromise secondary to treatment.

10. Concluding remarks

Neurosarcoidosis can range from mild to life threatening; and can affect any part of the central and peripheral nervous systems. It can present at any point during the course of the disease process. Many patients do not experience neurological symptoms until the disease has progressed for some time, and systemic symptoms are present. Other patients have neurological manifestations of the disease at the time of initial presentation. Overall, however, neurosarcoidosis only represents a small portion of the total population of patients with a diagnosis of sarcoidosis - about 5%. If patients present with neurological symptoms, with no prior diagnosis of sarcoidosis, it might prove difficult for clinicians to make a diagnosis. This is because these symptoms are quite general and can be seen with a multitude of other diseases. Patients have been reported to have not only general cranial nerve palsies and peripheral neuropathies, but also have been known to present with meningeal symptoms, hydrocephalus, seizures, and even psychosis.

Since the exact cause of neurosarcoidosis is not known, it is important to be aware of any clinical signs early on. It is also important to differentiate it from other diseases with similar manifestations, such as multiple sclerosis due to differences in management and treatment. There are many clinical and lab tests available, as well as imaging that can help determine if one has neurosarcoidosis. Although there is no pathgnomonic sign, brain contrast MRI is a vital tool along with CSF analysis that can give a presumptive diagnosis. They are highly sensitive, although lack specificity, which makes it difficult to definitively diagnose it. Gullapalli and Phillips found a sensitivity of brain MRI of about 82–97% for MS; for CSF abnormality and CSF ACE, sensitivity was 50–80% and 50%, respectively [34]. The most definitive diagnosis can be made from histological analysis of neural tissue via biopsy if there is still doubt despite the other tests or at autopsy. However, it is used as a last resort due to being the most invasive method.

As with other sarcoidosis patients, corticosteroids are the main treatment for neurosarcoidosis. However, some manifestations are more responsive to steroids than others. Additionally, many patients taking corticosteroids for an extended period of time often experience serious side effects; and there are also several contraindications to taking these medications. For this reason, several alternative therapies have been proposed for sarcoidosis patients, and several studies have found methotrexate and cyclophosphamide to be especially effective in treatment of neurological symptoms. Many other immunomodulatory medications have also been shown to be effective along with various symptom- specific treatments.

While many studies have been conducted with regards to the long term outcomes of neurosarcoidosis patients, no definitive conclusions can be made as yet. However, the prognosis for these patients is mainly dependent on the neurological manifestations they experience. Patients with cranial nerve palsies, and particularly optic neuropathies, have been shown in many cases to respond well to corticosteroid treatment. More serious symptoms on the other hand, such as seizures and spinal cord involvement generally suggest a poor prognosis. However, one must also keep in mind, that various disease patterns have been reported in neurosarcoidosis patients. Neurosarcoidosis may present as a monophasic, relapsing-remitting, or chronic progressive pattern. Thus, additional studies need to be conducted before any conclusive statements can be made regarding the outlook for patients with neurosarcoidosis.

Nomenclature

CNS: central nervous system

CD4: cluster of differentiation 4

Th1: type 1 helper cells

HLA: human leukocyte antigen

MS: multiple sclerosis

ACE: angiotensin converting enzyme

CSF: cerebrospinal fluid

LP: lumbar puncture

MRI: magnetic resonance imaging

HIV: human immunodeficiency virus

EEG: electroencephalogram

CT: computed tomography

DTPA: diethylene triamine pentaacetic acid

Mg: milligrams

Kg: kilograms

IV: intravenous

TNF: tumor necrosis factor

Author details

Mohankumar Kurukumbi[1], Preema Mehta[2], Isha Misra[2] and Jayam-Trouth Annapurni[1]

*Address all correspondence to: mohan311@gmail.com

1 Department of Neurology, Howard University Hospital, Washington, DC, USA

2 Howard University College of Medicine, Washington, DC, USA

References

[1] Fitzgerald PA. Chapter 26. Endocrine Disorders. In: McPhee SJ, Papadakis MA, Rabow MW, eds. CURRENT Medical Diagnosis & Treatment 2012. New York: McGraw-Hill; 2012.

[2] Smith JK, Matheus MG, Castillo M. Imaging manifestations of neurosarcoidosis. AJR 2004; 182:289-95.

[3] Vinas F, Rengachary S. Diagnosis and Management of Neurosarcoidosis. Journal of Clinical Neuroscience (2001) 8(6), 505-513

[4] Hunninghake GW, Costabel U, Ando M, et al. ATS/ERS/WASOG statement on sarcoidosis. Sarcoidosis Vasc Diffuse Lung Dis 1999; 16: 149–73.

[5] Mochizuki T, Negoro K, Morimatsu M, Arita K. Two siblings with sarcoidosis diagnosed by younger sister's central nervous symptoms. Rinsho Shinkeigaku 1996; 36: 1249-1255.

[6] Hoitsma E. Neurosarcoidosis: a clinical dilemma. Lancet Neurol. 2004 Jul;3(7): 397-407).

[7] Burns TM. Neurosarcoidosis. Arch Neurol 2003; 60:1166. Stern BJ, Krumholz A, Johns C, et al. Sarcoidosis and its neurological manifestations.

[8] Joseph FG and Scolding NJ. Neurosarcoidosis: a study of 30 new cases. J Neurol Neurosurg Psychiatry. 2009; 80(3):297.

[9] Lacomis D. Neurosarcoidosis. Curr Neuropharmacol. 2011; 9(3):429-436.

[10] Bopp FP et al. Heerfordt syndrome: a cause of facial paralysis. J La State Med Soc. 1990; 142(2):13-5

[11] Speigel DR et al. Neurosarcoidosis and the Complexity in its Differential Diagnoses. Innov Clin Neurosci. 2012 ; 9(4) :10-16.

[12] Afshar K et al. Sarcoidosis : a rare cause of Kleine Levine Critchley syndrome. Sarcoidosis Vasc Diffuse Lung Dis. 2008 ; 25(1) :60-3.

[13] Fried ED, Landau AJ, Sher JH, Rao C. Spinal cord sarcoidosis: a case report and review of the literature. J Assoc Acad Min Phys 1993; 4:132-137.

[14] Scott TF. A new cause of cerebrospinal fluid eosinophilia: Neurosarcoidosis. Am J Med 1988; 84: 973-974.

[15] Defendini R, Hunter SB, Schlemingi EB, Leifer E, Rowland LP. Eosinophilic meningitis in a case of disseminated glioblastoma. Arch Neurol 1981; 38: 52-53.

[16] Glaser GH. Neurologic complications of internal disease. In: Baker AB, Baker LH (eds) Clinical Neurology. Hagerstown: Maryland Harper & Row,1979: 3(44): 1-53.

[17] Stuart CA, Neelon FA, Lebovitz HE. Hypothalamic insufficiency: the cause of hypopituitarism in sarcoidosis. Ann Intern Med 1978; 88: 589-594.

[18] Winnacker JL, Becker KL, Katz S. Endocrine aspects of sarcoidosis. N Engl J Med 1968; 278: 427-434.

[19] Peeples DM, Stern BJ, Jiji V, Sahni KS. Germ cell tumors masquerading as central nervous system sarcoidosis. Arch Neurol 1991; 48:554.

[20] Bihan H, Christozova V, Dumas JL, et al. Sarcoidosis: clinical, hormonal, and magnetic resonance imaging (MRI) manifestations of hypothalamic-pituitary disease in 9 patients and review of the literature. Medicine (Baltimore) 2007; 86:259.

[21] Zajicek JP et al. Central nervous system sarcoidosis – diagnosis and management. Association of Physicians of Great Britain and Ireland. QJM 1999; 92(2):103-117.

[22] Khaw KT, Manji H, Britton J, Schon F. Neurosarcoidosis – demonstration of meningeal disease by gadolinium enhanced magnetic resonance imaging. J Neurol Neurosurg Psychiatry. 1991 Jun;54(6):499-502.

[23] Pawate S, Moses H, Sriram S. Presentations and outcomes of neurosarcoidosis: a study of 54 cases. QJM 2009; 102:449.

[24] Stern BJ and Corbett J. Neuro-opthalmologic Manifestations of Sarcoidosis. Curr Treat Opinions Neurol 2007; 9(1):63.

[25] Boumpas DT et al. Glucocorticoid therapy for immune related diseases: basic and clinical correlates. Ann Intern Med. 1993; 119(12):1198-208.

[26] Lower EE et al. Diagnosis and Management of Neurological Sarcoidosis. Arch Intern Med. 1997; 157 (16): 1864-1868.

[27] Scott TF et al. Aggressive therapy for neurosarcoidosis: long-term follow-up of 48 treated patients. Arch Neurol 2007; 64:691.

[28] Androdias G et al. Mycophenolate mofetil may be effective in CNS sarcoidosis but not in sarcoid myopathy. Neurology 2011; 76:1168.

[29] Baughman RP, Lower EE. Chapter 329. Sarcoidosis. In: Longo DL, Fauci AS, Kasper DL, Hauser SL, Jameson JL, Loscalzo J, eds. Harrison's Principles of Internal Medicine. 18th ed. New York: McGraw-Hill; 2012. http://www.accessmedicine.com/content.aspx?aID=9138725. Accessed August 14, 2012.

[30] Menninger MD et al. Role of Radiotherapy in the treatment of neurosarcoidosis. Am J Clin Oncol. 2003; 26(4):e 115.

[31] Luke RA, Stern BJ, Krumholz A, Johns CJ. Neurosarcoidosis: the long-term clinical course. Neurology 1987; 37:461.

[32] MR of CNS Sarcoidosis : Correlation of Imaging Features to Clinical Symptoms and Response to Treatment. GA Christoforidis et al. AJNR Am J Neuroradiol 20 :655-669, April 1999.

[33] Zajicek JP, Scolding NJ, Foster O, et al. Central nervous system sarcoidosis--diagnosis and management. QJM 1999; 92:103.

[34] Gullapalli D, Phillips LH. Neurologic manifestations of sarcoidosis. Neurol Clin 2002;20: 59–83.

[35] Joseph FG, Scolding NJ, Sarcoidosis of the nervous system: Review. Pract Neurol 2007;7:234-244

Diagnosis

Chapter 9

Endobronchial Ultrasound in the Diagnostic Evaluation of Sarcoidosis

Abiramy Jeyabalan and Andrew RL Medford

Additional information is available at the end of the chapter

1. Introduction

Endobronchial ultrasound-guided transbronchial needle aspiration (EBUS-TBNA) is a minimally invasive mediastinal sampling technique which combines the use of ultrasound with conventional bronchoscopy in order to visualise and sample structures adjacent to the tracheo-bronchial tree such as mediastinal and hilar lymph nodes. The technique is commonly used in the staging and diagnosis of lung cancers but can also be used for the diagnosis of benign conditions affecting the mediastinum including sarcoidosis.

In asymptomatic stage I sarcoidosis (bilateral hilar adenopathy) with evidence of arthritis and erythema nodosum (Lofgren's syndrome) it may be possible to make a presumptive diagnosis based on clinical and radiological findings however in symptomatic patients and particularly where immunosuppressive therapy is being considered or exclusion of other causes of mediastinal lymphadenopathy is required (e.g. tuberculosis, histoplasmosis, silicosis or lymphoma) a tissue diagnosis may be sought. A diagnosis of sarcoidosis can be made in the presence of pathological evidence demonstrating non-caseating granulomata, in the absence of positive mycobacterial and fungal cultures and with supporting clinical and radiological evidence. Tissue for diagnosis should be obtained from the most accessible involved organ. Since pulmonary sarcoidosis is the most frequent form, bronchoscopic techniques are often the first line investigation.

Conventional flexible bronchoscopy is frequently performed in the diagnosis of sarcoidosis but is of limited use when central or peripheral airways are not affected. Endobronchial biopsy (EBB) where there is evidence of disease affecting the airways may assist with the diagnosis. Transbronchial lung biopsy (TBLB) can be performed where there is evidence of parenchymal disease however this technique carries a risk of bleeding and pneumothorax. Transbronchial needle aspiration (TBNA) can be useful in the context of mediastinal lymphadenopathy however this is a "blind" technique and as such diagnostic accuracy is variable and further more there is risk of bleeding and damage to vascular structures. There are also limitations in terms of which nodes can be sampled using conventional TBNA. Mediastinoscopy remains the gold standard approach for sampling the mediastinal glands, particularly when other sampling techniques are non-diagnostic however this is an invasive procedure which requires a general anesthetic and is associated with morbidity. Many of the limitations associated with the aforementioned techniques can be overcome by the use of EBUS-TBNA. The following chapter describes the technique, its application in the diagnosis of sarcoidosis and the advantages of EBUS-TBNA over alternative mediastinal sampling techniques.

2. EBUS –TBNA - Technical issues

2.1. The EBUS scope

There are two probes available. The radial probe was initially developed in 1992. This is a high frequency probe (20-30MHz) which achieves a high resolution image but has limited depth penetration (4-5cm) and provides a 360 degree view. The radial probe is particularly useful for imaging of the airway wall however it does not allow real time identification of structures during sampling (table 1). The convex or linear probe EBUS scope integrates a convex transducer probe at the tip of a flexible bronchoscope (figure 1). The transducer has a frequency of 7.5 MHz and scans through the airway wall in a plane which is parallel to the insertion direction of the bronchoscope. Although images using the convex probe are of lower resolution there is improved depth of penetration (up to 9cm) and most importantly this probe enables real time imaging of the EBUS-TBNA needle throughout the sampling process thus reducing the risk of damage to vascular structures. The endoscopic image is viewed at an angle of 30 degrees forward oblique and the operator needs to compensate accordingly. The ultrasonic image is viewed at an angle of 90 degrees to the bronchoscope. The ultrasonic image of mediastinal structures is obtained by making direct contact between the probe and the airway wall. Improved image quality can be achieved by increasing the contact between the transducer and the airway wall using a balloon attached to the tip of the ultrasound which is filled with normal saline. The ultrasound image is processed and visualized with the conventional bronchoscopic image, on the same monitor (figure 2). The ultrasonic image can be frozen and the size of lesions or nodes can be measured in two dimensions. The use of colour flow and power Doppler also allows accurate identification of vascular structures adjacent to or within the area of interest. The linear probe is most commonly used in the sampling of mediastinal lymph nodes. Unless specified, the term EBUS in this chapter refers to linear probe EBUS.

	Radial Probe	Convex Probe
Frequency	20-30MHz	7.5MHz
Penetration (cm)	4-5	9
Applications	Assessment of airway wall Sampling of peripheral lesions	Sampling of mediastinal lesions e.g. lymph nodes

Table 1. Comparison of radial probe vs convex probe

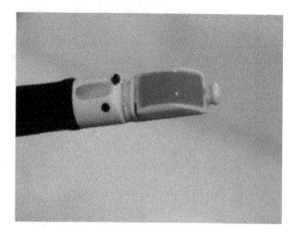

Figure 1. Linear EBUS probe

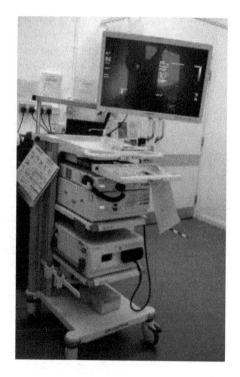

Figure 2. EBUS Scope Processor and Monitor

EBUS-TBNA is sometimes performed at the same time as flexible bronchoscopy which may be necessary when more detailed examination of the distal tracheobronchial tree or endobronchial biopsies are required. The external diameter of the EBUS-TBNA scope is wider than a conventional bronchoscope (6.9mm compared with 5-6mm) however endobronchial biopsies of more proximal airways can be carried out via the EBUS bronchoscope. As with flexible bronchoscopy, EBUS-TBNA procedure is commonly performed under light conscious sedation using intravenous midazolam and fentanyl as well as topical anaesthesia however some centres prefer to use deep sedation with propofol or a remifentanil infusion with a laryngeal mask airway in order to minimize coughing. Typically the procedure is carried out as a day case. Adequate sedation is essential as EBUS-TBNA takes longer than a flexible bronchoscopy, particularly if multiple nodal stations are sampled. The patient is positioned in a supine position and the bronchoscopist stands behind the patient. In view of the wider diameter of the EBUS-TBNA scope, oral intubation is preferred. As described above the endoscopic view is 30 degrees forward oblique, therefore the bronchoscope needs to be flexed down in order to obtain a straight view. In order to pass the bronchoscope through the vocal cords the anterior angle of the glottis should be visualized with the bronchoscope in the neutral position. The mediastinal lymph nodes are examined by positioning the bronchoscope in the correct anatomical position and then by flexing and pressing the ultrasound probe onto the airway wall. The bronchoscope is adjusted so that the area for sampling is viewed in its maximum diameter at the centre of the ultrasound image. The Doppler mode is used to visualize vascular landmarks and can be used to identify vessels within lymph nodes. The size of the lymph node is measured using the calipers.

2.2. The sampling technique

For a more detailed review of this aspect, the reader is directed to other sources [1]. Sampling using the dedicated single use TBNA needle is ideally performed by two operators however it is possible for the technique to be carried out with a single operator. Currently 2 sizes of dedicated EBUS-TBNA sampling needles (21-gauge and 22-gauge) are available. The needle is housed within a sheath which is inserted into the 2.0mm working channel of the EBUS bronchoscope. The sampling needle has multiple small dimples along its shaft in order to increase the echogenicity and screen visualisation. 21 gauge needles are often preferred for suspected granulomatous disease as there is evidence to suggest that the histological structure of specimens is better preserved using the larger needle [2, 3].

Following intubation, lymph nodes are identified according to the International Staging System [4] with the aid of vascular landmarks and the Doppler mode. Mediastinal lymph nodes at stations 2-4, 7, 10 and 11 can be accessed for EBUS-TBNA (figure 3). The EBUS-TBNA sampling needle is inserted through the working channel and is positioned so that the tip of the needle sheath is just visible on the endoscopic image. This is extremely important in order to avoid damage to the bronchoscope channel when the needle exits. The needle is locked on to the working channel and the internal stylet is withdrawn slightly. The depth for sampling is determined (0.5-4 cm) and this distance is set using the safety calibrator (figure 4). Holding the bronchoscope against the airway wall the needle is then inserted using a "jabbing" movement. The needle exits the working channel at angle of 20 degrees to the sheath of the insertion tube (figure 5). Following insertion of the needle the internal stylet is advanced and withdrawn within the needle lumen to clear any airway wall debris before it is completely removed. A 3-way vacuum syringe is attached to the needle and sampling commences by advancing and withdrawing the needle approximately 15 times within the node under direct vision (figure 6). Once sampling is complete the 3-way syringe is disconnected and then the needle is removed from the working channel. The internal stylet is used to expel the histological core tissue sample from the needle lumen onto a specimen collecting system. The stylet is removed and cleaned with saline and air is injected though the needle lumen to remove any remaining particles. The same node is usually sampled 2 to 3 times assuming a good sample is obtained at each pass. For benign disease such as granulomatous disease it may be preferable to do a limited number of passes in a greater number of lymph nodes in order to limit the total length of the procedure if conscious sedation is being used rather than general anaesthesia [5].

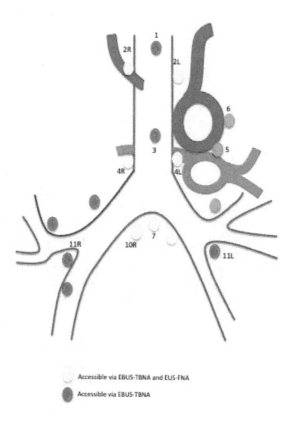

Accessible via EBUS-TBNA and EUS-FNA

Accessible via EBUS-TBNA

Figure 3. Diagrammatic representation of lymph node stations accessed via EBUS-TBNA/ EUS-FNA. EUS-FNA = endoscopic ultrasound-guided fine needle aspiration.

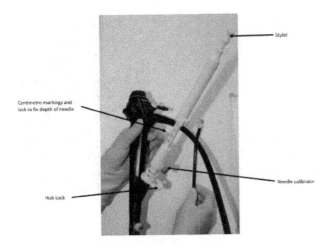

Figure 4. Sampling Needle inserted into working channel of EBUS scope

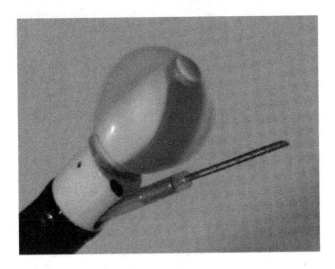

Figure 5. Tip of EBUS scope with balloon inflated and TBNA needle exiting

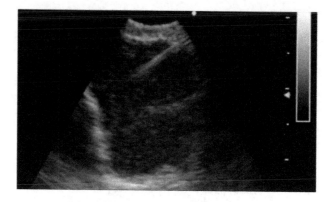

Figure 6. Ultrasound image of lymph node with EBUS-TBNA sampling needle in situ

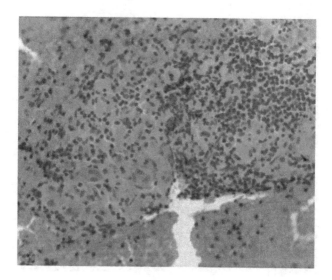

Figure 7. Histological sample obtained using EBUS-TBNA showing non-caseating granuloma

2.3. The specimen

The handling of the histological and cytological samples is extremely important. The diagnosis of sarcoidosis is established when clinical and radiological findings are supported by histological or cytological evidence of non-caseating epithelioid cell granulomas. Granulomas are defined by loose collections of non-pigmented epithelioid or spindle cell histiocytes with lymphocytes, necrotic material and neutrophils. In sarcoidosis numerous granulomas can be seen in FNA samples without evidence of necrosis [7]. It is important to exclude local sarcoid-like reactions and infective causes.

Many centres choose to utilise rapid on-site evaluation (ROSE) of cytology samples in order to confirm the adequacy of specimens however resources and cost are limiting factors. ROSE of specimens has been shown to increase diagnostic yield in some circumstances, however a recent meta-analysis examining the use of ROSE in cases of suspected sarcoidosis did not demonstrate a statistically significant increase (p = 0.66) in yield in studies where ROSE was carried out (165/206; 80.1% vs 282/347; 81.3%) [6]. ROSE allows a smaller number of passes to be carried per node. Once a diagnosis of granulomatous disease or malignancy is reached sampling of that particular node can be stopped. In order to minimize the number of false negative results, if no malignancy or granulomatous inflammation is seen, further sampling should be performed. Gross examination of the specimen can be helpful as adequate samples often appear creamy (rather than bloody, watery or mucoid) or may be black as a result of anthracosis [7].

Typically the EBUS-TBNA samples are smeared on to glass slides and air dried then fixed however some centres prefer to use liquid cytology bottles. Tissue cores are fixed in formalin or saline depending on whether culture for Mycobacterial disease is required. It has recently been reported that cell block analysis in addition to the Diff-Quick smear examination can reduce the false negative rate by 33%. Furthermore, Wang et al [8], found that of 37 patients who had EBUS-TBNA carried out, 100% of cell blocks contained non-necrotizing granulomas compared to 27% of smears. This may be because smearing samples between two slides disrupts the epithelioid groups in FNA samples which does not tend to occur during cell block preparation.

There is debate regarding the definition of an adequate tissue sample. In the absence of malignant cells or granulomatous cells it is clearly important to confirm that an adequate amount of lymphoid tissue is present in the sample. The negative predictive value of samples is far superior when lymphocytes are detected. Attempts have been made to quantify the number of cells required to define the adequacy of a sample. For example, [see 7] state that a sample containing at least 40 benign-appearing lymphocytes in a high-power field in the areas of highest cellularity of the smear constitutes an adequate sample. Likewise the identification of large numbers of anthracotic pigment and macrophages or large clusters of admixed lymphocytes and pigmented macrophages may further indicate an adequacy. If malignancy or granulomatous disease is seen with small numbers of lymphocytes this can also be considered to be adequate. The interpretation of adequacy is somewhat subjective and development of a standardised approach may help to reduce the number of false negative or positive results.

Sarcoid-like granulomata may be visualized in the context of malignancy such as non-small cell lung cancer, lymphoid and germ cell neoplasms and are thought to be a result of a local T cell-mediated immune reaction. It is therefore important to continue to attempt to exclude malignancy even if granulomatous inflammation is seen. Similarly granulomatous inflammation can be seen as a result of fungal or mycobacterial infections particularly in immunosuppressed patients and appropriate culture should be considered. The implication of EBUS-TBNA detection of granulomatous inflammation in patients with previously treated cancer and new mediastinal lymphadenopathy has been examined [9]. In this study, 17/153 (11%) of patients referred for EBUS-TBNA were found to have non-caseating granuloma. A subgroup of patients had a previous history of cancer and presented with mediastinal lymphadenopathy suspicious of cancer recurrence. All these patients had granulomatous inflammation confirmed via EBUS-TBNA and remained clinically stable during follow-up. The study highlights the importance of obtaining a tissue diagnosis in this subgroup of patients and supports the utility of EBUS-TBNA as a diagnostic tool in this circumstance. The differentiation between true sarcoidosis and sarcoid-like reaction must be made through clinical and radiological correlation.

2.4. Diagnostic yield of EBUS-TBNA

The diagnostic yield of EBUS-TBNA in sarcoid has been reported between 80-90% [10]. It is important to note that the highest sensitivity (92%) of EBUS-TBNA has been demonstrated in patients with stage I and II disease with nodes of >10mm however even in patients with nodes of <10mm and all stages of sarcoidosis the sensitivity is still adequate (85%) [11,12]. A recent meta-analysis of 15 studies of EBUS-TBNA in sarcoidosis described a yield between 54-93% with a pooled diagnostic accuracy of 79% (95% CI, 71-86%) however there was heterogeneity between studies included. There was also variability regarding the experience of the operators in these studies [6].

2.5. Contraindications

EBUS-TBNA is a well tolerated procedure. Patients should be fit enough to undergo flexible bronchoscopy in accordance with local guidelines [13]. Biopsies should not be carried out in patients who are currently taking warfarin and the international normalized ratio (INR) should be less than 1.4. Clopidogrel is normally withheld at least one week prior to the procedure although a small series of patients who had EBUS-TBNA whilst still taking clopidogrel (and a significant proportion also taking aspirin) did not report any bleeding complications [14]. The procedure should be avoided for 6 weeks after myocardial infarction and should not carried out in patients with arrhythmia or severe hypoxaemia at rest [15].

2.6. Complications

EBUS-TBNA has been shown to be a safe, minimally invasive technique. Only 5 minor complications (minimal pneumothorax, minor bleeding, airway oedema/hypoxaemia, prolonged coughing) were reported in a recent systematic review of 532 patients undergoing EBUS-TBNA for suspected sarcoidosis [6]. Compared to mediastinoscopy which carries a 0.5%

risk of major complications and 1.4-2.3% risk of significant complications the risk of compli-cations with EBUS-TBNA is lower [15]. Routine chest radiograph is not required following the procedure unless the patient reports specific symptoms (e.g. chest pain) during or after the procedure although some centres do a chest radiograph after sampling the hilar stations routinely [16].

2.7. Costs

The main costs of setting up an EBUS-TBNA service are due to equipment costs such as the EBUS bronchoscope, ultrasound processor and also the disposable EBUS needles (which are more expensive than conventional TBNA needles) and accessories (approximately £150-175). As the procedure takes longer than a conventional flexible bronchoscopy, the cost of additional staff time must be considered. If ROSE is required this is a further cost. Repair and servicing of the EBUS bronchoscope is more expensive than a flexible bronchoscope. Similar to conven-tional TBNA there is a risk of damage to the biopsy channel of the bronchoscope if the sheath of the EBUS-TBNA needle is not positioned correctly when the needle is advanced. Having taken into account the additional costs of EBUS-TBNA, since the technique has a higher sensitivity than conventional TBNA (particularly where distal or smaller node sampling is required, the overall cost saving potential from avoiding a mediastinoscopy is likely to be greater with this technique than with conventional TBNA [15].

2.8. Training and learning curve

EBUS-TBNA can be performed by pulmonologists. Training requires the operator to have had sufficient experience in all standard bronchoscopic techniques, including conventional TBNA. Experience with the interpretation of ultrasound is also useful e.g. thoracic ultrasound. Training of nursing staff is also required. The American College of Chest Physicians (ACCP) recommends that in order to achieve competence in EBUS-TBNA, 50 supervised procedures must be carried out. Furthermore in order to maintain competence it is recommended that a minimum of 20 procedures per year are carried out [17]. The learning curve and the number of procedures required to produce optimal results is high [18]. In fact a recent prospective study has demonstrated improving results up to 120 procedures [19].

3. Other diagnostic bronchoscopic techniques

3.1. Conventional TBNA

The use of TBNA in the diagnosis of sarcoidosis has been described since the 1980's. The technique of sampling lymph nodes using this method is a blind technique and diagnostic accuracy is likely to be dependant on the skill of the operator. The reported sensitivity of TBNA is variable, ranging from 46-90% [3]. It is also a technique which is underutilised by pulmo-nologists (10-30% uptake) because of concerns regarding diagnostic yield and fear of vascular injury [10]. There is also a belief that it is not useful (reported by 30% pulmonologists in one study) and concerns about performing the technique without onsite pathology support [20]. EBUS-TBNA carries a lower risk of complications compared with conventional TBNA. Several studies have directly compared EBUS-TBNA with conventional TBNA. In one, small prospective study of patients with suspected sarcoidosis EBUS-TBNA was followed by conventional TBNA. The two techniques were found to be of similar efficacy with a positive diagnosis established in 93% of patients using EBUS-TBNA and/ or conventional TBNA [3]. Only one randomised controlled trial has directly compared EBUS-TBNA with conventional TBNA. This study demonstrated a superior diagnostic yield with EBUS-TBNA compared to conventional TBNA (using a 19-gauge needle) in patients with suspected sarcoidosis. An absolute increase in yield of 29.5% was demonstrated with EBUS-TBNA (p <0.05; 95% confidence interval 8.6 to 55.4%). Sensitivity and specificity in the conventional TBNA group was 60.9% and 100% respectively compared with 83.3% and 100% in the EBUS-TBNA group. Of note, more lymph nodes were sampled in the EBUS-TBNA group but more passes were required in the TBNA group [21].

3.2. Bronchoalveolar Lavage (BAL)

BAL is a safe, minimally invasive and low cost technique which can be performed during flexible bronchoscopy but can also be performed via the EBUS bronchoscope. BAL samples can be used to support a diagnosis of sarcoidosis if a characteristic cytological predominance of lymphocytes is seen. A CD4+/CD8+ ratio of greater than 3.5 in the lymphocyte population has a high specificity (94%) for sarcoidosis. However a low ratio cannot be used to exclude a diagnosis of sarcoidosis [22]. BAL is also of use for microbiological testing particularly where mycobacterial disease is suspected.

3.3. Endobronchial and transbronchial lung biopsy

In patients with suspected sarcoidosis with evidence of parenchymal disease transbronchial lung biopsy (TBLB) can be used to obtain a diagnosis however the reported diagnostic yield is variable (44-90%) dependent on the number of sites sampled and the extent of the parenchymal disease [23]. TBLB has limited value in stage I disease and unlike EBUS-TBNA, TBLB carries a risk of pneumothorax and a higher risk of bleeding.

Endobronchial biopsy (EBB) can be carried out where there is evidence of airway involvement and even if the airways do not appear grossly abnormal EBB can further increase the yield with a 30% yield even in normal airways [24]. In practice EBB is typically performed when macroscopic disease is visible. EBUS-TBNA has been demonstrated to have superior diagnostic utility when compared with TBLB and endobronchial biopsy [3,25,26].

3.4. Endoscopic ultrasound-guided fine needle aspiration (EUS-FNA)

Transoesophageal EUS-FNA was first introduced in the early 1990s and was most commonly used by gastroenterologists to obtain tissue from pancreatic lesions. Subsequently this technique has been applied in the diagnosis of both intrabdominal and intrathoracic lesions. EUS-FNA enables access to lymph node stations 2L, 4L and most importantly the lower mediastinum (7, 8, and 9). Nodes in the aortopulmonary window (5) and para-aortic nodes (6) can be visualized however sampling is limited by the proximity of vascular structures. The left adrenal gland and the left lobe of the liver can also be sampled. The accuracy of EUS-FNA is greater with ROSE. The technique can be combined with EBUS-TBNA and pulmonologists can train to carry out both procedures or (if appropriately trained) alternatively intubate the oesophagus with the EBUS bronchoscope, as described in some centres, EUS-B-FNA [27, 28]. The disadvantage of EUS-FNA without EBUS-TBNA is the range of nodes which can be accessed is more limited and it is not possible to sample hilar nodes. This is of particular relevance in sarcoidosis as hilar nodes and nodes anterolateral to the trachea are more commonly involved [7].

Diagnostic yield is high with EUS-FNA and has been reported as 82%, sensitivity 89% and specificity 96% [29]. When combined with EBUS-TBNA the yield is improved further and the range of nodes which can be sampled is greater.

3.5. Mediastinoscopy

Mediastinoscopy has been considered to be the gold standard mediastinal sampling method of choice particularly if other techniques such as TBLB are non-contributory. Mediastinoscopy is an invasive technique which requires a general anaesthetic and an overnight hospital stay. There are several approaches which allow access to different nodal stations and areas of the mediastinum. Cervical mediastinoscopy (via an incision at the suprasternal notch) allows access to the pretracheal, upper paratracheal (2R, 2L), lower paratracheal (4R, 4L), subcarinal (7) and hilar (10) nodes. The extended cervical mediastino-scopy also allows access to the anterior mediastinum including pre-aortic (6) and aortopul-monary window (5) nodes. There are currently no studies comparing EBUS-TBNA with mediastinoscopy in suspected sarcoidosis. Successful diagnosis with EBUS-TBNA may obviate the need for mediastinoscopy. This is not only likely to be more preferable to patients who may avoid an invasive procedure but there are also cost saving benefits as discussed previously.

3.6. Peripheral lymph node biopsy

Sarcoidosis involving peripheral lymph nodes is frequently asymptomatic. The incidence of peripheral lymph node involvement has been reported between 2-25%. High diagnos-tic yield with sampling of peripheral lymph nodes has been reported. In one study, at least one enlarged peripheral lymph node was found in 14.5% (79/546) of patients with a diagnosis of sarcoidosis [30]. The diagnostic yield of peripheral lymph node biopsy in these patients was 93% with no associated complications and significantly a lower cost com-pared to other techniques. The most common sites of involvement were the cervical nodes (31.3%) and supraclavicular nodes (29.9%). Ultrasound guided peripheral lymph node biopsy may be an option in patients who have contraindications to mediastinal sampling techniques.

The advantages and disadvantages of all these techniques are summarised in table 2.

Technique	Advantages over EBUS-TBNA	Disadvantages over EBUS-TBNA
Conventional TBNA	Lower cost More commonly performed by pulmonologists Shorter procedure time	Risk of complications/ injury ("blind" technique) Shorter needle throw therefore smaller tissue core Lower diagnostic yield Less extensive range of node sampling
EBB	Performed by pulmonologists Lower cost	Lower diagnostic yield
TBLB	Performed by pulmonologists Lower cost	Risk of complications Less useful in the absence of parenchymal disease
EUS-FNA	Improved access to some lymph node stations	Unable to access hilar nodes More commonly performed by gastroenterologists /radiologists
Mediastinoscopy	Larger histological tissue sample obtained High negative predictive value	Invasive procedure with risk of significant complications Generally performed by thoracic surgeons Requires general anaesthetic and overnight hospital stay Higher cost
Peripheral lymph node biopsy	Low cost (especially if ultrasound-guided without theatre) Low complication rate	Small proportion of patients with enlarged nodes

Table 2. Pros and cons of other non-EBUS sampling techniques in sarcoidosis involving mediastinum/nodal tissue and/or lung

4. Advantages and disadvantages of EBUS-TBNA

4.1. Compared to conventional TBNA

Unlike conventional TBNA, EBUS-TBNA allows access to a wider range of lymph nodes stations (2-4,7, 10 and 11) and therefore provides access to more distal locations. This is of particular relevance in granulomatous disease where sampling of multiple nodal stations can further increase diagnostic yield. This advantage is augmented further by combining EBUS-TBNA with EUS-FNA thereby enabling access to even more lymph node stations.

Conventional TBNA is a blind technique and therefore carries a risk of bleeding through potential damage to vascular structures. EBUS-TBNA carries a lower bleeding risk as it is performed under real time ultrasound guidance. The use of Doppler mode imaging allows accurate visualisation of vessels prior to sampling. Furthermore because sampling is carried out under direct vision it is possible for the EBUS-TBNA needle to be inserted further into the sampling area with each pass compared with sampling during conventional TBNA. Larger cores of tissue can therefore be obtained compared with conventional TBNA. Once again this is particularly important in granulomatous disease.

The cost of equipment and additional staff time required in order to carry out EBUS-TBNA makes it a more expensive technique when compared with conventional TBNA, however as discussed earlier the overall cost saving gained from avoiding the need for mediastinoscopy is likely to be greater for EBUS-TBNA than with conventional TBNA.

4.2. Compared to mediastinoscopy

Mediastinoscopy has been considered to be the gold standard mediastinal sampling method of choice particularly if other techniques such as TBLB are non-contributory. Mediastinoscopy is an invasive technique which requires a general anaesthetic and an overnight hospital stay unlike EBUS-TBNA which is typically carried out under light conscious sedation as a day case procedure. Clearly there are financial advantages to a less invasive approach and it is likely to be more preferable to patients. Mediastinoscopy carries a risk of major complications (0.5%) and 1.4-2.3% risk of significant complications such as supraventricular arrhythmias. It also results in a neck scar and the development of adhesions following mediastinoscopy may hinder future attempts at lymph node sampling [16]. Previous neck surgery is a relative contraindication to mediastinoscopy. As discussed previously, the risk of complications with EBUS-TBNA is lower than with mediastinoscopy. The range of nodes which are accessible via EBUS-TBNA is greater than with mediastinoscopy particularly the hilar nodes. This is of relevance in granulomatous disease as the hilar nodes are frequently affected.

Smaller tissue samples are obtained with EBUS-TBNA compared to mediastinoscopy and as discussed earlier this can affect the adequacy of tissue samples obtained. For this reason the negative predictive value of EBUS-TBNA is lower. This is particularly relevant when sampling for malignancy. If there is concern that malignancy such as lymphoma is a possible cause for lymphadenopathy, mediastinoscopy should be the sampling technique of choice. Alternatively, a non-diagnostic EBUS-TBNA result should be considered for further investigation with mediastinoscopy. In experienced centres where adequate tissue samples are obtained through EBUS-TBNA the technique may be an alternative option for patients who have been deemed not fit for invasive mediastinoscopy.

5. Comparative studies of EBUS-TBNA with other mediastinal sampling techniques

Combining EBUS-TBNA with standard bronchoscopic techniques has been shown to improve diagnostic yield further. This is important as improved accuracy in non-invasive techniques may obviate the need for mediastinoscopy. A number of studies have evaluated combining EBUS-TBNA.

A prospective study carried out in an experienced centre examining the safety and efficacy of combining EBUS-TBNA with TBLB and EBB for the diagnosis of sarcoidosis in an unselected group of patients [26] demonstrate a sensitivity of standard bronchoscopic techniques (TBLB and EBB) of 35% (P<0.001) compared with 85% with EBUS-TBNA. Combining the two techniques resulted in a diagnostic yield of 93% (P<0.0001). In this study the relatively low sensitivity with TBLB and EBB was attributed to the fact that the majority of patients had stage I sarcoidosis without evidence of parenchymal disease.

Another study in which patients with clinical and radiological evidence of sarcoidosis underwent EBUS-TBNA, TBLB and BAL also supports a combined approach. The diagnostic accuracy was superior with EBUS-TBNA compared with TBLB (p<0.001). Analysis of BAL samples demonstrated that the CD4/CD8 ratio was >3.5 in 65.7% of patients with a final diagnosis of sarcoidosis. The diagnostic yield for all modalities of sampling was very high (100%) in patients with stage II sarcoidosis, however EBUS-TBNA was superior to all other modalities for stage I disease. Of note, all patients underwent cross sectional imaging prior to the procedure and had nodes measuring >10mm diameter. ROSE was also utilized [31].

There is evidence to support the use of combined flexible bronchoscopy and EUS-FNA +/-EBUS-TBNA in order to increase diagnostic yield. Tournoy et al, confirmed this in a study of patients with suspected sarcoidosis who did not have a definite diagnosis following standard bronchoscopic techniques (TBNA, TBLB and EBB) [32]. These patients were sent for EBUS-TBNA and/ or EUS-FNA. A definite diagnosis of sarcoidosis was established in 45% patients following standard flexible bronchoscopic procedures. However diagnostic yield increased by a further 39% with the addition of EBUS-TBNA and/ or EUS-FNA.

5.1. Newer techniques

EBUS-guided forceps or transbronchial needle forceps are currently under evaluation. This sampling tool is a combination of a needle and forceps which can be passed through the working channel of the EBUS scope. These forceps can potentially allow larger histological cores of tissue to be obtained. An initial pilot study has shown this tool to be safe and specific diagnosis was established in 86% of patients [33].

6. Conclusion

EBUS-TBNA is a safe, well tolerated and effective mediastinal sampling tool which can be used in the diagnosis of suspected sarcoidosis. As with all mediastinal sampling techniques, histological samples should be interpreted in the context of clinical and radiological findings. EBUS-TBNA has been shown to have a higher diagnostic yield compared to conventional bronchoscopic techniques such as EBB, TBLB and TBNA. Combining EBUS-TBNA with other modalities such as EUS-FNA may further increase diagnostic yield as may the use of newer sampling tools such as the transbronchial needle forceps. Improved accuracy and yield with this technique may obviate the need for further invasive sampling attempts such as mediasti-noscopy. This consequently reduces the overall cost compared to other techniques and importantly reduces the potential for procedure related complications. Future studies are required to further evaluate this technique in sarcoidosis as compared to existing sampling techniques.

Author details

Abiramy Jeyabalan and Andrew RL Medford*

*Address all correspondence to: andrewmedford@hotmail.com

North Bristol Lung Centre, Southmead Hospital, Westbury-on-Trym, Bristol, UK

References

[1] Medford AR. Convex probe endobronchial ultrasound: pitfalls, training and service issues. Br J Hosp Med (Lond). 2011;72(6):312

[2] Nakajima T, Yasufuku K, Takahashi, Shingyoji M, Hirata T, Itami M, Matsui Y, Ita-kura M, Ilzasa T, Kimura H. Comparison of 21-gauge and 22-gauge aspiration needle during endobronchial ultrasound-guided transbronchial needle aspiration. Respirology 2011;16: 90-94

[3] Oki M, Saka H, Kitagawa C, Kogure Y, Murata N, Ichihara, Mortamni S, Ando M. Randomized study of 21-gauge versus 22-gauge endobronchial ultrasound-guided transbronchial aspiration needles for sampling histology specimens. J Bronchol Intervent Pulmonol 2011;18: 306-310

[4] Mountain CF, Dresler CM. Regional lymph node classification for lung cancer staging. Chest 1997; 111: 1718-23

[5] Tremblay A, Stather DR, MacEachern P, Khalil M, Field S. A randomized controlled trial of standard vs endobronchial ultrasonography-guide transbronchial needle aspiration in patients with suspected sarcoidosis. Chest 2009;136(2): 340-346

[6] Agrawal R, Srinivasan, A, Aggarwal AN, Gupta D. Efficacy and safety of convex probe EBUS-TBNA in sarcoidosis: A systematic review and meta-analysis. Respiratory Medicine 2012;106: 883-892

[7] Cameron SHE, Andrade RS, Pambuccian. Endobronchial ultrasound-guided transbronchial needle aspiration cytology: a state of the art review. Cytopathology 2010; 21:6-26

[8] Wang H, Rao A, Lafranco A, Vachani A, Haas A, Gupta P. Cell block examination is critical for sarcoidosis diagnosis by endobronchial ultrasound-guided mediastinal

lymph node fine needle aspiration. North American Journal of Medicine and Science 2012;5(4): 198-202

[9]   Kennedy MP, Jimenez CA, Mhatre AD, Morice RC, Eapen GA. Clinical implications of granulomatous inflammation detected by endobronchial ultrasound transbronchial needle aspiration on patients with suspected cancer recurrence in the mediastinum. Journal of Cardiothoracic Surgery 2008;3:8

[10] Fielding D, Bashirzadeh F, Nguyen P, Hodgson A, James, D. Review of the role of EBUS-TBNA for the pulmonologist including lung cancer staging. Thoracic Cancer 2010 doi: 10.1111/j.1759-7714.2010.00007.x

[11] Wong M, Yasufuku K, Nakajima T, Herth FJ, Sekine Y, Shibuya K et al. Endobronchial ultrasound: a new insight for the diagnosis of sarcoidosis. Eur Respir J 2007;29: 1182-6

[12] Garwood S, Judson MA, Silvestri G, Hoda R, Fraid M, Doelken P. Endobronchial ultrasound for the diagnosis of pulmonary sarcoidosis. Chest 2007; 132:1298-1304

[13] British Thoracic Society Bronchoscopy Guidelines Committee, a Subcommittee of the Standards of Care Committee of the British Thoracic Society. Thorax (2001);56:(suppl I) i1–i21 British Thoracic Society guidelines on diagnostic flexible bronchoscopy

[14] Stather DR, MacEachern P, Chee A, Tremblay A. Safety of endobronchial ultrasound-guided transbronchial needle aspiration in patients taking clopidogrel: a report of 12 consecutive cases. Respiration 2012; 83(4):330-4

[15] Medford ARL, Bennett JA, Free CM and Agrawal S. Endobronchial ultrasound guided transbronchial needle aspiration. Postgrad Med J 2010; 86:106-115

[16] Pillai A and Medford ARL. Upcoming endoscopic techniques: endobronchial ultrasound-guided transbronchial needle aspiration. Minerva Pneumol 2011;50:67-82

[17] Ernst A, Silvestri GA, Johnstone D. American College of Chest Physicians. Interventional pulmonary procedures: Guidelines from the American College of Chest Physicians. Chest 2003; 123: 1969-1717

[18] Medford AR. Learning curve for endobronchial ultrasound-guided transbronchial needle aspiration. Chest 2012;141(6):1643-4.

[19] Fernandez-Villar A, Leiro-Fernandez V, Botana-Rial M, Represas-Represas C, Nunez-Delgado M. The endobronchial ultrasound-guided transbronchial needle biopsy learning curve for mediastinal and hilar lymph node diagnosis. Chest 2012;1411: 278-279

[20] Haponik EF, Shure D. Underutilization of transbronchial needle aspiration: experiences of current pulmonary fellows. Chest. 1997;112(1):251

[21] Tremblay A, Stather DR, MacEachern P, Khalil M, Field SK. A randomized controlled trial of standard vs endobronchial ultrasonography-guided transbronchial needle aspiration in patients with suspected sarcoidosis. Chest 2009;136(2): 340-346

[22] Costabel U. CD4/CD8 ratios in bronchoalveolar lavage fluid: of value for diagnosing sarcoidosis (comment). Eur Respir J 1997;10: 2699-2700

[23] de Boer S, Wilsher M. Sarcoidosis. Chronic respiratory disease 2010;7(4): 247-258

[24] Shorr AF, Torrington KG, Hnatiuk OW. Endobronchial biopsy for sarcoidosis: a prospective study. Chest 2001;120(1):109-14

[25] Plit M, Perason R, Da Costa J, Glanville AR. The diagnostic utility of endobronchial ultrasound-guided transbronchial needle aspiration compared to transbronchial and endobronchial biopsy for suspected sarcoidosis. Internal Medicine Journal 2011;42(4): 434-8

[26] Navani N, Booth HL, Kocjan G, Falzon M, Capitanio A, Brown JM et al. Combination of endobronchial ultrasound guided transbronchial needle aspiration with standard bronchoscopic techniques for the diagnosis of stage I and stage II pulmonary sarcoidosis. Respirology 2011;16(3): 467-72

[27] Medford AR, Agrawal S. Single bronchoscope combined endoscopic-endobronchial ultrasound guided fine-needle aspiration for tuberculous mediastinal nodes. Chest 2010;138(5):1274

[28] Hwangbo B, Lee GK, Lee HS, Lim KY, Lee SH, Kim HY, Lee HS, Kim MS, Lee JM, Nam BH, Zo JL. Transbronchial and transoesophageal fine-needle aspiration using an ultrasound bronchoscope in mediastinal staging of potentially operable lung cancer. Chest 2010;138(4):795-802

[29] Wildi SM, Judson MA, Friag M, Fickling E, Schmulewitz N, Varadarajulu S, Roberts SS, Prasad P, Hawes RH, Wallace MB, Hoffman BJ. Is endosonography guided fine needle aspiration (EUS-FNA) for sarcoidosis as good as we think. Thorax 2004; 59: 794-799

[30] Yanardag H, Caner M, Papila I, Uygun S, Demirci S, Karayel T. Diagnostic value of peripheral lymph node biopsy in sarcoidosis: A report of 67 cases. Can Respir J 2007; 14(4): 209-211

[31] Nakajima T, Yasufuku K, Kurisu K, Takiguchi Y, Fugiwara T, Chiyo M, Shibuya K, Hiroshima K, Nakatani Y, Yoshino I. The role of EBUS-TBNA for the diagnosis of sarcoidosis – comparisons with other bronchoscopic diagnostic modalities. Respiratory Medicine 2009;103: 1796-1800

[32] Tournoy KG, Bolly A, Aerts JG, Pierard P, De Pauw R, Leduc D et al. The value of endoscopic ultrasound after bronchoscopy to diagnose thoracic sarcoidosis. Eur Respir J 2010; 35(6): 1329-35

[33] Herth H, Gompelmann D, Kahn N, Gasparini S, Ernst A, Schuhmann M, Eberhardt R. Endobronchial ultrasound-guided lymph node biopsy with transbronchial needle forceps: a pilot study. Eur Respir J 2012;39(2): 373-7

Chapter 10

Laboratory Investigations and Immunological Testing in Sarcoidosis

Hasib Ahmadzai, Paul S. Thomas and
Denis Wakefield

Additional information is available at the end of the chapter

1. Introduction

Sarcoidosis is a systemic granulomatous disease of unknown aetiology, which can affect virtually any organ and is thus characterised by a variable clinical presentation and course. The disease is generally considered to be a T helper-1 (T_H1) type of reaction, although T_H2 and T_H17 features have also been identified. Approximately 90% of patients demonstrate disease involvement of the lungs and thoracic lymph nodes and although sarcoidosis is usually subacute and self-limiting, progressive inflammation can lead to pulmonary fibrosis and death. Despite these features, there is currently no definitive single laboratory investigation used to identify sarcoidosis, indicating the need for improved understanding of the immuno-pathogenesis and identification of disease-specific biomarkers. Currently, sarcoidosis is generally a diagnosis of exclusion that is best confirmed by clinical and radiological findings and tissue biopsies revealing non-caseating granulomas in the absence of known granuloma-genic agents. Laboratory testing is nonetheless beneficial in further supporting a diagnosis of sarcoidosis and assessing disease severity.

In this chapter, we focus on the laboratory and immunological testing used in sarcoidosis, including biomarkers that have been proposed as measures of the immunological response, as well as cellular markers present in blood and bronchoalveolar lavage. Comparisons will also be made with older immunological investigations including the Kveim-Siltzbach test and recent evidence of potential sarcoid antigens. Novel methods of sampling disease biomarkers, including the technique of exhaled breath analysis will be explored. Immunological testing and measurement of various biomarkers in body tissues has been a useful research tool in understanding sarcoid pathophysiology. There may be a useful role for some of these laboratory investigations as future clinical tools, improving diagnostic sensitivity and identifying novel targets for treatment [1].

2. Serum chemistries and other initial investigations

The diagnosis of sarcoidosis is based on a compatible clinical and radiological picture, histological evidence of non-caseating granulomas and exclusion of other diseases which show a similar clinical or histological picture [2]. The clinical, radiological and histological features of sarcoidosis are discussed elsewhere in this book. The recommended initial clinical and laboratory investigations for a patient suspected of having sarcoidosis are listed in Table 1. The rationale for these investigations is to detect frequent manifestations of the disease, as well as identification of serious, although rare complications of sarcoidosis such as cardiac disease.

	Routine testing	Additional testing
Peripheral blood	Peripheral blood counts: white blood cells, red blood cells, platelets	Angiotensin-converting enzyme (ACE)
	Serum chemistry: calcium, creatinine, renal function, liver enzymes, CRP, ESR	Glucose
Radiological procedures	Chest radiography	High resolution CT scan
Pulmonary function studies	Spirometry	Lung volumes and diffusing capacity of carbon monoxide. Six-minute walk with oximetry
Other testing	Urinalysis	24-hour urinary calcium
	Electrocardiogram (ECG)	
	Routine ophthalmologic examination	
	Tuberculin skin test	IFN-γ release assays
	Other tests depending on clinical manifestations and suspicion of specific organ involvement	

Table 1. Recommended initial clinical and laboratory investigations of patients with suspected sarcoidosis. *Source:* reference [11].

Simple baseline blood tests are useful to identify the presence and severity of specific organ involvement, including hepatic or renal impairment. Peripheral blood lymphopenia is a common finding in patients with sarcoidosis [3], as the activated T cells accumulate at the sites of granulomatous inflammation [4]. This may contribute to the systemic immunological abnormalities observed in sarcoidosis, with exaggerated local immune responses, but suppressed delayed-type hypersensitivity (DTH) skin tests and peripheral blood immune responses [5-7]. Other haematological abnormalities such as neutropenia or auto-immune haemolytic anaemia and/or thrombocytopenia appear very infrequently [8]. Approximately 10-20% of all patients with sarcoidosis have elevated serum aminotransferase and alkaline phosphatase levels [2, 9]. A cholestatic picture of hepatic impairment from granulomatous cholangitis can also occur with a syndrome of pruritis and jaundice. Hepatic failure or portal hypertension can also develop, although liver involvement is usually clinically silent [10].

Although renal disease is uncommon, increased serum creatinine and urea levels can reflect renal impairment related to chronic hypercalcemia, hypercalciuria, nephrolithiasis, nephro-calcinosis or granulomatous interstitial nephritis [12-14]. Hypercalciuria is observed in over 40% of patients with sarcoidosis and hypercalcemia in 5-10% of cases and occurs mainly in males over 40 years of age [8, 10]. Hypercalcemia and hypercalciuria in sarcoidosis are attributed to increased levels of serum 1,25-dihydroxyvitamin D_3 (also known as calcitriol), which increases serum calcium levels via increased intestinal calcium absorption and osteo-clastic bone resorption. The kidney is normally the only organ that can hydroxylate vitamin D_3 to its biologically active form of 1,25-dihydroxyvitamin D_3. Sarcoid macrophages have also been shown to posses the enzyme 25-hydroxyvitamin D_3-1α-hydroxylase, which converts 25-hydroxyvitamin D_3 to its active form, which is produced in excess in sarcoid granulomas [12, 15, 16] and is not inhibited by normal negative feedback from hypercalcemia [15]. Alveolar macrophages have been shown to be the source of excess calcitriol in sarcoidosis, through elevated mRNA expression of the 25-hydroxyvitamin D_3-1α-hydroxylase gene [17]. It has been found that even anephric patients with sarcoidosis can develop hypercalcemia, through this alternative extrarenal source of the hydroxylase enzyme to create calcitriol [18]. Hypercalciuria is common in sarcoidosis and results from an increased calcium load filtered at the glomerulus, along with suppression of parathyroid hormone secretion by calcitriol, which diminishes renal tubular calcium reabsorption [12]. In an evaluation of 736 newly diagnosed sarcoidosis patients in the United States, 3.7% of all patients had abnormalities with calcium metabolism, with hypercalcaemia being more common in Caucasians than African Americans [9]. Therefore monitoring of serum calcium, as well as 24-hour urinary excretion of calcium should be measured in all patients with sarcoidosis [12]. As chronic hypercalcemia is a common and treatable cause of renal failure in sarcoidosis, it is important not to miss this complication. Hypercalcemia and increased calcitriol have also been described in infectious granulomatous disorders [19-22], again resulting from abnormal extrarenal metabolism of vitamin D_3.

The erythrocyte sedimentation rate (ESR) and the acute phase reactant C-reactive protein (CRP) have been used as nonspecific markers of inflammation in a wide variety of diseases. They are simple initial investigations for assessing the severity of systemic inflammation. In sarcoidosis very high levels of ESR and CRP have been observed in some patients with active disease [23]. The ESR level is more likely to be increased in patients with arthritis [24] and in those with erythema nodosum [25] than for other manifestations of the disease. CRP has been found to be associated with fatigue in sarcoidosis [26]. Levels of CRP are generally lower in patients with sarcoidosis compared with tuberculosis [27] and CRP measurement is less sensitive and specific for sarcoidosis compared to ACE [28].

3. Lymphocytic aspects, cytokines and chemokines in sarcoidosis

Sarcoidosis is characterised by an "immune paradox" of exaggerated T_H1 lymphocyte processes causing localised inflammation, although there is peripheral anergy to common antigens [29]. In patients with sarcoidosis total numbers of peripheral blood lymphocytes are normal or slightly reduced, but at disease sites there is a marked increase characterised by ratios of CD4+ to CD8+ T-cells ranging between 3.5:1 to 15:1 in about 50% of cases, compared to normal ratios of 2:1 [1, 30]. Peripheral anergy in sarcoidosis as displayed by suppression of delayed-type hypersensitivity (DTH) responses may be explained by expansion of a subgroup of $CD25^{bright}$ $FOXP3^+$ regulatory T-cells (Treg) in active sarcoidosis [6, 29]. The initial stimulus which induces local inflammation arises when an unknown insoluble antigen is presented on MHC class II molecules to CD4+ T_H1 lymphocytes. This leads to exaggerated activation and clonal proliferation of these lymphocytes, which produce increased amounts of interleukin-2 (IL-2), a local growth, survival and differentiation factor for T-lymphocytes [31]. These lymphocytes also release interferon-γ, together with cytokines and chemokines produced by mononuclear phagocytes (namely TNF-α, IL-12, IL-18, monocyte chemotactic protein-1 (MCP-1), macrophage inflammatory protein-1α (MIP1α)) into the local milieu [1, 31), which leads to activation of blood monocytes that form non-caseating granulomas. The likely outcomes following granuloma formation are either resolution or fibrosis, which may be dependent on predominance of T_H1 or T_H2 T cell responses respectively.

T_H1 cytokines including IFN-γ promote granulomatous inflammation and inhibit fibrosis development, with Bronchoalveolar lavage (BAL) fluid IFN-γ levels being inversely related to progression to pulmonary fibrosis and are higher than BAL IFN-γ levels in healthy controls [1]. T_H2 type cytokines (e.g. IL-4, IL-5, IL-10, IL-13) and macrophage derived factors including fibronectin, platelet-derived growth factor, insulin-like growth factor-1 (IGF-1) and transforming growth factor-β_1 (TGF-β_1) promote fibroblast proliferation leading to either healing or progressive fibrosis [10]. The IL-17 producing T_H17 cells, considered developmentally distinct from T_H1 and T_H2 cells, have also recently been implicated in the pathogenesis of sarcoidosis. T_H17 cells are associated with autoimmune disease processes, granuloma formation and have a role in host defence against extracellular pathogens [32]. Recent findings from flow cytometry indicate that there are increased $IL-17^+$ and $IL-23R^+$ peripheral blood and BAL CD4+ T-cells from patients with active sarcoidosis compared to those with inactive disease or healthy controls and increased IL-17 and IL-23R expression in lung and lymph node specimens [33]. This was also confirmed with an increased presence of $IL-17A^+$, $IL-17A^+$ $IFN-\gamma^+$ and IL-17A $^+$ $IL-4^+$ memory T-cells in peripheral blood and BAL of patients with sarcoidosis and increased $IL-22^+$ cells in granuloma containing biopsies [34]. Gene profiling studies using sarcoid skin biopsies have also showed upregulated T_H1 and T_H17 gene expression along with increased IL-23 and IL-23R expression in patients with sarcoidosis compared with healthy volunteers [35]. Other groups found conflicting results using enzyme-linked immunospot (ELISPOT) assays [36], as well as finding reduced IL-17A gene expression in BAL CD4+ T-cells in patients with Löfgren's syndrome compared to controls [37]. These data indicate that the T_H17 subset may have a systemic role in active non-Löfgren's disease and may be involved in disease progression [1].

Some of the principal cytokines and chemokines involved in sarcoidosis are summarised in Table 3. Sarcoidosis is also characterised by a polyclonal hypergammaglobulinaemia and circulating immune complexes, which is observed in 20-80% of cases. This may result from non-specific B-cell activation by activated T-helper lymphocytes in lymphoid organs [38].

Monocytes/macrophages	Lymphocytes
ACE	IL-2, IFN-γ
Lysozyme	TNF-α, TNF-β
Neopterin	TGF-β
Chitotriosidase	IL-6, IL-10, IL-12, IL-17
TGF-β	CCL-5
TNF-α, IL1-1β, IL-12, IL-18	GM-CSF
CCL2, CCL3, CCL4, CCL10, CCL18	
CXCL10	
GM-CSF	

Table 2. Summary of key cytokines, chemokines and factors expressed by activated lymphocytes and macrophages in the pathogenesis of sarcoidosis, which have be measured in biological samples. *Abbreviations*: CCL: C-C motif ligand; CXCL: C-X-C motif ligand; GM-CSF: granulocyte macrophage colony stimulating factor.

3.1. Lymphocyte markers: Soluble IL-2 receptor (sIL-2R)

Lung T-cells from patients with pulmonary sarcoidosis express both early and late activation cell surface markers, with IL-2R (CD25) being one of the most widely studied. The soluble form of the IL-2 receptor (sIL-2R) is a T-cell receptor for IL-2, which is used to monitor graft rejection after solid organ transplantation and can be elevated in a number of conditions including infection and autoimmune disease [39]. Its concentrations are elevated and easily detectable in the serum and BAL of patients with sarcoidosis and arises as a result of increased numbers and enhanced activation of macrophages and T-cells from granulomatous inflammation [40, 41]. In some studies, elevated serum sIL-2R falls during therapy or with spontaneous remission [42, 43]. Recent studies indicate that sIL-2R may have prognostic value as a marker of disease activity as the levels are significantly higher in patients with active sarcoidosis compared with inactive disease, correlating with BAL CD4+ T-cell numbers [41, 44]. Patients with extrapulmonary sarcoidosis excluding Löfgren's syndrome have also demonstrated greater serum sIL-2R levels compared to those with isolated pulmonary involvement [41], with sIL-2R appearing to be an independent marker for worse disease. sIL-2R has been compared with serum CRP, serum amyloid A and ACE activity indicating that only sIL-2R was predictive of sarcoidosis severity and could be used for patient follow-up [23].

3.2. β_2-microglobulin

β_2-microglobulin is a low molecular weight protein and a marker of lymphocyte activation. It has been described in a variety of infectious, inflammatory and neoplastic diseases and is used to monitor patients with lymphoma. Various studies have identified that approximately 25% of patients with sarcoidosis have elevated serum β_2-microglobulin concentrations [30, 45, 46]. Initial findings in sarcoidosis patients indicated that the levels were elevated at the time of diagnosis, rose during relapse and fell with corticosteroid therapy [47]. In a study of 107 patients with sarcoidosis, β_2-microglobulin levels were found to correlate with granuloma formation in the initial phases, whilst ACE activity reflected later phases. It was also noted that in patients with acute sarcoidosis and erythema nodosum, β_2-microglobulin was elevated and ACE was usually normal [46]. Another study of 132 sarcoidosis patients did not find an association between β_2-microglobulin and ACE [45], indicating that lymphocyte and macrophage activation are not always concurrently present. This is one limitation of this marker in that it only assesses lymphocyte activation, compared to sIL-2R which reflects both macrophage and lymphocyte activation. β_2-microglobulin concentrations have also been measured in the cerebrospinal fluid (CSF) and were found to be elevated in 68% of patients with neurosarcoidosis, although it was not elevated in patients who did not have neurological involvement [48]. As it has low specificity and sensitivity, serum β_2-microglobulin has limited use in clinical practice.

4. Immunological studies of alveolitis: BAL and induced sputum

BAL fluid analysis is a useful investigation for the diagnosis of pulmonary sarcoidosis by detecting a lymphocytosis with elevated ratios of CD4+/CD8+ cells, typically >3.5:1, in the absence of other causes [1]. BAL lymphocytosis with elevated CD4/CD8 ratios, normal percentages of eosinophils and neutrophils and the absence of plasma cells suggest a diagnosis of sarcoidosis. Cellular analysis of T-lymphocyte subsets and cytokine levels from BAL fluid and peripheral blood using flow cytometry have been compared and can provide useful diagnostic information on sarcoid alveolitis. Costabel et al. reported on the clinical utility of BAL CD4/CD8 ratios in the diagnosis of sarcoidosis. Ratios greater than 3.5 have a sensitivity of 53%, specificity of 94%, positive predictive value of 76% and a negative predictive value of 85% for sarcoidosis, and with higher ratios the specificity nearly reaches 100% [49]. For individual cases, CD4/CD8 ratios may not always be useful as some patients may have either decreased, normal or increased ratios, or in rare cases may present with a CD8 alveolitis, such as in sarcoid patients with HIV-1 infection [50].

Ex vivo studies in patients with sarcoidosis with flow cytometry identified greater activation of non-stimulated BAL CD4+ and CD8+ T cells when compared with peripheral blood lymphocytes [51], demonstrating compartmentalisation of the immune response. A large number of BAL lymphocytes from patients with active sarcoidosis express cell surface activation markers including CD26, CD54, CD69, CD95 and HLA-DR [51, 52]. CD4+/HLA-DR + T-cells spontaneously release IL-2. Some investigators identified the possibility of using the number of CD4+/HLA-DR$^+$ cells for evaluating the activation state of the IL-2 system and defining different phases of sarcoidosis, as numbers decrease in inactive disease [53]. It is also interesting to note studies with BAL fluid from sarcoidosis patients who have the HLA-DRB1*0301-positive genotype predominantly express the Vα2.3 (AV2S3+) T-cell receptor. The increase in AV2S3+ CD4+ T-cells may be very significant during acute disease in these patients and constitute more than 30% of BAL T-cells, as well as expressing cell surface activation markers including CD26, CD28, CD69 and HLA-DR [54], indicating acute clonal expansion and proliferation in response to inciting antigen(s) [55].

Intracellular cytokine expression has been compared in activated BAL and peripheral blood lymphocytes using non-specific lymphocyte mitogens in patients with sarcoidosis and healthy controls. Some studies suggest compartmentalised shifts in the T_H1/T_H2 cytokine balance modulate granulomatous lung inflammation and its evolution towards disease resolution or development of pulmonary fibrosis [1]. BAL T-cells from patients with pulmonary sarcoidosis show a dominant T_H1 cytokine expression, with elevated mRNA and protein levels of IFN-γ and IL-2, as well as TNF-α but not IL-4 [52, 56-59]. Additionally, BAL alveolar macrophages have been shown to be important regulators of the T_H1 response by producing IL-12 and IL-18, which stimulate IFN-γ production and differentiation of naïve T-cells into a T_H1 phenotype [60]. Following stimulation, significantly more BAL CD4+ cells express T_H1 receptors CXCR3, CCR5, IL-12R and IL-18R, but fewer T_H2 chemokine receptors (CXCR4, CCR4) when compared with paired peripheral blood CD4+ T-cells [61]. A recent study of 52 sarcoidosis patients and 21 healthy controls identified that circulating levels of the T_H1 chemokine IFN-inducible protein (IP-10/CXCL10) and the T_H2 chemokine CCL17 were both elevated in the serum of patients compared to controls [62]. They additionally found that there was significantly greater IP-10 production by BAL cells in patients with active sarcoidosis compared to controls but no difference in BAL CCL17 levels. Interestingly, increased numbers of CD4+ CD25^{bright} FOXP3$^+$ Treg cells have been identified in the peripheral blood and BAL fluid of patients with active sarcoidosis. These cells exhibit powerful anti-proliferative ability but are unable to completely down-regulate production of pro-inflammatory cytokines including IFN-γ and TNF-α, thus allowing granuloma formation [6, 29]. Further investigations are needed to evaluate the $T_H1/T_H2/T_H17$ network in sarcoidosis, during different disease stages and the regulatory mechanisms which may be involved.

A CD4+ IFN-γ^+ T-cell alveolitis with elevated ratios of CD4+/CD8+ T-cells has also been confirmed in patients with active pulmonary disease using induced sputum, a relatively less-invasive technique compared with BAL [63]. A strong correlation has been confirmed between T-cell subsets in BAL fluid and induced sputum in patients with sarcoidosis, although the proportion of alveolar macrophages was significantly lower in induced sputum [64]. Increased levels of regulatory CD4+ CD25^{bright} CD127^{low} T-cells have also been confirmed in induced sputum of patients with active pulmonary sarcoidosis [65]. This indicates that induced sputum may be a less invasive yet useful method of investigating the immunology of pulmonary disorders.

5. Exclusion of granulomatous diseases mimicking sarcoidosis

There has been an increase in the armamentarium of specific immunological and microbiological tests to identify granulomatous disorders which would have previously been mistakenly labelled as sarcoidosis. Table 3 lists common granulomatous conditions, some of which need to be considered in the differential diagnosis of a patient with suspected sarcoidosis.

Some investigations which can be used depending on the clinical context to identify other causes of granulomatous inflammation include: the beryllium lymphocyte proliferation test, which can be performed on peripheral blood or BAL mononuclear cells to test for chronic beryllium disease [66], tests for anti-neutrophil cytoplasmic antibodies for Wegener's granulomatosis and related vasculitides, anti-mitochondrial antibodies for primary biliary cirrhosis and serological and culture methods for infectious diseases. Investigations of special interest are discussed in detail below.

5.1. Tuberculin skin test, delayed-type hypersensitivity and interferon-γ release assays

Although patients with sarcoidosis exhibit an exaggerated T_H1 immune response at sites of disease, they commonly have depressed peripheral blood responses to common antigens [5, 67], are unresponsive to vaccinations [7, 68] and demonstrate suppression of DTH to tuberculin. Impaired DTH is a clinical feature of sarcoidosis, with skin anergy demonstrated to recall antigens and polyclonal mitogens including mumps virus, *Trichophyton*, *Candida*, streptokinase/streptodornase, dinitrochlorobenzene [5, 69-71] but not phytohaemagglutinin (PHA) [72]. Similarly, patients exhibit cutaneous anergy to the tuberculin skin test, which is considered as part of the diagnostic criteria for sarcoidosis [73]. It has also been determined that in populations with a high incidence of tuberculosis, the presence of tuberculin skin test anergy is less reliable in making a diagnosis of sarcoidosis, compared with the use of interferon-γ release assays (IGRA). In these populations and in patients with immune deficiencies, IGRA is more accurate in unmasking an actual case of latent tuberculosis infection, in patients who were labelled as having "sarcoidosis" [74, 75]. IGRAs have a higher sensitivity and specificity for detecting *Mycobacterium tuberculosis* (MTB) than the conventional tuberculin skin test, as they utilise antigens specific for MTB complex [76, 77]. The recent QuantiFERON-TB Gold IGRA is based on the principle that T-cells from a whole blood sample of a patient previously exposed to specific MTB complex antigens, including Culture Filtrate Protein-10 (CFP-10), Early Secretory Antigenic Target-6 (ESAT-6) and purified protein-derivative (PPD) will produce IFN-γ, which is measured using enzyme-linked immunosorbent assay (ELISA). These proteins are absent from BCG strains and most non-tuberculous mycobacteria, hence providing specific testing for *M. tuberculosis*. Screening for prior tuberculosis infection, with a detailed history, tuberculin skin testing or use of IGRAs is also required prior to starting anti-TNF therapy, as these drugs are associated with serious infection risk from reactivation of latent tuberculosis [78].

Disease associations	Characterisation
Infectious	Mycobacteria: tuberculosis, leprosy, Bacillus Calmette-Guérin (BCG) and atypical mycobacteria
	Propionibacterium acnes, P. granulosum; Borrelia burgdorferi; Yersinia spp.;Brucella spp., Cat-Scratch disease (*Bartonella henselae*)
	Protozoal: Toxoplasmosis, Leishmaniasis
	Spirochaetes: *Treponema pallidum* (secondary or tertiary syphilis), *T. carateum, T. pertunue* (yaws)
	Invasive fungal infections: histoplasmosis, sporotrichosis, aspergillosis, cryptococcosis, blastomycosis, coccidioidomycosis
	Pseudomycoses: actinomycoses, nocardiosis, botryomycosis
	Herpes simplex virus, Epstein-Barr virus, cytomegalovirus
	Helminth infections: Schistosomiasis, *Ascaris lumbricoides*
	Demodicidosis (*Demodex* species)
	Other sexually transmitted: Chancre (*Haemophilus ducreyi*); donovanosis (*Calymmatobacterium granulomatis*); lymphogranuloma venereum
	Whipple's disease (*Tropheryma whipplei*)
Inflammatory/unknown cause	Sarcoidosis
	Crohn's disease
	Granulomatous vasculitis: Wegener's, Churg-Strauss disease, bronchocentric granulomatosis, polyarteritis nodosa
	Primary biliary cirrhosis, hepatic granulomatosis
	Giant cell arteritis
	Granuloma annulare and actinic granuloma
	Granulomatous rosacea, Granulomatous cheilitis
	Necrobiosis lipoidica, Necrobiosis xanthogranuloma
	Langerhans cell histiocytosis (histiocytosis X)
	Granulomatous lesions of unknown significance (GLUS) syndromes
Identifiable inflammatory aetiology	Hypersensitivity pneumonitis- (e.g. farmer's lung, bird fancier's lung, hot tub lung, metal workers lung). Foreign body granulomas: beryllium, aluminium, titanium, zirconium, talc, paraffin, pine tree pollen, clay, interferon-α injections, tattoos
Neoplastic	Granulomatous mycosis fungoides
	Lymphomas with histiocytic infiltration (Lennert's disease)
Other causes	Blau's syndrome, chalazion, chronic granulomatous disease of childhood

Table 3. Some causes of granulomatous inflammation, table modified from references [79, 80].

IFN-γ production in response to PPD stimulation of BAL lymphocytes has been shown to distinguish *M. tuberculosis* infection from sarcoidosis in a patient with sarcoid-associated optic neuropathy [77]. The QuantiFERON TB Gold has also been investigated in a cohort of 90 Japanese patients with sarcoidosis and was found to be positive in 3 patients (3.3%), which is similar to the false-positive rate in healthy non-sarcoidosis subjects. In these 3 patients, their specimens were negative for *M. tuberculosis* by acid fast staining, culture and PCR evaluation of tissues and none developed tuberculosis infection at 1-year follow-up [81]. A recent study compared the release of IFN-γ by BAL mononuclear cells and PBMC following *ex vivo* stimulation with whole PPD, ESAT-6 and CFP-10 from German patients with sarcoidosis, tuberculosis and healthy controls. They similarly found that BAL and PBMC IFN-γ release was comparable amongst patients with sarcoidosis and controls, but less compared to patients with tuberculosis [82]. Hence IGRAs such as the QuantiFERON TB Gold are specific for tuberculosis infection and results are negative in patients with sarcoidosis.

Recent investigations have indicated that certain undegradable *M. tuberculosis* antigens (which are not present in tuberculosis-specific IGRAs) may be potential pathogenic antigens in sarcoidosis. Investigations utilising IFN-γ ELISPOT and flow cytometry indicated greater PBMC and BAL T_H1 responses to recombinant *M. tuberculosis* catalase-peroxidase (mKatG) [83] and mKatG peptides in patients with sarcoidosis compared to healthy controls, but no difference with PPD-positive (PPD+) control subjects, which profiles a possible pathogenic antigen in sarcoidosis [67, 84-88]. A greater frequency of peripheral blood T_H1 responses have also been shown in patients with sarcoidosis compared with healthy PPD- controls following stimulation with mycobacterial heat shock proteins [86, 89, 90] and *M. tuberculosis* peptides from ESAT-6 [67, 84-88], mycolyl-transferase Antigen 85A [86, 91] and superoxide dismutase A [86, 92]. Cellular immune responses against mycobacterial antigens were detected in cells from patients with sarcoidosis that did not react to *Trypanosoma brucei* lysates [88] or the neoantigen keyhole limpet hemocyanin [84], as well as Cytomegalovirus cell lysate and Cytomegalovirus, Epstein-Barr virus and Influenza (CEF) peptides [67]. Recent findings with flow cytometry have also shown significantly greater BAL CD4+ and CD8+ IFN-γ+ immune responses to *M. tuberculosis* ESAT-6 and *Propionibacterium acnes* proteins in sarcoidosis patients compared with healthy controls. This study also utilised matrix-assisted laser desorption ionisation mass spectrometry (MALDI-IMS) to localise ESAT-6 and *P. acnes* signals within sarcoidosis and control specimens. The authors identified localised signals consistent with ESAT-6 in sarcoid granulomas, although there was no specific localisation of *P. acnes* in sarcoid tissues [93]. This demonstrates specific mycobacterial antigen specificity inducing the immune response in some patients with sarcoidosis.

5.2. Histopathological testing and Polymerase-Chain Reaction (PCR)

In sarcoidosis tissue micro-organisms are not detected through conventional staining techniques or cultures of non-caseating granulomas. Important differential diagnoses, including infectious diseases must be excluded with histopathological testing using special stains for acid-fast bacilli, fungi and microbial cultures. This is especially important if the patient has a fever or when granulomas exhibit focal necrosis. Granulomas can also be found in regional lymph nodes of carcinomas or in primary tumours such as breast carcinoma and seminoma. However, with immunohistochemical techniques, granulomas associated with neoplastic processes are generally B-cell positive, whilst in sarcoidosis they are B-cell negative [94].

With the use of special stains or culture methods some investigators have also been able to identify micro-organisms in sarcoid tissues, most commonly those resembling mycobacteria [95]. Bacilli-like structures have also been observed using immunofluorescence techniques [96]. Schaumann bodies, are a type of inclusion body found in sarcoidal giant cells, which consist of small calcifications of calcium carbonate, iron and oxidised lipid with a lamellar morphology. They are identified in up to 88% of cases of sarcoidosis and arise from lysosomes [97]. They have interestingly been identified as sites of mycobacterial degradation by demon-strating the localisation of lysosomal components and mycobacterial antigens in immunohis-tologically stained sarcoidosis tissues [98]. Other investigators identified bacterial structures in skin and lymph node biopsies [99], as well as blood, bronchial washings, ocular anterior chamber fluid and cerebrospinal fluid from patients with sarcoidosis [100-104]. These organ-isms were identified as 'L-form' cell-wall deficient bacteria, which can occur during the life-cycle of mycobacteria or in response to inhospitable conditions [95, 103, 105]. However, in a larger multicentre study with 197 sarcoidosis cases and 150 controls an equal frequency of cell-wall deficient forms were observed in blood specimens [101]. Sarcoidosis can also be histo-logically similar to lesions in atypical mycobacterial infections, including *Mycobacterium avium-intracellulare* complex (MAC), *Mycobacterium marinum* and following BCG vaccination [95, 104]. Sarcoidosis is also an important differential diagnosis of *M. marinum* infection, where the acid-fast bacilli are detected in 22% of active cases and use of polymerase chain reaction (PCR) is more useful for diagnosis [106, 107].

In an attempt to improve the diagnostic sensitivity of traditional culture techniques, many investigators have used DNA amplification techniques to search for mycobacterial or propio-nibacterial infection in sarcoidosis. Investigations have used PCR and nested PCR techniques to identify mycobacterial and propionibacterial DNA or RNA in sarcoid tissue specimens, including fresh tissues, paraffin-embedded tissues, granulomas, lymph nodes, lung and BAL sediments and archival biopsy specimens. Several reports emerged indicating the presence of mycobacterial DNA in some sarcoid tissues using DNA primers for *M. tuberculosis* complex organisms [108-113], which could also suggest cell wall deficient mycobacterial infection. The results have been inconsistent, however, as other groups did not find fluorescent in situ hybridisation or PCR evidence of mycobacterial DNA or RNA in sarcoid tissues [114-116]. A recent meta-analysis of 31 such studies identified that 231 out of 874 (26.4%) sarcoidosis biopsy specimens had evidence of mycobacterial DNA, which is 9- to 19-fold higher than control tissue samples, supporting an association between mycobacterial infection and sarcoidosis [117]. However, it is important to note that these results are not reproducible in all sarcoidosis patients and that treatment of sarcoidosis with corticosteroids does not show reactivation of tuberculosis- indicating the lack of a direct role of mycobacterial infection in sarcoidosis [118]. In a patient with negative microscopy, culture and PCR for tuberculosis; in the presence of compatible clinical features and histology, a diagnosis of sarcoidosis can be made with confidence.

Propionibacterium acnes has also been isolated from sarcoid lesions [119] which has suggested a role for this commensal organism in sarcoidosis. Using PCR to amplify segments of the 16S rRNA of *P. acnes* or *P. granulosum*, several authors reported isolation of propionibacterial DNA from sarcoid tissues [120-123], with a DNA signal intensity greater than surrounding non-granulomatous tissue. These initial studies were followed by a cooperative study from Japanese and European investigators that confirmed the presence of *P. acnes* and *P. granulosum* DNA in all but two of 108 sarcoidosis specimens obtained from both Japanese and European biopsies [113]. However, *P. acnes* DNA was also reported in 57% of control tissues including from healthy controls, suggesting that it is a common commensal organism in peripheral lung tissues and mediastinal lymph nodes [124].

5.3. Exclusion of other infectious agents

A history of previous possible environmental exposure, or travel to endemic areas is important to exclude infectious granulomatous diseases. Apart from culture and microscopy of specimens with special stains for fungi and acid-fast bacilli, other investigations can be performed to exclude infection. These depend on the clinical context and may include serologic analyses. Some specialised investigations may be used including identification of the histoplasmosis urinary antigen and skin tests for fungi and protozoa (e.g. the Leishmanin test) [125]. In patients with leprosy the *ex vivo* lymphocyte proliferation test in response to *M. leprae* as well as the Mitsuda type of lepromin skin test [126] have been shown useful to differentiate leprosy from cutaneous sarcoidosis [127]. Tissue must also be analysed for presence of metals, and foreign bodies need to be excluded on microscopy.

5.4. Beryllium lymphocyte proliferation testing

The granulomas formed as a result of chronic beryllium exposure closely resembles that of sarcoidosis, such that some investigators have suggested berylliosis defines a sarcoidosis subset [128]. It is possible that in genetically susceptible individuals, distinct antigens can precipitate sarcoidosis or sarcoidosis-like diseases [129]. A history of occupational or environmental exposure to beryllium is important when considering a diagnosis of sarcoidosis, in patients who have been exposed to the metal dust or fumes. The beryllium lymphocyte proliferation test has been used in the diagnosis of chronic beryllium disease to distinguish it from sarcoidosis and other granulomatous diseases [128]. This laboratory investigation involves the addition of beryllium salts to a sample of peripheral blood or BAL fluid, which can lead to mononuclear cell proliferation, only in patients with berylliosis [66]. Beryllium sulphate stimulation of BAL from patients with chronic beryllium disease induced greater T_H1 immune responses, with markedly elevated numbers of CD4+ INF-γ and IL-2 secreting beryllium-specific lymphocytes, as well as *ex vivo* lymphocyte proliferation compared to healthy controls [130, 131], making it a useful investigation to distinguish berylliosis from sarcoidosis. Patients with chronic beryllium disease can also have preserved skin test-reactivity to common recall antigens such as candida, tetanus and mycobacteria, as well as hyperresponsive DTH to beryllium with the beryllium patch test, unlike sarcoidosis, where patients demonstrate cutaneous anergy [132]. Interestingly, patients with severe chronic beryllium disease may have lymphopenia, calcium metabolism abnormalities, elevation of serum ACE and elevated CD4+ T-cells at sites of inflammation- similar to sarcoidosis, but have negative Kveim test reactions [132].

6. The Kveim-Siltzbach test

Before the use of fibre-optic bronchoscopy and BAL, the Kveim-Siltzbach test was used as the diagnostic test for sarcoidosis, although now it remains of historical importance only. It was performed by intradermal injection of Kveim-reagent, a validated suspension of allogeneic human sarcoid tissue, typically sarcoid spleen or lymph nodes homogenised in phosphate-buffered saline, pasteurised, resuspended with 0.25% phenol, while later preparations were irradiated [133, 134]. The resultant papule at the injection site was biopsied three to six weeks later and presence of non-caseating granulomas indicated sarcoidosis [135, 136]. Kveim reactions can also be induced from similar preparations made from sarcoidosis BAL cells or peripheral blood monocytes, suggesting systemic dissemination of the inciting agent by mononuclear phagocytes [38, 137, 138]. Ansgar Kveim was the first to report in the 1940s that biopsy of these papules demonstrated the presence of epithelioid granulomas that were histologically identical to granulomas observed in sarcoid tissues [135]. In 1967 Siltzbach demonstrated that >80% of sarcoid patients worldwide reacted positively to a single batch of Kveim reagent, with <1% false positive rate of non-specific reactions in control subjects, indicating the possibility of a common antigen in the aetiology of sarcoidosis [139]. The test was very useful in distinguishing sarcoidosis from other granulomatous diseases [140]. A medical centre that performed >10,000 Kveim-Siltzbach tests over fifty years identified a true positive rate of >50% and false negative rate of nearly zero [10]. This test is now rarely used as no commercially available preparation of the reagent exists, with the additional problem that each new Kveim-Siltzbach preparation requires validation *in vivo* [136]. Furthermore, use of human tissue extracts for clinical purposes presents constraints, including risks of transmitting infections such as Creutzfeldt-Jakob disease even after heating, phenol and irradiation [141].

Because of the four week delay in response and need for biopsies, attempts were made to develop a rapid *in-vitro* Kveim-Siltzbach test [142, 143]. These have been based on examining morphology of lymphoblastic transformation or macrophage activation in response to Kveim reagent, which was identified but most results were controversial and negative [144-146]. A study investigating stimulation of BAL and blood lymphocytes from sarcoidosis patients using Kveim antigen did not show any significant increase in lymphocyte responses to Kveim antigen as measured by lymphocyte DNA synthesis [147]. Hence no comprehensive *in vitro* Kveim-Siltzbach test has been developed that could be used for diagnostic purposes. Nevertheless, Kveim reagent or sarcoid tissues can theoretically be utilised as a lymphocyte stimulus *ex vivo*. Improvements to *in vitro* Kveim tests could include purer validated preparations [148], addition of macrophages for enhanced antigen presentation and reactivity, avoidance of sarcoid sera known to inhibit lymphocyte function and advanced immunological techniques [149].

It was later identified that the granulomagenic factor was an insoluble undegradable particulate, devoid of a consistently identifiable infectious agent by electron microscopy that aggregated in phagolysosomes of antigen presenting cells [38]. The Kveim reaction is characterised by an influx of mainly CD4+ T cells which express a restricted variable-β (Vβ) region of the T-cell receptor (TCR), indicating oligoclonal expansion in response to a limited number of antigens [150]. This may also indicate that the aetiological agent may be present in Kveim reagent as Vα and Vβ specific TCR oligoclonality has also been identified in T-cells from sites of sarcoid inflammation [150, 151]. Based on hypotheses that pathogenic antigens in sarcoidosis have similar physicochemical properties as Kveim reagent (including poor solubility in neutral detergent and resistance to acidity and protease digestion) [152], this led to a limited proteomics approach to determine potential antigens with these characteristics in sarcoidosis tissue homogenates [153]. Using matrix-assisted laser desorption/ionisation time of flight (MALDI-TOF) mass spectroscopy and protein immunoblotting, mycobacterial catalase-peroxidase (KatG) protein was identified in 55% of samples that was also a target of circulating IgG in 48% of sarcoidosis subjects [153]. This suggested that this remnant mycobacterial protein is one target of the adaptive immune response driving granulomatous inflammation in at least a subset of sarcoidosis tissues. Subsequently, investigations with IFN-γ ELISPOT and flow cytometry following intracellular staining for IFN-γ indicated greater peripheral blood mononuclear cell (PBMC) and BAL T_H1 responses to recombinant *Mycobacterium tuberculosis* KatG [83] and KatG peptides in patients with sarcoidosis compared to healthy controls. However, there was no difference when compared with PBMC from PPD+ control subjects, which profiles a pathogenic antigen in some patients with sarcoidosis [84,86-88]. We also determined that stimulation with pooled peptides from *M. tuberculosis* Early-Secretory Antigen Target-6 (ESAT-6) and KatG induced greater numbers of IFN-γ producing T-cells and elevated IL-2, IL-6 and TNF-α in sarcoidosis compared to PPD- healthy control subjects [67]. Since these mycobacterial antigens do not induce immune responses in all patients with sarcoidosis, newer, more specific approaches are thus needed to identify other potential antigens in Kveim reagent.

7. Important markers of granulomatous inflammation

7.1. Angiotensin Converting Enzyme (ACE)

Most clinicians are familiar with ACE, as it is the glycoprotein enzyme responsible for converting angiotensin I to angiotensin II, for which ACE inhibitors are used to treat hypertension and congestive heart failure. ACE is typically measured using a functional assay which measures ACE activity rather than ACE concentrations [154]. As the test is a functional biological assay, the presence of ACE inhibitors in the patient's serum can affect measurements [155]. ACE activity levels also tend to be higher in younger subjects [156].

ACE is a ubiquitous enzyme secreted by monocytes and macrophages, as well as pulmonary endothelial cells into the bloodstream where it exerts its actions. Serum ACE was first reported by Lieberman in 1975 as being elevated in patients with untreated active sarcoidosis [157, 158]. Sarcoid granulomas produce ACE, with the source being epithelioid and giant cells from the macrophage line [159]. Serum ACE activity is elevated in ~60% of patients with sarcoidosis [10, 160, 161], although values can vary depending on the time of diagnosis, extent of disease, acute or chronic disease and radiological stage and corticosteroid treatment. It is a useful diagnostic and prognostic tool, but normal levels do not exclude sarcoidosis and false positives are not uncommon. Serum ACE may also be elevated in a variety of other granulomatous and non-granulomatous diseases such as pulmonary silicosis, asbestosis [162], chronic beryllium disease [163], histoplasmosis [164], miliary tuberculosis, leprosy [165, 166], diabetes mellitus [167], hyperthyroidism [168] and Gaucher's disease [169]. Hence serum ACE activity in sarcoidosis is a marker of granuloma formation but with limited sensitivity and specificity. It must be interpreted with other markers of sarcoidosis, along with clinical and radiological features, although serial values may be helpful in disease monitoring. One confounding factor is that ACE activity in biological fluids is also affected by insertion/deletion (I/D) polymorphisms of the ACE gene and the Angiotensin II receptor 1 (AT2R1) gene [170]. Patients can be classified into three groups based on the ACE gene polymorphisms, including II, ID and DD. Homozygous carriers of the deletion mutation (DD) or the insertion (II) are associated with the highest and lowest ACE levels respectively, which can lead to underestimation or overestimation [171]. Patient genotyping for ACE I/D polymorphisms may improve assessment of ACE activity, however, there is a need for genotype-corrected reference levels.

ACE activity is also measurable and elevated in BAL fluid of patients with sarcoidosis [172] and is considered to provide better prognostic information than serum ACE. ACE has also been measured in urine and cerebrospinal fluid (CSF) and other biological fluids. Elevated CSF ACE has been identified as a useful marker in patients with suspected neurosarcoidosis, with values ≥8nmol/mL/min having a specificity of 94% and sensitivity of 55% in one study [173].

7.2. Lysozyme

Lysozyme is another monocyte-macrophage derived enzyme that may be considered a potential marker of macrophage activity. It is normally found in the granules of monocytes, macrophages, and neutrophils, where it may be released and is readily detectable in tears, saliva, airway secretions and CSF. Elevated serum lysozyme has been found in patients with active sarcoidosis, in ~30% of patients at clinical onset [30, 174, 175] and had been identified before the ACE test became available [176]. In sarcoidosis and in the Kveim reaction, immunohistochemical studies have identified the source of lysozyme as macrophages and epithelioid giant cells involved in granuloma formation [177]. Several authors have compared serum lysozyme with ACE and have identified a positive correlation between them, as both tests are positive in the majority of patients with acute disease [178, 179]. Lysozyme may be used to aid in the diagnosis of sarcoidosis and monitor disease course. However, the use of serum lysozyme is limited in clinical practice by its low sensitivity and specificity compared to other biomarkers, as it is also elevated in several other diseases [30].

7.3. Neopterin

Neopterin is a metabolite of guanosine triphosphate released by activated macrophages in response to IFN-γ [30, 180] and is elevated in serum and urine of patients with sarcoidosis [181, 182]. Other groups have detected elevated neopterin in patients with active disease [40, 183, 184] and have noted that levels fall with disease resolution [185, 186]. Interestingly, comparing neopterin to other serum and BAL markers demonstrated that elevated neopterin and sIL-2R were present in patients who were more likely to have progressive disease requiring long-term treatment with corticosteroids [40, 44].

7.4. Chitotriosidase

Chitotriosidase is a member of a group of enzymes involved in the breakdown of chitins (polymers of N-acetylglucosamine- commonly found in cell walls of fungi and exoskeletal elements of some animals and arthropods) [187]. The role of chitotriosidase in the pathogenesis of sarcoidosis is not clearly understood. It is believed that chronic over-expression, along with CCL18 over-expression (a chemokine involved in fibrotic remodelling of diffuse lung diseases) may induce pro-fibrotic T_H2 cytokines and fibronectin, predisposing to development of fibrosis [188]. In situ hybridisation has confirmed that alveolar macrophages from BAL fluid of patients with sarcoidosis are the primary source of this mediator [188, 189]. Serum chitotriosidase has been identified to be elevated in the serum of >90% of patients with sarcoidosis [190]. Significantly greater chitotriosidase activity was also demonstrated in the BAL and serum of sarcoidosis patients than in controls and levels generally increase with disease progression. BAL chitotriosidase activity also correlated with sarcoidosis radiological stages, serum ACE activity and radiological CT findings of fibrotic lung involvement [191]. Levels also decrease significantly with therapeutic interventions indicating that it may be a suitable marker of disease severity and granulomatous inflammation in sarcoidosis [187] and that it may have potential for identifying patients at risk of developing chronic fibrotic disease [191].

7.5. Other markers

Serum amyloid A is an amyloid precursor protein related to the high-density lipoprotein and is an innate receptor ligand with some physicochemical properties seen in the Kveim reagent [152]. It has been found to regulate granulomatous inflammation through Toll-like receptor-2 in experimental models of mKatG induced granulomatous lung inflammation and using alveolar macrophages from sarcoid patients [192]. Serum amyloid A is also an acute phase protein that is released together with C-reactive protein by the liver under systemic IL-1 and IL-6 stimulation and is hence also regarded as a nonspecific inflammatory marker of sarcoidosis, although it is less sensitive and specific than other markers such as sIL-2R [23].

Adenosine deaminase is an enzyme for purine metabolism that is important for differentiation of T lymphocytes. It has been studied in sarcoidosis and tuberculosis and is elevated in BAL fluid and serum in some cases of sarcoidosis [193]. Some studies have found serum adenosine deaminase to be useful, finding elevated levels in active sarcoidosis compared to inactive disease and healthy controls [194], whilst others found conflicting results indicating no relationship with disease activity [179].

Endothelin-1 is a vasoactive bronchoconstrictive peptide identified in pulmonary fibroproliferative processes and has been assessed in the serum, BAL, urine and lung tissues in sarcoidosis [195-197]. Elevated endothelin-1 levels have been associated with the clinical course of sarcoidosis and the degree of lymphocytic alveolitis and number of BAL macrophages [196, 197]. It is hypothesised that endothelin-1 may be involved in the development of pulmonary hypertension and fibrosis, although further studies are needed to confirm this in sarcoidosis.

Other markers studied in sarcoidosis include neutrophils and neutrophil-associated markers, which have been noted to be associated with chronic disease in sarcoidosis with progressive fibrosis and diffuse fibrotic lung disease. Important neutrophil markers studied in sarcoidosis include elastase and collagenase. Elastase appears to have a limited role in monitoring sarcoidosis although is elevated in those with chronic Stage III radiological disease [198]. Collagenase is elevated in the serum of some patients with sarcoidosis and elevated BAL collagenase has also been measured in conjunction with elevated fibronectin and is associated with more progressive and fibrotic disease [199].

8. A proteomics approach

Proteomics is emerging as a useful method of simultaneously analysing large numbers of proteins, including protein structure and functions in biological samples, as well as identifying profiles characteristic of disease processes. This approach has the potential to make new discoveries as the findings are usually independent of any earlier specific protein biomarkers. In sarcoidosis various proteomic techniques have been used for profiling protein patterns in BAL fluid and serum. Two-dimensional electrophoresis and mass spectrometry identified a total of 85 proteins in BAL fluid, of which 38 were newly identified in BAL from patients with sarcoidosis and idiopathic pulmonary fibrosis [200]. Proteins identified included locally secreted, plasma derived, proteolytic or cell damage products that have pro-inflammatory, anti-inflammatory and anti-protease activity. Compared with systemic sclerosis and idiopathic pulmonary fibrosis, BAL from patients with sarcoidosis also had greater acute phase proteins including ceruloplasmin, haptoglobin β, β_2-microglobulin and α_1-antichymotrypsin [59]. Other techniques have included applying narrow range pH gradients, which also identified new groups of proteins in the BAL and serum of patients with sarcoidosis, many of which are proteins involved in inflammatory and oxidative stress processes [201, 202]. This same group also applied difference gel electrophoresis proteomics to the analysis of BAL from patients at risk of developing chronic sarcoidosis (with a HLA-DRB1*15 genotype) compared with patients with chronic beryllium disease and controls. The investigators identified differing protein patterns between the three groups including increased peroxiredoxin 5, heat shock protein 70, complement C3, annexin A2 and transthyretin in sarcoidosis patients compared to the control group [203]. Other novel approaches have utilised surface-enhanced laser desorption ionization-time of flight-mass spectrometry (SELDI-TOF-MS) and have found different disease-related proteins and protein patterns in serum; identifying the α_2 chain of haptoglobin as a potential serologic marker [204]. This was also performed in BAL fluid of patients with sarcoidosis identifying proteins that may related to clinical course, including α_1-antitrypsin, protocadherin-2 precursor and albumin [205]. Proteomic analysis has provided a large-scale of novel data identifying protein biomarkers in sarcoidosis, which are different to those of healthy controls and patients with other interstitial lung diseases. However, much still needs to be done in identifying their role in the pathogenesis and validating the clinical utility of these markers in patients with sarcoidosis through further large-scale studies.

9. Exhaled breath analysis

Approximately 90% of patients with sarcoidosis have pulmonary disease involvement. It has hence been proposed that exhaled biomarkers from the lungs of patients with sarcoidosis could potentially be used to provide novel insights into the immunopathogenesis of the disease as well as for diagnosis and disease monitoring [1]. Initial studies investigating exhaled breath in sarcoidosis identified increased exhaled nitric oxide (FENO) in patients with sarcoidosis compared to healthy controls, which then reduced significantly after 6 weeks of treatment with corticosteroids [206]. Increased exhaled nitric oxide possibly reflects disease activity, and is associated with increased T_H1 immune responses. This may arise through up-regulation of nitric oxide synthase, which is induced (iNOS) by increased IFN-γ and TNF-α in active disease [206]. Other investigators however, found conflicting results, identifying that FENO from 59 patients with sarcoidosis did not differ significantly from 44 healthy controls and were not related to the extent of individual CT scan abnormalities or pulmonary function impairment [207]. Similar results have been obtained in a recent study examining multiple flow rates measurement of exhaled nitric oxide in patients with sarcoidosis and healthy controls, as well as patients treated with corticosteroids [208], which indicated that exhaled nitric oxide measurement did not appear to be a clinically useful method of monitoring disease progression in sarcoidosis. One study recently investigated the use of exhaled carbon monoxide (CO) in sarcoidosis, an oxidative stress biomarker for alveolar macrophage heme oxygenase activity. The authors identified a significantly elevated exhaled CO in patients with sarcoidosis compared to healthy controls and patients with miscellaneous interstitial lung disease [209]. However, the prognostic value of this measurement remains undefined and may be affected by cigarette smoke.

Exhaled breath condensate (EBC) analysis is a simple method of sampling airway lining fluids that has been shown to be useful for analysing exhaled breath markers [210-212] and is less invasive compared with induced sputum and BAL. Total protein levels are much higher in BAL than EBC [213], but nevertheless, the presence of a few biomarkers has been demonstrated in the EBC of patients with sarcoidosis. Levels of inflammatory markers e.g. TNF-α, Insulin-like growth factor-1 (IGF-1), and plasminogen activator inhibitor-1 (PAI-1) have been shown to be comparable and closely correlated in EBC and BAL samples, however, EBC IL-6 concentration was significantly lower when compared with that in BAL fluid in patients with sarcoidosis [214]. This study concluded that besides IL-6, EBC reflects cytokine production in the lung as effectively as BAL and may allow for a simplified sampling method. Hepatocyte growth factor (HGF) is produced by fibroblasts, causing strong epithelial proliferative responses and has been found to be elevated in EBC of patients with pneumonia [215]. However, levels of HGF are comparable in both EBC and BAL fluid of patients with sarcoidosis and healthy controls, suggesting it is not useful as an EBC biomarker in sarcoidosis [216]. Transforming growth factor-β_1 (TGF-β_1) has also recently been identified in the EBC of patients with sarcoidosis, along with vascular endothelial growth factor (VEGF), PAI-1, TNF-α and IL-8 but not urokinase-type plasminogen activator (uPA) [217]. TGF-β is implicated in fibrosis by inducing extracellular matrix synthesis and has been detected in *ex vivo* BAL cell cultures from patients with sarcoidosis [30], suggesting it may be a useful sarcoid EBC marker. Markers of granulomatous inflammation identified in our laboratory at greater levels in the EBC of patients with sarcoidosis compared to healthy controls include neopterin and TGF-β_1 (H. Ahmadzai, D. Wakefield, P.S. Thomas; unpublished observations), which could potentially be measured as airway markers of sarcoid activity.

Recent investigations have identified exhaled eicosanoids including 8-isoprostane and cysteinyl leukotrienes as being elevated in the EBC and BAL fluid of sarcoidosis patients [218]. A correlation has been identified between the levels of 8-isoprostane and leukotriene B_4 in BAL fluid and EBC of patients with sarcoidosis [219]. EBC levels of 8-isoprostane also positively correlate with the percentage of eosinophils in BAL and negatively with neutrophils [220, 221]. 8-isoprostane levels are increased in active sarcoidosis compared to healthy subjects, which may serve as a marker of disease severity and indicate increased oxidation [220]. Increased markers of oxidative stress including elevated hydrogen peroxide levels have also been demonstrated in EBC and BAL of sarcoidosis patients, as well as end-products of lipid peroxidation [222]. Growth factors, reactive oxygen species and products of oxidative stress in BAL and exhaled breath cannot yet be considered specific prognostic markers in sarcoidosis. Further research is needed into their potential clinical applications for disease monitoring.

10. Novel and experimental testing and conclusions

Laboratory and immunological testing has provided significant advances in the understanding of sarcoid immunopathogenesis and has allowed for easier diagnosis. Important recent findings have included the investigation of the immunology of the disease, through the $T_H1/T_H2/T_H17$ paradigm, which could provide further new insights into immunopathogenesis and potential treatments. Novel methods of identifying peripheral blood T-cell activation, such as with an in vitro Kveim reaction, could identify causative antigenic peptides. Large-scale studies validating initial proteomics findings from BAL and serum need to be conducted to identify the different clinical phenotypes of sarcoidosis and recognise patients at risk of chronic disease and pulmonary fibrosis. Simple, less invasive investigations such as exhaled breath analysis also need to be improved for clinical use. There is also potential for advanced immunological investigations including multiplex protein and gene expression technology to further investigate this intriguing disease. Although various biomarkers have been identified and proposed for diagnosis and monitoring, there is still no sufficiently specific or sensitive disease marker for clinical practice and much is yet to be understood.

Author details

Hasib Ahmadzai[1,2*], Paul S. Thomas[1,2,3] and Denis Wakefield[1,3,4]

*Address all correspondence to: h.ahmadzai@unswalumni.com

1 Inflammation and Infection Research Centre (IIRC), Faculty of Medicine, University of New South Wales, Sydney, NSW, Australia

2 Department of Respiratory Medicine, Prince of Wales Hospital, Randwick, NSW, Australia

3 Multidisciplinary Sarcoidosis Clinic, Prince of Wales Hospital, Randwick, NSW, Australia

4 Immunology of the Eye Clinic, St. Vincent's Clinic, Darlinghurst, NSW, Australia

References

[1] Ahmadzai H, Wakefield D, Thomas PS. The potential of the immunological markers of sarcoidosis in exhaled breath and peripheral blood as future diagnostic and monitoring techniques. Inflammopharmacology. 2011;19(2):55-68.

[2] Statement on Sarcoidosis. Joint Statement of the American Thoracic Society (ATS), the European Respiratory Society (ERS) and the World Association of Sarcoidosis and other Granulomatous Disorders (WASOG), adapted by the ATS Board of Directors and by the ERS Executive Committee. American Journal of Respiratory and Critical Care Medicine. 1999;160(2):736-55.

[3] Gerke AK, Hunninghake G. The Immunology of Sarcoidosis. Clinics in Chest Medicine. 2008;29(3):379-90.

[4] Hunninghake GW, Fulmer JD, Young RC Jr, Gadek JE, Crystal RG. Localization of the immune response in sarcoidosis. The American Review of Respiratory Disease. 1979;120(1):49-57.

[5] Mathew S, Bauer KL, Fischoeder A, Bhardwaj N, Oliver SJ. The Anergic State in Sarcoidosis is Associated with Diminished Dendritic Cell Function. The Journal of Immunology. 2008;181:746-55.

[6] Grunewald J, Eklund A. Role of CD4+ T cells in Sarcoidosis. Proceedings of the American Thoracic Society. 2007;4(5):461-4.

[7] Mert A, Bilir M, Ozaras R, Tabak F, Karayel T, Senturk H. Results of Hepatitis B Vaccination in Sarcoidosis. Respiration. 2000;67(5):543-5.

[8] Nunes H, Soler P, Valeyre D. Pulmonary sarcoidosis. Allergy. 2005;60(5):565-82.

[9] Baughman RP, Teirstein AS, Judson MA, Rossman MD, Yeager H Jr, Bresnitz EA, et
al. Clinical characteristics of patients in a case control study of sarcoidosis. American
Journal of Respiratory and Critical Care Medicine. 2001;164(10 Pt 1):1885-9.

[10] Iannuzzi MC, Rybicki BA, Teirstein AS. Sarcoidosis. The New England Journal of
Medicine. 2007;357(21):2153-65.

[11] Hunninghake GW, Costabel U, Ando M, Baughman R, Cordier JF, du Bois R, et al.
ATS/ERS/WASOG statement on sarcoidosis. American Thoracic Society/European
Respiratory Society/World Association of Sarcoidosis and other Granulomatous Dis-
orders. Sarcoidosis, Vasculitis & Diffuse Lung Diseases. 1999;16(2):149-73.

[12] Berliner AR, Haas M, Choi MJ. Sarcoidosis: the nephrologist's perspective. American
Journal of Kidney Diseases. 2006;48(5):856-70.

[13] Ponce C, Gujral JS. Renal failure and hypercalcemia as initial manifestations of extrapulmonary sarcoidosis. Southern Medical Journal. 2004;97(6):590-2.

[14] Rizzato G, Colombo P. Nephrolithiasis as a presenting feature of chronic sarcoidosis:
a prospective study. Sarcoidosis, Vasculitis & Diffuse Lung Diseases. 1996;13(2):
167-72.

[15] Reichel H, Koeffler HP, Barbers R, Norman AW. Regulation of 1,25-dihydroxyvita-
min D3 production by cultured alveolar macrophages from normal human donors
and from patients with pulmonary sarcoidosis. Journal of Clinical Endocrinology
and Metabolism. 1987;65(6):1201-9.

[16] Clavel S, Garabedian M, Tau C, Orgiazzi J. Extrarenal synthesis of calcitriol in sarcoidosis. [Article in French]. Presse médicale. 1987;16(3):107-10.

[17] Inui N, Murayama A, Sasaki S, Suda T, Chida K, Kato S, et al. Correlation between
25-hydroxyvitamin D3 1 alpha-hydroxylase gene expression in alveolar macrophages and the activity of sarcoidosis. The American Journal of Medicine. 2001;110(9):
687-93.

[18] Barbour GL, Coburn JW, Slatopolsky E, Norman AW, Horst RL. Hypercalcemia in an
anephric patient with sarcoidosis: evidence for extrarenal generation of 1,25-dihy-
droxyvitamin D. The New England Journal of Medicine. 1981;305(8):440-3.

[19] Richmond BW, Drake WP. Vitamin D, innate immunity, and sarcoidosis granulomatous inflammation: insights from mycobacterial research. Current Opinion in Pulmonary Medicine. 2010;16(5):461-4.

[20] Playford EG, Bansal AS, Looke DF, Whitby M, Hogan PG. Hypercalcaemia and elevated 1,25(OH)(2)D(3) levels associated with disseminated Mycobacterium avium infection in AIDS. The Journal of Infection. 2001;42(2):157-8.

[21] Liu JW, Huang TC, Lu YC, Liu HT, Li CC, Wu JJ, et al. Acute disseminated histoplasmosis complicated with hypercalcaemia. The Journal of Infection. 1999;39(1):88-90.

[22] Caldwell JW, Arsura EL, Kilgore WB, Reddy CM, Johnson RH. Hypercalcemia in patients with disseminated coccidioidomycosis. The American Journal of the Medical Sciences. 2004;327(1):15-8.

[23] Rothkrantz-Kos S, van Dieijen-Visser MP, Mulder PG, Drent M. Potential usefulness of inflammatory markers to monitor respiratory functional impairment in sarcoidosis. Clinical Chemistry. 2003;49(9):1510-7.

[24] Shorr AF, Murphy FT, Gilliland WR, Hnatiuk W. Osseous disease in patients with pulmonary sarcoidosis and musculoskeletal symptoms. Respiratory Medicine. 2000;94(3):228-32.

[25] Greenberg G, James DG, Feizi T, Bird R. Serum-proteins in sarcoidosis. The Lancet. 1964;2(7373):1315-5.

[26] Drent M, Wirnsberger RM, de Vries J, van Dieijen-Visser MP, Wouters EF, Schols AM. Association of fatigue with an acute phase response in sarcoidosis. European Respiratory Journal. 1999;13(4):718-22.

[27] Hind CR, Flint KC, Hudspith BN, Felmingham D, Brostoff J, Johnson NM. Serum C-reactive protein concentrations in patients with pulmonary sarcoidosis. Thorax. 1987;42(5):332-5.

[28] Peros-Golubicić T. Serum C-reactive protein measurement in the detection of intercurrent infection in patients with sarcoidosis. Acta Medica Croatica. 1995;49(1):1-3.

[29] Miyara M, Amoura Z, Parizot C, Badoual C, Dorgham K, Trad S, et al. The immune paradox of sarcoidosis and regulatory T cells. The Journal of Experimental Medicine. 2006;203(2):359-70.

[30] Bargagli E, Mazzi A, Rottoli P. Markers of Inflammation in sarcoidosis: Blood, Urine, BAL, Sputum, and Exhaled Gas. Clinics in Chest Medicine. 2008;29(3):445- 58.

[31] Ziegenhagen MW, Muller-Quernheim J. The cytokine network in sarcoidosis and its clinical relevance. Journal of Internal Medicine. 2003;253:18-30.

[32] Betelli E, Kom T, Oukka M, Kuchroo VK. Induction and effector functions of TH17 cells. Nature. 2008;453(1051-1057).

[33] Facco M, Cabrelle A, Teramo A, Olivieri V, Gnoato M, Teolato S, et al. Sarcoidosis is a Th1/Th17 multisystem disorder. Thorax. 2010;66(2):144-50.

[34] Ten Berge B, Paats MS, Bergen IM, van den Blink B, Hoogsteden HC, Lambrecht BN, et al. Increased IL-17A expression in granulomas and in circulating memory T cells in sarcoidosis. Rheumatology. 2012;51(1):37-46.

[35] Judson MA, Marchell RM, Mascelli M, Piantone A, Barnathan ES, Petty KJ, et al. Molecular profiling and gene expression analysis in cutaneous sarcoidosis: the role of interleukin-12, interleukin-23, and the T-helper 17 pathway. Journal of the American Academy of Dermatology. 2012;66(6):901-10.

[36] Meloni F, Solari N, Cavagna L, Morosini M, Montecucco CM, Fietta AM. Frequency of Th1, Th2 and Th17 producing T lymphocytes in bronchoalveolar lavage of patients with systemic sclerosis. Clinical and experimental Rheumatology. 2009;27(5):765-72.

[37] Wikén M, Idali F, Al Hayja MA, Grunewald J, Eklund A, Wahlström J. No evidence of altered alveolar macrophage polarization, but reduced expression of TLR2 in bronchoalveolar lavage cells in sarcoidosis. Respiratory Research. 2010;11(1):121-33.

[38] Kataria YP, Holter JF. Immunology of sarcoidosis. Clinics in Chest Medicine. 1997;18(4):719-39.

[39] Olejniczak K, Kasprzak A. Biological properties of interleukin 2 and its role in pathogenesis of selected diseases--a review. Medical Science Monitor. 2008;14(10):RA179-89.

[40] Ziegenhagen MW, Rothe ME, Schlaak M, Müller-Quernheim J. Bronchoalveolar and serological parameters reflecting the severity of sarcoidosis. European Respiratory Journal. 2003;21(3):407-13.

[41] Grutters JC, Fellrath JM, Mulder L, Janssen R, van den Bosch JM, van Velzen-Blad H. Serum soluble interleukin-2 receptor measurement in patients with sarcoidosis: a clinical evaluation. Chest. 2003;124(1):186-95.

[42] Lawrence EC, Brousseau KP, Berger MB, Kurman CC, Marcon L, Nelson DL. Elevated concentrations of soluble interleukin-2 receptors in serum samples and bronchoalveolar lavage fluids in active sarcoidosis. American Review of Respiratory Disease. 1988;137(4):759-64.

[43] Keicho N, Kitamura K, Takaku F, Yotsumoto H. Serum concentration of soluble interleukin-2 receptor as a sensitive parameter of disease activity in sarcoidosis. Chest. 1990;98(5):1125-9.

[44] Prasse A, Katic C, Germann M, Buchwald A, Zissel G, Müller-Quernheim J. Phenotyping sarcoidosis from a pulmonary perspective. American Journal of Respiratory and Critical Care Medicine. 2008;177(3):330-6.

[45] Parrish RW, Williams JD, Davies BH. Serum beta-2-microglobulin and angiotensin-converting enzyme activity in sarcoidosis. Thorax. 1982;37(12):936-40.

[46] Selroos O, Klockars M. Relation between clinical stage of sarcoidosis and serum values of angiotensin converting enzyme and beta2-microglobulin. Sarcoidosis. 1987;4(1):13-7.

[47] Mornex JF, Revillard JP, Vincent C, Deteix P, Brune J. Elevated serum beta 2-microglobulin levels and C1q-binding immune complexes in sarcoidosis. Biomedicine. 1979;31(7):210-3.

[48] Oksanen V. New cerebrospinal fluid, neurophysiological and neuroradiological examinations in the diagnosis and follow-up of neurosarcoidosis. Sarcoidosis. 1987;4(2):105-10.

[49] Costabel U, Bonella F, Ohshimo S, Guzman J. Diagnostic modalities in sarcoidosis: BAL, EBUS, and PET. Seminars in Respiratory and Critical Care Medicine. 2010;31(4): 404-8.

[50] Agostini C, Trentin L, Zambello R, Bulian P, Siviero F, Masciarelli M, et al. CD8 alveolitis in sarcoidosis: incidence, phenotypic characteristics, and clinical features. The American Journal of Medicine. 1993;95(5):466-72.

[51] Wahlström J, Berlin M, Sköld CM, Wigzell H, Eklund A, Grunewald J. Phenotypic analysis of lymphocytes and monocytes/macrophages in peripheral blood and bronchoalveolar lavage fluid from patients with pulmonary sarcoidosis. Thorax. 1999;54:339-46.

[52] Hill TA, Lightman S, Pantelidis P, Abdallah A, Spagnolo P, du Bois RM. Intracellular cytokine profiles and T cell activation in pulmonary sarcoidosis. Cytokine. 2008;42:289-92.

[53] Saltini C, Spurzem JR, Lee JJ, Pinkston P, Crystal RG. Spontaneous release of interleukin 2 by lung T lymphocytes in active pulmonary sarcoidosis is primarily from the Leu3+DR+ T cell subset. Journal of Clinical Investigation. 1986;77(6):1962-70.

[54] Katchar K, Wahlström J, Eklund A, Grunewald J. Highly activated T-cell receptor AV2S3(+) CD4(+) lung T-cell expansions in pulmonary sarcoidosis. American Journal of Respiratory and Critical Care Medicine. 2001;163(7):1540-5.

[55] Wahlström J, Dengjel J, Persson B, Duyar H, Rammensee HG, Stevanović S, et al. Identification of HLA-DR-bound peptides presented by human bronchoalveolar lavage cells in sarcoidosis. Journal of Clinical Investigation. 2007;117(11):3576-82.

[56] Inui N, Chida K, Suda T, Nakamura H. TH1/TH2 and TC1/TC2 profiles in peripheral blood and bronchoalveolar lavage fluid cells in pulmonary sarcoidosis. Journal of Allergy and Clinical Immunology. 2001;107(2):337-44.

[57] Mllers M, Aries SP, Drmann D, Mascher B, Braun J, Dalhoff K. Intracellular cytokine repertoire in different T cell subsets from patients with sarcoidosis. Thorax. 2001;56:487-93.

[58] Wahlström J, Katchar K, Wigzell H, Olerup O, Eklund A, Grunewald J. Analysis of Intracellular Cytokines in CD4+ and CD8+ Lung and Blood T cells in Sarcoidosis. American Journal of Respiratory and Critical Care Medicine. 2001;163:115-21.

[59] Rottoli P, Magi B, Perari MG, Liberatori S, Nikiforakis N, Bargagli E, et al. Cytokine profile and proteome analysis in bronchoalveolar lavage of patients with sarcoidosis, pulmonary fibrosis associated with systemic sclerosis and idiopathic pulmonary fibrosis. Proteomics. 2005;5:1423-30.

[60] Shigehara K, Shijubo N, Ohmichi M, Takahashi R, Kon S, Okamura H, et al. IL-12 and IL-18 Are Increased and Stimulate IFN-γ Production in Sarcoid Lungs. The Journal of Immunology. 2001;166:642-9.

[61] Katchar K, Eklund A, Grunewald J. Expression of Th1 markers by lung accumulated T cells in pulmonary sarcoidosis. Journal of Internal Medicine. 2003;254:564-71.

[62] Nureki S, Miyazaki E, Ando M, Ueno T, Fukami T, Kumamoto T, et al. Circulating levels of both Th1 and Th2 chemokines are elevated in patients with sarcoidosis. Respiratory Medicine. 2008;102:239-47.

[63] Tsiligianni I, Antoniou KM, Kyriakou D, Tzanakis N, Chrysofakis G, Siafakas NM, et al. Th1/Th2 cytokine pattern in bronchoalveolar lavage fluid and induced sputum in pulmonary sarcoidosis. BMC Pulmonary Medicine. 2005;5:8-13.

[64] Sobiecka M, Kus J, Demkow U, Filewska M, Jozwik A, Radwan-Rohrenschef P, et al. Induced sputum in patients with interstitial lung disease: a non-invasive surrogate for certain parameters in bronchoalveolar lavage fluid. Journal of Physiology and Pharmacology. 2008;59(Suppl 6):645-57.

[65] Mroz RM, Korniluk M, Stasiak-Barmuta A, Ossolinska M, Chyczewska E. Increased levels of Treg cells in bronchoalveolar lavage fluid and induced sputum of patients with active pulmonary sarcoidosis. European Journal of Medical Research. 2009;14(Suppl 4):165-9.

[66] Mroz MM, Kreiss K, Lezotte DC, Campbell PA, Newman LS. Reexamination of the blood lymphocyte transformation test in the diagnosis of chronic beryllium disease. The Journal of Allergy and Clinical Immunology. 1991;88(1):54-60.

[67] Ahmadzai H, Cameron B, Chui JJ, Lloyd A, Wakefield D, Thomas PS. Peripheral blood responses to specific antigens and CD28 in sarcoidosis. Respiratory Medicine. 2012;106(5):701-9.

[68] Seyhan EC, Günlüoǒlu G, Altin S, Çetinkaya E, Sökücü S, Uzun H, et al. Results of teanus vaccination in sarcoidosis. Sarcoidosis, Vasculitis & Diffuse Lung Diseases. 2012;29(1):3-10.

[69] Friou GJ. A study of the cutaneous reactions to oidomycin, trichopytin and mumps skin test antigens in patients with sarcoidosis. Yale Journal of Biology and Medicine. 1952;24:533-9.

[70] Jones JV. Development of sensitivity to dinitrochlorobenzene in patients with sarcoidosis. Clinical and Experimental Immunology. 1967;2:477-87.

[71] Daniele RP, Dauber JH, Rossman MD. Immunologic abnormalities in sarcoidosis. Annals of Internal Medicine. 1980;92(3):406-16.

[72] Kataria YP, LoBuglio AF, Helentjaris T, Bromberg PA. Phytohemagglutinin (PHA) skin test in patients with sarcoidosis. American Review of Respiratory Disease. 112(4):575-8.

[73] Gupta D, Chetty M, Kumar N, Aggarwal AN, Jindal SK. Anergy to tuberculin in sarcoidosis is not influenced by high prevalence of tuberculin sensitivity in the population. Sarcoidosis, Vasculitis & Diffuse Lung Diseases. 2003;20(1):40-5.

[74] Amicosante M. IGRAs for tuberculosis in sarcoidosis patients: is the immune response to mycobacteria helpful in the differential diagnosis or still a confounding factor? Sarcoidosis, Vasculitis & Diffuse Lung Diseases. 2011;28(2):85-6.

[75] Gupta D, Kumar S, Aggarwal AN, Verma I, Agarwal R. Interferon gamma release assay (QuantiFERON-TB Gold In Tube) in patients of sarcoidosis from a population with high prevalence of tuberculosis infection. Sarcoidosis, Vasculitis & Diffuse Lung Diseases. 2011;28(2):95-101.

[76] Luetkemeyer AF, Charlebois ED, Flores LL, Bangsberg DR, Deeks SG, Martin JN, et al. Comparison of an interferon-gamma release assay with tuberculin skin testing in HIV-infected individuals. American Journal of Respiratory and Critical Care Medicine. 2007;175(7):737-42.

[77] Mori T, Sakatani M, Yamagishi F, Takashima T, Kawabe Y, Nagao K, et al. Specific detection of tuberculosis infection: an interferon-gamma-based assay using new antigens. American Journal of Respiratory and Critical Care Medicine. 2004;170(1):59-64.

[78] Iannuzzi MC, Fontana JR. Sarcoidosis: clinical presentation, immunopathogenesis, and therapeutics. Jorunal of the Aerican Medical Association. 2011;305(4):391-9.

[79] James GD, Williams WJ. 2. Classification of granulomatous disorders: a clinicopathological synthesis. In: James GD, Zumla, A., editor. The Granulomatous Disorders. Cambridge: Cambridge University Press; 1999.

[80] Ezzie ME, Crouser ED. Considering an infectious etiology of sarcoidosis. Clinics in Dermatology. 2007;25(3):259-66.

[81] Inui N, Suda T, Chida K. Use of the QuantiFERON-TB Gold test in Japanese patients with sarcoidosis. Respiratory Medicine. 2008;102:313-5.

[82] Hörster R, Kirsten D, Gaede KI, Jafari C, Strassburg A, Greinert U, et al. Antimycobacterial immune responses in patients with pulmonary sarcoidosis. The Clinical Respiratory Journal. 2009;3(4):229-38.

[83] Chen ES, Wahlström J, Song Z, Willett MH, Wikén M, Yung RC, et al. T Cell Responses to Mycobacterial Catalase-Peroxidase Profile a Pathogenic Antigen in Systemic Sarcoidosis. The Journal of Immunology. 2008;181(8784-8796).

[84] Oswald-Richter K, Culver DA, Hawkins C, Hajizadeh R, Abraham S, Shepherd BE, et al. Cellular Responses to Mycobacterial Antigens Are Present in Bronchoalveolar Lavage Fluid Used in the Diagnosis of Sarcoidosis. Infection and Immunity. 2009;77(9):3740-8.

[85] Oswald-Richter K, Sato H, Hajizadeh R, Shepherd BE, Sidney J, Sette A, et al. Mycobacterial ESAT-6 and katG are Recognized by Sarcoidosis CD4+ T Cells When Presented by the American Sarcoidosis Susceptibility Allele, DRB1*1101. Journal of Clinical Immunology. 2010;30:157-66.

[86] Oswald-Richter K, Beachboard DC, Zhan X, Gaskill CF, Abrahams S, Jenkins C, et al. Multiple mycobacterial antigens are targets of the adaptive immune response in pulmonary sarcoidosis. Respiratory Research. 2010;11:161.

[87] Drake WP, Dhason MS, Nadaf M, Shepherd BE, Vadivelu S, Hajizadeh R, et al. Cellular Recognition of Mycobacterium tuberculosis ESAT-6 and KatG Peptides in Systemic Sarcoidosis. Infection and Immunity. 2007;75(1):527-30.

[88] Carlisle J, Evans W, Hajizadeh R, Nadaf M, Shepherd B, Ott RD, et al. Multiple Mycobacterium antigens induce interferon-γ production for sarcoidosis peripheral blood mononuclear cells. Clinical and Experimental Immunology. 2007;150:460-8.

[89] Dubaniewicz A, Trzonkowski P, Dubaniewicz-Wybieralska M, Dubaniewicz A, Singh M, Myśliwski A. Mycobacterial heat shock protein-induced blood T lymphocytes subsets and cytokine pattern: Comparison of sarcoidosis with tuberculosis and healthy controls. Respirology. 2007;12:346-54.

[90] Dubaniewicz A. Mycobacterium tuberculosis heat shock proteins and autoimmunity in sarcoidosis. Autoimmunity Reviews. 2010;9(6):419-24.

[91] 91. Hajizadeh R, Sato H, Carlisle J, Nadaf MT, Evans W, Shepherd BE, et al. Mycobacterium tuberculosis Antigen 85A Induces Th-1 Immune Responses in Systemic Sarcoidosis. Journal of Clinical Immunology. 2007;27(4):445-54.

[92] Allen SS, Evans W, Carlisle J, Hajizadeh R, Nadaf M, Shepherd BE, et al. Superoxide dismutase A antigens derived from molecular analysis of sarcoidosis granulomas elicit systemic Th-1 immune responses. Respiratory Research. 2008;9:36-47.

[93] Oswald-Richter KA, Beachboard DC, Seeley EH, Abraham S, Shepherd BE, Jenkins CA, et al. Dual Analysis for Mycobacteria and Propionibacteria in Sarcoidosis BAL. Journal of Clinical Immunology. 2012;32(5):1129-40.

[94] Brincker H, Pedersen NT. Immunohistologic separation of B-cell-positive granulomas from B-cell-negative granulomas in paraffin-embedded tissues with special ref-

erence to tumor-related sarcoid reactions. Acta Pathologica, Microbiologica et Immunologica Scandinavica. 1991;99(3):282-90.

[95] Brownell I, Ramírez-Valle F, Sanchez M, Prystowsky S. Evidence for mycobacteria in sarcoidosis. American Journal of Respiratory Cell and Molecular Biology. 2011;45(5): 899-905.

[96] Richter J, Bartak F, Halova R. Detection of mycobacteria by fluorescent microscopy in sarcoidosis. In: Levinsky L, Macholda F, editors. 5th International Conference on Sarcoidosis; June 16-21, 1969; Prague: University Karlova; 1971. p 83-4.

[97] Ma Y, Gal A, Koss MN. The pathology of pulmonary sarcoidosis: update. Seminars in Diagnostic Pathology. 2007;24(3):150-61.

[98] Alavi HA, Moscovic EA. Immunolocalization of cell-wall-deficient forms of Mycobacterium tuberculosis complex in sarcoidosis and in sinus histiocytosis of lymph nodes draining carcinoma. Histology and Histopathology. 1996;11(3):683-94.

[99] Cantwell ARJ. Histologic observations of variably acid-fast pleomorphic bacteria in systemic sarcoidosis: a report of 3 cases. Growth. 1982;46(2):113-25.

[100] Kon OM, du Bois RM. Mycobacteria and sarcoidosis. Thorax. 1997;52(Supp 3):S47-S51.

[101] Brown ST, Brett I, Almenoff PL, Lesser M, Terrin M, Teirstein AS. Recovery of cell wall-deficient organisms does not distinguish between patients with sarcoidosis and control subjects. Chest. 2003;123(413-417).

[102] Almenoff PL, Johnson A, Lesser M, Mattman LH. Growth of acid fast L forms from the blood of patients with sarcoidosis. Thorax. 1996;51(5):530-3.

[103] Moscovic EA. Sarcoidosis and mycobacterial L-forms. A critical reappraisal of pleomorphic chromogenic bodies (Hamazaki corpuscles) in lymph nodes. Pathology Annual. 1978;13(Pt 2):69-164.

[104] el-Zaatari FA, Naser SA, Markesich DC, Kalter DC, Engstand L, Graham DY. Identification of Mycobacterium avium complex in sarcoidosis. Journal of Clinical Microbiology. 1996;34(9):2240-5.

[105] Onwuamaegbu ME, Belcher RA, Soare C. Cell wall-deficient bacteria as a cause of infections: a review of the clinical significance. The Journal of International Medical Research. 2005;33(1):1-20.

[106] Hess CL, Wolock BS, Murphy MS. Mycobacterium marinum infections of the upper extremity. Plastic and Reconstructive Surgery. 2005;115(3):55e-9e.

[107] Moling O, Sechi LA, Zanetti S, Seebacher C, Rossi P, Rimenti G, et al. Mycobacterium marinum, a further infectious agent associated with sarcoidosis: the polyetiology hypothesis. Scandinavian Journal of Infectious Diseases. 2006;38(2):148-52.

[108] Saboor SA, Johnson NM, McFadden J. Detection of mycobacterial DNA in sarcoido-
       sis and tuberculosis with polymerase chain reaction. The Lancet. 1992;339(1012-1015).

[109] Fidler HM, Rook GA, Johnson NM, McFadden J. Mycobacterium tuberculosis DNA
       in tissue affected by sarcoidosis. British Medical Journal. 1993;306(6877):546-9.

[110] Grosser M, Luther T, Muller J, Schuppler M, Brickhardt J, Matthiessen W, et al. De-
       tection of M. tuberculosis DNA in Sarcoidosis: correlation with T-cell response. Labo-
       ratory Investigation. 1999;79(7):775-84.

[111] Klemen H, Husain AN, Cagle PT, Garrity ER, Popper HH. Mycobacterial DNA in re-
       current sarcoidosis in the transplanted lung- a PCR-based study on four cases. Virch-
       ows Archiv. 2000;436(4):365-9.

[112] Drake WP, Pei Z, Pride DT, Collins RD, Cover TL, Blaser MJ. Molecular analysis of
       sarcoidosis tissues for mycobacterium species DNA. Emerging Infectious Diseases.
       2002;8(11):1334-41.

[113] Eishi Y, Suga M, Ishige I, Kobayashi D, Yamada T, Takemura T, et al. Quantitative
       analysis of mycobacterial and propionibacterial DNA in lymph nodes of Japanese
       and European patients with sarcoidosis. Journal of Clinical Microbiology. 2002;40(1):
       198-204.

[114] Svendsen CB, Milman N, Rasmussen EM, Thomsen VØ, Andersen CB, Krogfelt KA.
       The continuing search for Mycobacterium tuberculosis involvement in sarcoidosis: a
       study on archival biopsy specimens. The Clinical Respiratory Journal. 2011;5(2):
       99-104.

[115] Lisby G, Milman N, Jacobsen GK. Search for Mycobacterium paratuberculosis DNA
       in tissue from patients with sarcoidosis by enzymatic gene amplification. Acta Patho-
       logica, Microbiologica et Immunologica Scandinavica. 1993;101(11):876-8.

[116] Vokurka M, Lecoissier D, du Bois RM, Wallaert B, Kambouchner M, Tazi A, et al.
       Absence of DNA from mycobacteria of the M, tuberculosis complex in sarcoidosis.
       American Journal of Respiratory and Critical Care Medicine. 1997;156(1000-1003).

[117] Gupta D, Agarwal R, Agarwal AN, Jindal SK. Molecular evidence for the role of my-
       cobacteria in sarcoidosis: A meta-analysis. European Respiratory Journal. 2007;30(3):
       508-16.

[118] Milman N. From Mycobacteria to Sarcoidosis - Is the Gate Still Open? Respiration.
       2006;73:14-5.

[119] Abe C, Iwai K, Mikami R, Hosoda Y. Frequent isolation of Propionibacterium acnes
       from sarcoidosis lymph nodes. Zentralbl Bakteriol Mikrobiol Hyg A. 1984;256(4):
       541-7.

[120] Ebe Y, Ikushima S, Yamaguchi T, Kohno K, Azuma A, Sato K, et al. Proliferative re-
       sponse of peripheral blood mononuclear cells and levels of antibody to recombinant

protein from Propionibacterium acnes DNA expression library in Japanese patients with sarcoidosis. Sarcoidosis, Vasculitis & Diffuse Lung Diseases. 2000;17(3):256-65.

[121] Ishige I, Usui Y, Takemura T, Eishi Y. Quantitative PCR of mycobacterial and propionibacterial DNA in lymph nodes of Japanese patients with sarcoidosis. The Lancet. 1999;354(9173):120-3.

[122] Gazouli M, Ikonomopoulos J, Trigidou R, Foteinou M, Kittas C, Gorgoulis V. Assessment of mycobacterial, propionibacterial, and human herpesvirus 8 DNA in tissues of Greek patients with sarcoidosis. Journal of Clinical Microbiology. 2002;40:3060-3.

[123] Yamada T, Eishi Y, Ikeda S, Ishige I, Suzuki T, Takemura T, et al. In situ localization of Propionibacterium acnes DNA in lymph nodes from sarcoidosis patients by signal amplification with catalysed reporter deposition. The Journal of Pathology. 2002;198(4):541-7.

[124] Ishige I, Eishi Y, Takemura T, Kobayashi I, Nakata K, Tanaka I, et al. Propionibacterium acnes is the most common bacterium commensal in peripheral lung tissue and mediastinal lymph nodes from subjects without sarcoidosis. Sarcoidosis, Vasculitis and Diffuse Lung Diseases. 2005;22(1):33-42.

[125] Newman LS, Rose CS, Maier LA. Sarcoidosis. The New England Journal of Medicine. 1997;336(17):1224-34.

[126] Yamada M, Fujimoto, F. Lymphocyte transformation using Mitsuda antigen (lepromin). The Journal of Dermatology. 1975;2(4):175-8.

[127] Proença NG. Interpretation of the Mitsuda and Kveim tests in the differential diagnosis of tuberculoid hanseniasis and cutaneous sarcoidosis. [Article in Portuguese]. Medicina cutánea ibero-latino-americana. 1989;17(3):163-5.

[128] Rossman MD, Kreider ME. Is chronic beryllium disease sarcoidosis of known etiology? Sarcoidosis, Vasculitis & Diffuse Lung Diseases. 2003;20:104-9.

[129] Newman KL, Newman LS. Occupational causes of sarcoidosis. Current Opinion in Allergy and Clinical Immunology. 2012;12(2):145-50.

[130] Pott GB, Palmer BE, Sullivan AK, Silviera L, Maier LA, Newman LS, et al. Frequency of beryllium-specific, TH1-type cytokine-expressing CD4+ T cells in patients with beryllium-induced disease. Journal of Allergy and Clinical Immunology. 2005;115(5):1036-42.

[131] Tinkle SS, Kittle LA, Schumacher BA, Newman LS. Beryllium induces IL-2 and IFN-gamma in berylliosis. Journal of Immunology. 1997;158(1):518-26.

[132] Glazer CS, Newman LS. 15. Beryllium as a model for sarcoidosis. In: Baughman RP, editor. Lung Biology in Health and Disease- Sarcoidosis. New York: Taylor and Francis Group; 2006.

[133] Siltzbach LE. The Kveim test in sarcoidosis: a study of 750 patients. Journal of the American Medical Association. 1961;178:476-82.

[134] Teirstein AS. The Kveim-Siltzbach test. Clinics in Dermatology. 1986;4(4):154-64.

[135] Kveim A. En ny og spesifikk kutan-reaksjon ved Boeck's sarcoid. Nordisk medicin. 1941;9:169-72.

[136] Parrish S, Turner JF. Diagnosis of Sarcoidosis. Disease-a-Month. 2009;55(11):693-703.

[137] Holter JF, Park, H.K., Sjoerdsma, K.W., Kataria, Y.P. Nonviable autologous bronchoalveolar lavage cell preparations induce intradermal epithelioid cell granulomas in sarcoidosis patients. American Review of Respiratory Disease. 1992;145(4 Pt 1): 864-71.

[138] Gaede KI, Kataria YP, Mamat U, Müller-Quernheim J. Analysis of differentially regulated mRNAs in monocytic cells induced by in vitro stimulation with Kveim-Siltzbach test reagent. Experimental Lung Research. 2004;30(3):181-92.

[139] Siltzbach LE, editor. An international Kveim test study in sarcoidosis. Proceedings of the Fourth International Conference on sarcoidosis; 1967; Paris: Mason.

[140] Mishra BB, Poulter LW, Janossy G, Sherlock S, James DG. The Kveim-Siltzbach granuloma. A model for sarcoid granuloma formation. Annals of the New York Academy of Sciences. 1986;465(164-75.).

[141] de Silva RN, Will RG. Moratorium on Kveim test. The Lancet. 1993;342(8864):173.

[142] Williams WJ, Price CD, Pugh A, Dighero M. In vitro (KMIF) Test. Zeitschrift für Erkrankungen der Atmungsorgane. 1977;149(2):226-30.

[143] Lyons DJ, Mitchell EB, Mitchell DN. Sarcoidosis: in search of Kveim reactivity in vitro. Biomedicine and Pharmacotherapy. 1991;45(4-5):187-92.

[144] Cowling DC, Quaglino D, Barrett PKM. Effect of Kveim Antigen and Old Tuberculin on Lymphocytes in Culture from Sarcoid Patients. British Medical Journal. 1964;1(5396):1481-2.

[145] Kurti V, Mankiewicz E. In vitro study of macrophages from patients with sarcoidosis. Canadian Medical Association Journal. 1972;107(6):509-15.

[146] Izumi T, Nilsson BS, Ripe E. In vitro lymphocyte reactivity to different Kveim preparations in patients with sarcoidosis. Scandinavian Journal of Respiratory Diseases. 1973;54(2):123-7.

[147] Lindahl M, Andersson O, Ripe E, Holm G. Stimulation of Bronchoalveolar (BAL) and blood lymphocytes by Kveim antigen, Tuberculin, and Concanavalin A in sarcoidosis. British Diseases of the Chest. 1988;82(4):386-93.

[148] Chase MW, Siltzbach LE, editor. Concentration of the active principle responsible for the Kveim reaction. Proceedings of the 4th International Conference on Sarcoidosis; 1967; Paris: Mason.

[149] James GD, Williams WJ. Kveim-Siltzbach Test Revisited. Sarcoidosis. 1991;8(1):6-9.

[150] Klein JT, Horn TD, Forman JD, Silver RF, Teirstein AS, Moller DR. Selection of Oligoclonal Vβ-specific T Cells in the Intradermal Response to Kveim-Siltzbach Reagent in Individuals with Sarcoidosis. The Journal of Immunology. 1995;154:1450-60.

[151] Moller DR, Konishi K, Kirby M, Balbi B, Crystal RG. Bias toward use of a specific T cell receptor beta-chain variable region in a subgroup of individuals with sarcoidosis. Journal of Clinical Investigation. 1988;82(4):1183-91.

[152] Lyons DJ, Donald S, Mitchell DN, Asherson GL. Chemical Inactivation of the Kveim Reagent. Respiration. 1992;59:22-6.

[153] Song Z, Marzilli L, Greenlee BM, Chen ES, Silver RF, Askin FB, et al. Mycobacterial catalase–peroxidase is a tissue antigen and target of the adaptive immune response in systemic sarcoidosis. The Journal of Experimental Medicine. 2005;201(5):755-67.

[154] Studdy PR, Bird R. Serum angiotensin converting enzyme in sarcoidosis - its value in present clinical practice. Annals of Clinical Biochemistry. 1989;26:13-8.

[155] Lieberman J, Zakria F. Effect of captopril and enalapril medication on the serum ACE test for sarcoidosis. Sarcoidosis. 1989;6(2):118-23.

[156] Rohrbach MS, DeRemee RA. Age dependence of serum angiotensin-converting enzyme activity. The Lancet. 1979;2(8135):196.

[157] Lieberman J. Elevation of serum angiotensin-converting-enzyme (ACE) level in sarcoidosis. The American Journal of Medicine. 1975;59(3):365-72.

[158] Studdy P, Bird R, James DG. Serum angiotensin-converting enzyme (SACE) in sarcoidosis and other granulomatous disorders. The Lancet. 1978;2(8104-5):1331-4.

[159] Pertschuk LP, Silverstein E, Friedland J. Immunohistologic diagnosis of sarcoidosis. Detection of angiotensin-converting enzyme in sarcoid granulomas. American Journal of Clinical Pathology. 1981;75(3):350-4.

[160] Loddenkemper R, Kloppenborg A, Schoenfeld N, Grosser H, Costabel U. Clinical findings in 715 patients with newly detected pulmonary sarcoidosis--results of a cooperative study in former West Germany and Switzerland. WATL Study Group. Wissenschaftliche Arbeitsgemeinschaft für die Therapie von Lungenkrankheitan. Sarcoidosis, Vasculitis & Diffuse Lung Diseases. 1998;15(2):178-82.

[161] Lieberman J, Nosal A, Schlessner A, Sastre-Foken A. Serum angiotensin-converting enzyme for diagnosis and therapeutic evaluation of sarcoidosis. American Review of Respiratory Disease. 1979;120(2):329-35.

[162] Gronhagen-Riska C, Kurppa K, Fyhrquist F, Selroos O. Angiotensin-converting en-
       zyme and lysozyme in silicosis and asbestosis. Scandinavian Journal of Respiratory
       Diseases. 1978;59(4):228-31.

[163] Newman LS, Orton R, Kreiss K. Serum angiotensin converting enzyme activity in
       chronic beryllium disease. The American Review of Respiratory Disease. 1992;146(1):
       39-42.

[164] Davies SF, Rohrbach MS, Thelen V, Kuritsky J, Gruninger R, Simpson ML, et al. Ele-
       vated serum angiotensin-converting enzyme (SACE) activity in acute pulmonary his-
       toplasmosis. Chest. 1984;85(3):307-10.

[165] Gupta SK, Chakraborty M, Mitra K. Serum angiotensin converting enzyme in respi-
       ratory diseases. The Indian Journal of Chest Diseases and Allied Sciences. 1992;34(1):
       19-24.

[166] Brice EA, Friedlander W, Bateman ED, Kirsch RE. Serum angiotensin-converting en-
       zyme activity, concentration, and specific activity in granulomatous interstitial lung
       disease, tuberculosis, and COPD. Chest. 1995;107(3):706-10.

[167] Lieberman J, Sastre A. Serum angiotensin-converting enzyme: elevations in diabetes
       mellitus. Annals of Internal Medicine. 1980;93(6):825-6.

[168] Smallridge RC, Rogers J, Verma PS. Serum angiotensin-converting enzyme: altera-
       tions in hyperthyroidism, hypothyroidism and subacute thyroiditis. Journal of the
       American Medical Association. 1983;250:2489-93.

[169] Lieberman J, Beutler E. Elevation of serum angiotensin-converting enzyme in Gauch-
       er's disease. The New England Journal of Medicine. 1976;294(26):1442-4.

[170] Biller H, Ruprecht B, Gaede KI, Müller-Quernheim J, Zissel G. Gene polymorphisms
       of ACE and the angiotensin receptor AT2R1 influence serum ACE levels in sarcoido-
       sis. Sarcoidosis, Vasculitis & Diffuse Lung Diseases. 2009;26(2):139-46.

[171] Kruit A, Grutters JC, Gerritsen WB, Kos S, Wodzig WK, van den Bosch JM, et al. ACE
       I/D-corrected Z-scores to identify normal and elevated ACE activity in sarcoidosis.
       Respiratory Medicine. 2007;101(3):510-5.

[172] Allen RK, Pierce RJ, Barter CE. Angiotensin-converting enzyme in bronchoalveolar
       lavage fluid in sarcoidosis. . Sarcoidosis. 1992;9(1):54-9.

[173] Tahmoush AJ, Amir MS, Connor WW, Farry JK, Didato S, Ulhoa-Cintra A, et al. CSF-
       ACE activity in probable CNS neurosarcoidosis. Sarcoidosis, Vasculitis & Diffuse
       Lung Diseases. 2002;19(3):191-7.

[174] Miyoshi S HH, Kadowaki T, Hamaguchi N, Ito R, Irifune K, et al. Comparative eval-
       uation of serum markers in pulmonary sarcoidosis. Chest. 2010;137(6):1391-7.

[175] Tomita H, Sato S, Matsuda R, Sugiura Y, Kawaguchi H, Niimi T, et al. Serum lyso-
       zyme levels and clinical features of sarcoidosis. Lung. 1999;177(3):161-7.

[176] Pascual RS, Gee JB, Finch SC. Usefulness of serum lysozyme measurement in diagnosis and evaluation of sarcoidosis. The New England Journal of Medicine. 1973;289(20):1074-6.

[177] Klockars M, Selroos O. Immunohistochemical demonstration of lysozyme in the lymph nodes and Kveim reaction papules in sarcoidosis. Acta Pathologica et Microbiologica Scandinavica, Section A. 1977;85A(2):169-73.

[178] Prior C, Barbee RA, Evans PM, Townsend PJ, Primett ZS, Fyhrquist F, et al. Lavage versus serum measurements of lysozyme, angiotensin converting enzyme and other inflammatory markers in pulmonary sarcoidosis. European Respiratory Journal. 1990;3(10):1146-54.

[179] Klockars M, Pettersson T, Weber TH, Froseth B, Selroos O. Angiotensin-converting enzyme, lysozyme, beta-2-microglobulin and adenosine deaminase in sarcoidosis. Archivio Monaldi. 1984;39(5-6):345-56.

[180] Homolka J, Lorenz J, Zuchold HD, Müller-Quernheim J. Evaluation of soluble CD 14 and neopterin as serum parameters of the inflammatory activity of pulmonary sarcoidosis. The Clinical Investigator. 1992;70(10):909-16.

[181] Eklund A, Blaschke E. Elevated serum neopterin levels in sarcoidosis. Lung. 1986;164(6):325-32.

[182] Lacronique J, Auzeby A, Valeyre D, Traore BM, Barbosa ML, Soler P, et al. Urinary neopterin in pulmonary sarcoidosis. Relationship to clinical and biologic assessment of the disease. American Review of Respiratory Disease. 1989;139(6):1474-8.

[183] Kollert F, Geck, B, Suchy R, Jörres RA, Arzt M, Heidinger D, et al. The impact of gas exchange measurement during exercise in pulmonary sarcoidosis. Respiratory Medicine. 2011;105(1):122-9.

[184] Blaschke E, Eklund A, Persson U. Relationship between serum neopterin and lymphocytic alveolitis in sarcoidosis. Sarcoidosis. 1988;5(1):25-30.

[185] Planck A, Eklund A, Grunewald J. Markers of activity in clinically recovered human leukocyte antigen-DR17-positive sarcoidosis patients. European Respiratory Journal. 2003;21(1):52-7.

[186] Prior C, Frank A, Fuchs D, Hausen A, Judmaier G, Reibnegger G, et al. Urinary neopterin excretion in pulmonary sarcoidosis: correlation to clinical course of the disease. Clinica Chimica Acta. 1988;177(3):211-20.

[187] Bargagli E, Maggiorelli C, Rottoli P. Human Chitotriosidase: a potential new marker of sarcoidosis severity. Respiration. 2008;76(234-38.).

[188] Boot RG, Hollak CE, Verhoek M, Alberts C, Jonkers RE, Aerts JM. Plasma chitotriosidase and CCL18 as surrogate markers for granulomatous macrophages in sarcoidosis. Clinica Chimica Acta. 2010;411(1-2):31-6.

[189] Korolenko TA, Zhanaeva SY, Falameeva OV, Kaledin VI, Filyushina EE, Buzueva II, et al. Chitotriosidase as a marker of macrophage stimulation. Bulletin of Experimental Biology and Medicine. 2000;130(10):948-50.

[190] Bargagli E, Bianchi N, Margollicci M, Olivieri C, Luddi A, Coviello G, et al. Chitotriosidase and soluble IL-2 receptor: comparison of two markers of sarcoidosis severity. Scandinavian Journal of Clinical and Laboratory Investigation. 2008;68(6):479-83.

[191] Bargagli E, Margollicci M, Perrone A, Luddi A, Perari MG, Bianchi N, et. Chitotriosidase analysis in bronchoalveolar lavage of patients with sarcoidosis. Sarcoidosis, Vasculitis & Diffuse Lung Diseases. 2007;24(1):59-64.

[192] Chen ES, Song Z, Willett MH, Heine S, Yung RC, Liu MC, et al. Serum Amyloid A Regulates Granulomatous Inflammation in Sarcoidosis through Toll-like Receptor-2. American Journal of Respiratory and Critical Care Medicine. 2010;181:360-73.

[193] Albera C, Mabritto I, Ghio P, Solidoro P, Marchetti L, Pozzi E. Adenosine deaminase activity and fibronectin levels in bronchoalveolar lavage fluid in sarcoidosis and tuberculosis. Sarcoidosis. 1993;10(1):18-25.

[194] Wetzel E, Müller-Quernheim J, Lorenz J. [Serum adenosine deaminase as a parameter for activity in sarcoidosis]. [Article in German]. Pneumologie. 1999;53(7):323-8.

[195] Sofia M, Mormile M, Faraone S, Alifano M, Carratù P, Carratù L. Endothelin-1 excretion in urine in active pulmonary sarcoidosis and in other interstitial lung diseases. Sarcoidosis. 1995;12(2):118-23.

[196] Terashita K, Kato S, Sata M, Inoue S, Nakamura H, Tomoike H. Increased endothelin-1 levels of BAL fluid in patients with pulmonary sarcoidosis. Respirology. 2006;11(2):145-51.

[197] Letizia C, Danese A, Reale MG, Caliumi C, Delfini E, Subioli S, et al. Plasma levels of endothelin-1 increase in patients with sarcoidosis and fall after disease remission. Panminerva Medica. 2001;43(4):257-61.

[198] Peros-Golubicić T, Ivicević A, Bekić A, Alilović M, Tekavec-Trkanjec J, Smojver-Jezek S. Lung lavage neutrophils, neutrophil elastase and albumin in the prognosis of pulmonary sarcoidosis. Collegium Antropologicum. 2001;25(1):349-55.

[199] O'Connor C, Odlum C, Van Breda A, Power C, Fitzgerald MX. Collagenase and fibronectin in bronchoalveolar lavage fluid in patients with sarcoidosis. Thorax. 1988;43(5):393-400.

[200] Magi B, Bini L, Perari MG, Fossi A, Sanchez JC, Hochstrasser D, et al. Bronchoalveolar lavage fluid protein composition in patients with sarcoidosis and idiopathic pulmonary fibrosis: a two-dimensional electrophoretic study. Electrophoresis. 2002;23(19):3434-44.

[201] Sabounchi-Schütt F, Aström J, Hellman U, Eklund A, Grunewald J. Changes in bron-choalveolar lavage fluid proteins in sarcoidosis: a proteomics approach. European Respiratory Journal. 2003;21(3):414-20.

[202] Sabounchi-Schütt F, Mikko M, Eklund A, Grunewald J, Aström J. Serum protein pattern in sarcoidosis analysed by a proteomics approach. Sarcoidosis, Vasculitis & Diffuse Lung Diseases. 2004;21(3):182-90.

[203] Silva E, Bourin S, Sabounchi-Schütt F, Laurin Y, Barker E, Newman L, et al. A quantitative proteomic analysis of soluble bronchoalveolar fluid proteins from patients with sarcoidosis and chronic beryllium disease. Sarcoidosis, Vasculitis & Diffuse Lung Diseases. 2007;24(1):24-32.

[204] Bons JA, Drent M, Bouwman FG, Mariman EC, van Dieijen-Visser MP, Wodzig WK. Potential biomarkers for diagnosis of sarcoidosis using proteomics in serum. Respiratory Medicine. 2007;101(8):1687-95.

[205] Kriegova E, Melle C, Kolek V, Hutyrova B, Mrazek F, Bleul A, et al. Protein profiles of bronchoalveolar lavage fluid from patients with pulmonary sarcoidosis. American Journal of Respiratory and Critical Care Medicine. 2006;173(10):1145-54.

[206] Moodley YP, Chetty R, Lalloo UG. Nitric oxide levels in exhaled air and inducible nitric oxide synthase immunolocalization in pulmonary sarcoidosis. European Respiratory Journal. 1999;14(4):822-7.

[207] Wilsher ML, Fergusson W, Milne D, Wells AU. Exhaled nitric oxide in sarcoidosis. Thorax. 2005;60(11):967-70.

[208] Choi J, Hoffman LA, Sethi JM, Zullo TG, Gibson KF. Multiple flow rates measurement of exhaled nitric oxide in patients with sarcoidosis: a pilot feasibility study. Sarcoidosis, Vasculitis & Diffuse Lung Diseases. 2009;26(2):98-109.

[209] Ciarleglio G, Refini RM, Pieroni MG, Martino VA, Bargagli E, Rottoli P, et al. Exhaled carbon monoxide in sarcoidosis. Sarcoidosis, Vasculitis & Diffuse Lung Diseases. 2008;25(1):46-50.

[210] Kharitonov SA, Barnes PJ. Exhaled Markers of Pulmonary Disease. American Journal of Respiratory and Critical Care Medicine. 2001;163:1693-722.

[211] Horváth I, Hunt J, Barnes PJ. Exhaled breath condensate: methodological recommendations and unresolved questions. European Respiratory Journal. 2005;26(3):523-48.

[212] Mutlu GM, Garey KW, Robbins RA, Danziger LH, Rubinstein I. Collection and Analysis of Exhaled Breath Condensate in Humans. American Journal of Respiratory and Critical Care Medicine. 2001;164:731-7.

[213] Jackson AS, Sandrini A, Campbell C, Chow S, Thomas PS, Yates DH. Comparison of Biomarkers in Exhaled Breath Condensate and Bronchoalveolar Lavage. American Journal of Respiratory and Critical Care Medicine. 2007;175(222-227).

[214] Rożyi A, Czerniawska J, Stępniewska A, Woźbińska B, Goljan A, Puścińska E, et al. Inflammatory markers in the exhaled breath condensate of patients with pulmonary sarcoidosis. Journal of Physiology and Pharmacology. 2006;57(4):335-40.

[215] Nayeri F, Millinger E, Nilsson I, Zetterström, Brudin L, Forsberg P. Exhaled breath condensate and serum levels of hepatocyte growth factor in pneumonia. Respiratory Medicine. 2002;96(2):115-9.

[216] Piotrowski WJ, Kurmanowska Z, Antczak A, Marczak J, Górski P. Hepatocyte growth factor in exhaled breath and BAL fluid in sarcoidosis. Pneumonologia i alergologia polska. 2010;78(3):187-91.

[217] Kowalska A, Puścińska E, Czerniawska J, Goljan-Geremek A, Czystowska M, Roży A, et al. Markers of fibrosis and inflammation in exhaled breathcondensate (EBC) and bronchoalveolar lavage fluid (BALF) of patients with pulmonary sarcoidosis- a pilot study [Polish]. Pneumonologia i alergologia polska. 2010;78(5):356-62.

[218] Psathakis K, Papatheodorou G, Plataki M, Panagou P, Loukides S, Siafakas NM, et al. 8-Isoprostane, a Marker of Oxidative Stress, Is Increased in the Expired Breath Condensate of Patients With Pulmonary Sarcoidosis. Chest. 2004;125:1005-11.

[219] Antczak A, Piotrowski W, Marczak J, Ciebiada M, Gorski P, Barnes PJ. Correlation between eicosanoids in bronchoalveolar lavage fluid and in exhaled breath condensate. Disease Markers. 2011;30(5):213-20.

[220] Piotrowski WJ, Kurmanowska Z, Antczak A, Marczak J, Górski P. Exhaled 8-isoprostane as a prognostic marker in sarcoidois. A short term follow up. BMC Pulmonary Medicine. 2010;10:23-9.

[221] Piotrowski WJ, Antczak A, Marczak J, Nawrocka A, Kurmanowska Z, Górski P. Eicosanoids in exhaled breath condensate and BAL Fluid of patients with Sarcoidosis. Chest. 2007;132:589-96.

[222] Kwiatkowska S, Luczynska M., Grzelewska-Rzymowska I, Nowak D, Zieba M. Comparison of oxidative stress markers in exhaled breath condensate and in serum of patients with tuberculosis and sarcoidosis. [Polish]. Polski Merkuriusz Lekarski. 2005;19(109):37-40.

Chapter 11

Pathological Diagnosis with Endobronchial Ultrasonography — Guided Transbronchial Needle Aspiration (EBUS-TBNA)

Atsushi Kitamura and Yuichi Takiguchi

Additional information is available at the end of the chapter

1. Introduction

The diagnosis of sarcoidosis is based on clinico-radiological findings and histological evidence of non-caseating epithelioid-cell granulomas [1]. Traditionally, if pulmonary sarcoidosis is suspected, pathological diagnostic materials are often obtained using conventional bronchoscopy together with procedures such as bronchoalveolar lavage (BAL) for evaluation of disease activity, transbronchial needle aspiration (TBNA) for hilar/mediastinal lymph node lesions, transbronchial lung biopsy (TBLB) for lung parenchymal lesions, and transbronchial biopsy (TBB) for endobronchial lesions. In most cases, however, definitive pathological diagnosis of this disease mainly depends on TBLB for lung parenchymal lesions because hilar/mediastinal lymph node lesions are often difficult to access and endobronchial lesions are uncommon. The diagnostic yield of TBLB in this disease is reportedly about 40–90% when several biopsy samples are obtained [2, 3]. When mediastinal or hilar lymphadenopathy is detected on computed tomography (CT) and cannot be diagnosed with conventional bronchoscopy, mediastinoscopy is performed to obtain histological samples. Although the diagnostic sensitivity of this procedures is >90% [4, 5], it is invasive and requires general anesthesia [5]. In this chapter, a newly developed bronchoscopic technique, endobronchial ultrasonography (EBUS)-guided transbronchial needle aspiration (EBUS-TBNA) for the definitive diagnosis of sarcoidosis is discussed.

2. EBUS-TBNA, a newly developed bronchoscopic technique

An endobronchial ultrasound, recently developed in Japan [6, 7], is a bronchoscope equipped with a convex-type ultrasound probe at the tip of the scope to simultaneously visualize endobronchial images with optical-wavelength light and images of peribronchial structures, such as lymph nodes and vessels, with ultrasound (Figure 1). By introducing a specialized TBNA needle into the forceps channel, it is possible to obtain cytological and even histological samples [6, 7]. This technique was developed primarily as a novel minimally invasive diagnostic technique for lymph node staging of lung cancer [6, 8- 17]. As summarized in Table 1, initial research disclosed its high sensitivity and diagnostic yields for this purpose. This new technique has obviated the need for classical and invasive mediastinoscopy in many cases, and a current European guideline for lymph node staging in lung cancer primarily recommends EBUS-TBNA over mediastinoscopy [18]. Recent reports also indicate that EBUS-TBNA is a valuable diagnostic method for pulmonary sarcoidosis with hilar/mediastinal lymphadenopathy [19 - 32]. The presence of non-caseating epithelioid-cell granulomas in the lymph nodes obtained by EBUS-TBNA suggests the diagnosis of granulomatous disease including sarcoidosis.

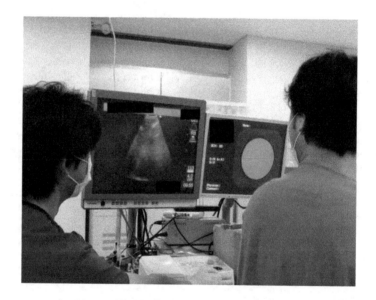

Figure 1. A bronchoscopic procedure with EBUS. The operator and assistants can view simultaneous real-time images of both endobronchus with natural light (right monitor) and peribronchial structures with ultrasonography (left monitor).

Author	Year	No. of patients	Study design	Sensitivity (%)	Specificity (%)
Yasufuku[6]	2005	108	Prospective	94.1	100
Yasufuku[10]	2006	102	Prospective	92.3	100
Herth[11]	2006	502	Prospective	94	100
Vincent[12]	2008	146	Retrospective	99.1	100
Wallace[13]	2008	138	Prospective	69	100
Herth[14]	2008	97	Prospective	88.9	100
Ernst[15]	2008	66	Prospective	88.1	100
Petersen[16]	2009	157	Retrospective	85	100
Yasufuku[17]	2011	102	Prospective	81	100

Table 1. Recent studies for staging of lung cancer with EBUS-TBNA

3. Technique to obtain histological and cytological materials with EBUS-TBNA

EBUS-TBNA is performed under local anesthesia with mild sedation, which is comparable to conventional bronchoscopy [7 - 11]. Contrast medium-enhanced CT images are used
to identify target lymph nodes. A convex-probe-equipped EBUS bronchoscope (CP-EBUS;
for example, BF-UC260F-OL8; Olympus, Tokyo, Japan) supported by an ultrasound image
processor (model EU-C2000; Olympus) and a dedicated 22- or 21-gauge aspiration needle
(NA-201SX-4022/NA-201SX-4021; Olympus) are used (Figures 2, 3). Although 21 G and 22
G needles yield similar sensitivity in the diagnosis of malignant diseases, 22 G needles are
more efficient than 21 G needles for obtaining materials from patients with sarcoidosis [33].
While the target lymph node is visualized with EBUS, a transbronchial puncture under
real-time ultrasound guidance is performed with a needle equipped with an internal sheath
(Figure 4). The internal sheath prevents clogging of the needle with bronchial epithelial
cells. On confirming that the tip of the needle has penetrated the target lymph node, the
internal sheath is removed, and rapid negative pressure is applied by aspirating with a 20-
mL syringe several times. After the needle is moved back and forth inside the lymph node
under real-time ultrasound guidance, it is retrieved and the internal sheath is used to expel
the material aspirated in the needle (Figure 5). A histological core is first obtained in many
cases; this material is placed on a small piece of filter paper for fixation in 10% buffered
formalin. The internal sheath is then removed, and positive pressure is applied using an
air-filled 20-mL syringe to expel the remaining material in the needle onto a glass slide,
which is then smeared against another glass slide by using the squash preparation
technique to yield cytological smears on 2 glass slides (Figure 6). Both histological cores
and cytological specimens are obtained in many cases with this method. In our institution, tentative on-site cytological diagnosis by a cytoscreener is available. One of the

cytological slides is placed in 95% ethanol for fixation and staining with the Papanicolaou technique. The other one is air-dried, stained with a Romanowsky-type stain (Diff-Quik®), and sent for on-site evaluation. The cytoscreener ensures that the specimen is of adequate quality. Tissue sampling is repeated until sufficient material is obtained. The aspirated materials can also be dispersed into sterile saline solution for microbiological examinations, including staining and culture for bacteria, fungi, and acid-fast bacilli. In addition, polymerase chain reaction examinations can be performed for acid-fast bacilli. Histological diagnoses are based on the results of hematoxylin and eosin (H-E) staining.

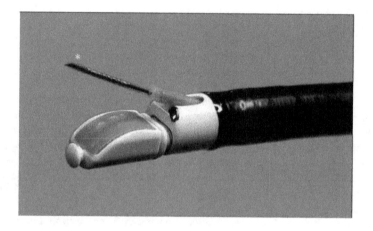

Figure 2. The tip of the endobronchial ultrasound equipped with an aspiration needle (asterisk). The needle is protruded for demonstration.

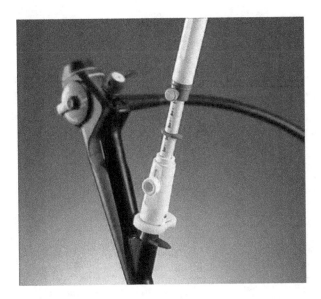

Figure 3. The control head of an endobronchial ultrasound is similar to that of a conventional bronchoscope except for a sophisticated needle aspiration kit that enables operators to control internal and outer sheaths separately.

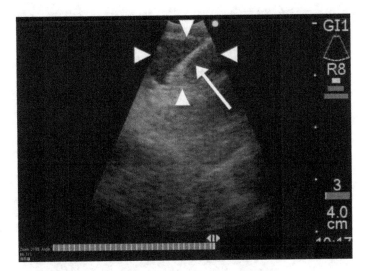

Figure 4. An ultrasound image showing an enlarged lymph node (hypoechoic area; arrowheads) and an aspiration needle (arrow) inserted into the lymph node. On ensuring that the tip of the needle is inside the target lymph node, negative pressure is applied and the needle is moved back and forth inside the lymph node to obtain material for pathological examination.

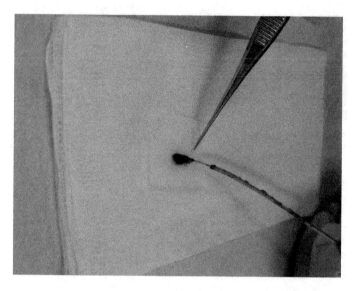

Figure 5. Aspirated material inside the needle is expelled by inserting the inner sheath. Usually a histological core is obtained, and the material is collected on a filter paper for fixation in formalin solution.

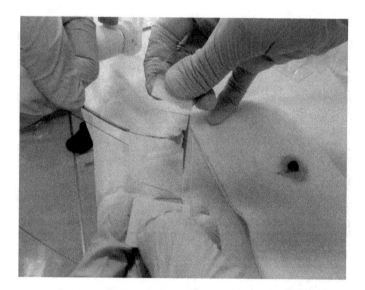

Figure 6. After obtaining the histological core, the inner sheath is removed. An abrupt positive pressure is used to expel remaining material inside the needle for cytological samples, which are obtained on 2 glass slides by using the squash preparation technique.

BAL followed by TBLB with conventional bronchoscopy is performed before EBUS-TBNA [22,28] when required.

4. Sensitivity and specificity of EBUS-TBNA in the diagnosis of sarcoidosis

Table 2 summarizes the results of recent reports and shows a diagnostic sensitivity for sarcoidosis of EBUS-TBNA ranging from 56% to 94% [19 - 32]. Non-caseating epithelioid-cell granulomas on histological examination of EBUS-TBNA specimens have high sensitivity and specificity for sarcoidosis at stages 1 and 2. Nakajima et al. [22], Oki et al. [28], and Kitamura et al. [29] reported that the sensitivity of EBUS-TBNA for stage 1 and 2 sarcoidosis is much higher than that of TBLB from the lung parenchyma.

Author	Year	No. of patients	Study design	Histology		Cytology		Histology & Cytology	
				Sensitivity (%)	Specificity (%)	Sensitivity (%)	Specificity (%)	Sensitivity (%)	Specificity (%)
Garwood[19]	2007	48	Prospective	-	-	-	-	85	-
Oki[20]	2007	14	Prospective	57	-	65	-	78	-
Wong[21]	2007	61	Prospective	-	-	-	-	92	-
Nakajima[22]	2009	32	Retrospective	63	-	71	-	91	-
Tremblay[23]	2009	24	Prospective	-	-	-	-	83	-
Eckardt[24]	2010	43	Retrospective	-	-	-	-	77	-
Tournoy[25]	2010	54	Prospective	-	-	-	-	56	-
Navani[26]	2011	27	Prospective	-	-	-	-	85	-
Plit[27]	2011	37	Retrospective	-	-	-	-	84	-
Oki[28]	2012	54	Prospective	-	-	-	-	94	-
Kitamura[29]	2012	72	Retrospective	72	97	65	94	88	92

- : not available

Table 2. Recent studies for diagnosis of sarcoidosis with EBUS-TBNA

5. Diagnostic validity for sarcoidosis of epithelioid-cell clusters on cytological examination

Cytological evaluation has been reported in the diagnosis of sarcoidosis with conventional TBNA, trans-esophageal ultrasound-guided biopsy [34 - 40], and EBUS-TBNA [41,42]; however, the validity of the diagnostic criteria has not been defined.

Epithelioid-cell clusters suggesting the presence of granulomas are defined by variably-sized loose collections of non-pigmented epithelioid or spindle-cell histiocytes that are usually accompanied by lymphocytes [31]. Typical cytological findings are shown in Figures 7 to 10, together with their corresponding histological findings obtained from the same aspiration. The validity of cytological evaluation in the diagnosis of sarcoidosis, however, was not well-defined. To elucidate the diagnostic validity of epithelioid-cell clusters on cytological examination, we performed a study in which cytological samples from 72 patients with sarcoidosis and 116 control patients with malignant lung diseases mainly of primary lung cancer (with lymphadenopathy eventually proven to be metastasis free) were evaluated independently by 2 cytoscreeners and a pathologist, all blinded to patient information. The results included excellent inter-observer variability and a high specificity of 94.0%, indicating validity of cytological diagnosis of sarcoidosis [29]. Our study also uncovered a very high rate (87.5% or 63/72) of pathological proof of epithelioid-cell granulomas when cytological and histological evaluations with EBUS-TBNA-obtained materials were combined. Validity of cytological diagnosis of sarcoidosis might be applicable to other organs.

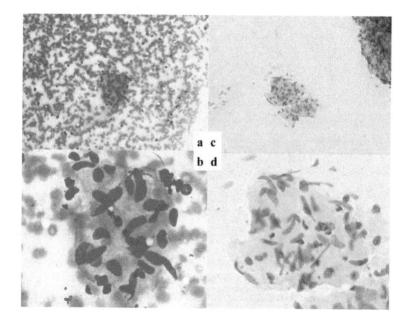

Figure 7. Typical epithelioid-cell clusters in a cytological specimen, with Diff-Quik staining (a and b) and Papanicolaou staining (c and d). They were obtained from the same lymph node in a patient with sarcoidosis. The original magnifications were ×100 (a and c) and ×400 (b and d).

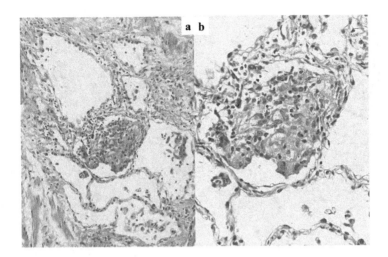

Figure 8. Histological findings of a histological core obtained from the same patient whose cytological findings are shown in Figure 7. Histological findings characteristic of a non-caseating epithelioid-cell granuloma are shown (H-E stain; original magnification of ×100 in a and ×200 in b).

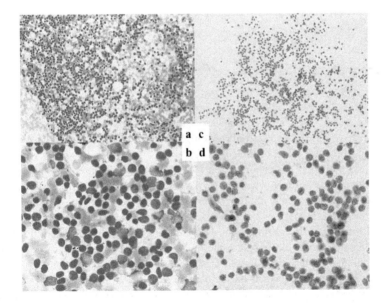

Figure 9. Normal lymph node findings shown in a cytological specimen, with Diff-Quik staining (a and b) and Papanicolaou staining (c and d). They were obtained from the same lymph node in a control patient. The original magnification were ×100 (a and c) and ×400 (b and d).

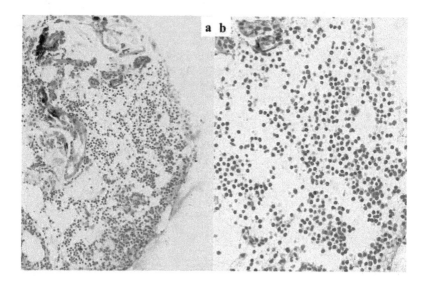

Figure 10. Histological findings of a histological core obtained from the same patient whose cytological findings are shown in Figure 9. Although the structure has partially disintegrated probably because of tissue damage inside the aspiration needle, normal lymph node architecture is observed without evidence of epithelioid-cell granuloma or malignant cells (H-E stain; original magnification of ×100 in a and ×200 in b).

6. Epithelioid-cell granulomas in lymphadenopathy with lung cancer

Non-caseating epithelioid-cell granulomas may be seen in draining lymph nodes in various malignant diseases. These relatively uncommon histological findings, which are not systemic sarcoidosis, have been termed sarcoid reactions [43]. Sarcoid reactions are also seen in lung malignancy with a reported incidence of 1.2–4.3% [44- 46]. This value was 6.0% in our study [29], that is, cytological evaluation of the EBUS-TBNA samples revealed epithelioid-cell clusters in lymph nodes from 7 patients out of the 116 patients with primary lung cancer whose lymphadenopathy was eventually proven to be metastasis free. Sarcoid reactions probably reflect an immune response to tumor antigens due to T-cell mediated immune responses [47]. The tumor antigens are thought to be carried by lymphatic vessels to the draining lymph nodes, causing sarcoid reactions in situ [43]. Although uncommon, it is very important that this is considered in the pathological diagnosis of sarcoidosis. There is no report on differentiating sarcoidosis from sarcoid reactions on the basis of histological and/or cytological findings. Clinical differentiation of sarcoid reaction from sarcoidosis, however, may not be difficult because of the presence of primary lesion and asymmetric distribution of the hilar/mediastinum lymphadenopathy. Nevertheless, it should be stressed that sarcoid reaction potentially misleads N staging of the lung cancer.

7. Future directions

As discussed in the above sections, EBUS-TBNA results in a very high rate (>80%) of patho-logical proof of sarcoidosis provided enlarged hilar/mediastinal lymph nodes are accessible. The technique has been reported to be very safe because target lymph nodes and surrounding vessels are easily visualized with ultrasound images. In contrast, the sensitivity of TBLB of pulmonary parenchymal lesions is reportedly much lower than that with EBUS-TBNA. In fact, it was 34.5% (or 20/58) in our study [29], where only 58 patients out of the 72 patients with sarcoidosis were evaluated with TBLB because of absent pulmonary lesions in the imaging studies and/or possible complications. TBLB is potentially invasive; consequently, the proce-dure may be complicated with massive bleeding or pneumothorax. These possible complica-tions may justify avoiding TBLB in the diagnosis of sarcoidosis when EBUS-TBNA is available. Excluding certain conditions where proof of pulmonary parenchymal lesions is required, prioritizing EBUS-TBNA over TBLB would be reasonable. Advances in this new technology might change the diagnostic practices in sarcoidosis.

In addition, easier access to involved lymph nodes with EBUS-TBNA may provide new opportunities to obtain biomarkers for elucidating pathogenesis of the disease. In fact, Nakajima et al. [48] and Sakairi et al. [49] were successful with this technique in detecting various gene mutations in patients with lung cancer. Similar advances with the same technique in the field of sarcoidosis and other granulomatous diseases would be realistic. We anticipate that sarcoidosis, an unpleasant refractory disease, will be conquered by applied investigation and personalized care in the future.

Author details

Atsushi Kitamura[1,2] and Yuichi Takiguchi[1]

*Address all correspondence to: takiguchi@faculty.chiba-u.jp

1 Department of Medical Oncology, Graduate School of Medicine, Chiba University, Japan

2 Department of Respiratory Medicine, St. Luke's International Hospital, Japan

References

[1] Statement on sarcoidosisJoint Statement of the American Thoracic Society (ATS), the European Respiratory Society (ERS) and the World Association of Sarcoidosis and Other Granulomatous Disorders (WASOG) adopted by the ATS Board of Directors and by the ERS Executive Committee, February 1999. Am J Respir Crit Care Med (1999). , 160, 736-755.

[2] Gilman, M. J, & Wang, K. P. Transbronchial lung biopsy in sarcoidosis. An approach to determine the optimal number of biopsies. Am Rev Respir Dis (1980). , 122, 721-724.

[3] De Boer, S, Milne, D. G, Zeng, I, et al. Does CT scanning predict the likelihood of a positive transbronchial biopsy in sarcoidosis? Thorax (2009). , 64, 436-439.

[4] Raghu, G. Interstitial lung disease: a diagnostic approach. Are CT scan and lung biopsy indicated in every patient? Am J Respir Crit Care Med (1995). , 151, 909-914.

[5] Gossot, D, Toledo, L, Fritsch, S, et al. Mediastinoscopy vs thoracoscopy for mediastinal biopsy. Results of a prospective nonrandomized study. Chest (1996). , 110, 1328-1331.

[6] Yasufuku, K, Chiyo, M, Koh, E, et al. Endobronchial ultrasound guided transbronchial needle aspiration for staging of lung cancer. Lung Cancer (2005). , 50, 347-354.

[7] Yasufuku, K, Chiyo, M, Sekine, Y, et al. Real-time endobronchial ultrasound-guided transbronchial needle aspiration of mediastinal and hilar lymph nodes. Chest (2004). , 126, 122-128.

[8] Gu, P, Zhao, Y. Z, Jiang, L. Y, et al. Endobronchial ultrasound-guided transbronchial needle aspiration for staging of lung cancer: a systematic review and meta-analysis. Eur J Cancer (2009). , 45, 1389-1396.

[9] Adams, K, Shah, P. L, Edmonds, L, et al. Test performance of endobronchial ultrasound and transbronchial needle aspiration biopsy for mediastinal staging in patients with lung cancer: systematic review and meta-analysis. Thorax (2009). , 64, 757-762.

[10] Yasufuku, K, Nakajima, T, Motoori, K, et al. Comparison of endobronchial ultrasound, positron emission tomography, and CT for lymph node staging of lung cancer. Chest (2006). , 130, 710-718.

[11] Herth, F. J, Ernst, A, Eberhardt, R, et al. Endobronchial ultrasound-guided transbronchial needle aspiration of lymph nodes in the radiologically normal mediastinum. Eur Respir J (2006). , 28, 910-914.

[12] Vincent, B. D, Bayoumi, E, Hoffman, B, et al. Real-time endobronchial ultrasound-guided transbronchial lymph node aspiration. Ann Thorac Surg (2008). , 85, 224-230.

[13] Wallace, M. B, Pascual, J. M, Raimondo, M, et al. Minimally invasive endoscopic staging of suspected lung cancer. JAMA (2008). , 299, 540-546.

[14] Herth, F. J, Eberhardt, R, Krasnik, M, et al. Endobronchial ultrasound-guided transbronchial needle aspiration of lymph nodes in the radiologically and positron emission tomography-normal mediastinum in patients with lung cancer. Chest (2008). , 133, 887-891.

[15] Ernst, A, Anantham, D, Eberhardt, R, et al. Diagnosis of mediastinal adenopathy-real-time endobronchial ultrasound guided needle aspiration versus mediastinoscopy. J Thorac Oncol (2008). , 3, 577-582.

[16] Omark Petersen HEckardt J, Hakami A, et al. The value of mediastinal staging with endobronchial ultrasound-guided transbronchial needle aspiration in patients with lung cancer. Eur J Cardiothorac Surg (2009). , 36, 465-468.

[17] Yasufuku, K, Pierre, A, Darling, G, et al. A prospective controlled trial of endobronchial ultrasound-guided transbronchial needle aspiration compared with mediastinoscopy for mediastinal lymph node staging of lung cancer. J Thorac Cardiovasc Surg (2011). e1391, 142, 1393-1400.

[18] De Leyn, P, Lardinois, D, Van Schil, P, et al. European trends in preoperative and intraoperative nodal staging: ESTS guidelines. J Thorac Oncol (2007). , 2, 357-361.

[19] Garwood, S, Judson, M. A, Silvestri, G, et al. Endobronchial ultrasound for the diagnosis of pulmonary sarcoidosis. Chest (2007). , 132, 1298-1304.

[20] Oki, M, Saka, H, Kitagawa, C, et al. Real-time endobronchial ultrasound-guided transbronchial needle aspiration is useful for diagnosing sarcoidosis. Respirology (2007). , 12, 863-868.

[21] Wong, M, Yasufuku, K, Nakajima, T, et al. Endobronchial ultrasound: new insight for the diagnosis of sarcoidosis. Eur Respir J (2007). , 29, 1182-1186.

[22] Nakajima, T, Yasufuku, K, Kurosu, K, et al. The role of EBUS-TBNA for the diagnosis of sarcoidosis--comparisons with other bronchoscopic diagnostic modalities. Respir Med (2009). , 103, 1796-1800.

[23] Tremblay, A, Stather, D. R, Maceachern, P, et al. A randomized controlled trial of standard vs endobronchial ultrasonography-guided transbronchial needle aspiration in patients with suspected sarcoidosis. Chest (2009). , 136, 340-346.

[24] Eckardt, J, Olsen, K. E, Jorgensen, O. D, et al. Minimally invasive diagnosis of sarcoidosis by EBUS when conventional diagnostics fail. Sarcoidosis Vasc Diffuse Lung Dis (2010). , 27, 43-48.

[25] Tournoy, K. G, Bolly, A, Aerts, J. G, et al. The value of endoscopic ultrasound after bronchoscopy to diagnose thoracic sarcoidosis. Eur Respir J (2010). , 35, 1329-1335.

[26] Navani, N, Booth, H. L, Kocjan, G, et al. Combination of endobronchial ultrasound-guided transbronchial needle aspiration with standard bronchoscopic techniques for the diagnosis of stage I and stage II pulmonary sarcoidosis. Respirology (2011). , 16, 467-472.

[27] Plit, M, & Pearson, R. Da Costa J, et al. The Diagnostic Utility of Endobronchial Ultrasound-guided Transbronchial Needle Aspiration Compared to Transbronchial and Endobronchial Biopsy for Suspected Sarcoidosis. Intern Med J (2012). , 42, 434-438.

[28] Oki, M, Saka, H, Kitagawa, C, et al. Prospective study of endobronchial ultrasound-guided transbronchial needle aspiration of lymph nodes versus transbronchial lung biopsy of lung tissue for diagnosis of sarcoidosis. J Thorac Cardiovasc Surg (2012). , 143, 1324-1329.

[29] Kitamura, A, Takiguchi, Y, Kurosu, K, et al. Feasibility of cytological diagnosis of sarcoidosis with endobronchial US-guided transbronchial aspiration. Sarcoidosis Vasc Diffuse Lung Dis (2012). in press)

[30] Poletti, V, & Tomassetti, S. Ultrasound endoscopy (EBUS, EUS) as a sophisticated tool for morphological confirmation of sarcoidosis: do we need to find new answers for an old quest? Sarcoidosis Vasc Diffuse Lung Dis (2010). , 27, 5-6.

[31] Cameron, S. E, Andrade, R. S, & Pambuccian, S. E. Endobronchial ultrasound-guided transbronchial needle aspiration cytology: a state of the art review. Cytopathology (2010). , 21, 6-26.

[32] Agarwal, R, Srinivasan, A, Aggarwal, A. N, et al. Efficacy and safety of convex probe EBUS-TBNA in sarcoidosis: A systematic review and meta-analysis. Respir Med (2012). , 106, 883-892.

[33] Nakajima, T, Yasufuku, K, Takahashi, R, et al. Comparison of 21-gauge and 22-gauge aspiration needle during endobronchial ultrasound-guided transbronchial needle aspiration. Respirology (2011). , 16, 90-94.

[34] Tambouret, R, Geisinger, K. R, Powers, C. N, et al. The clinical application and cost analysis of fine-needle aspiration biopsy in the diagnosis of mass lesions in sarcoidosis. Chest (2000). , 117, 1004-1011.

[35] Trisolini, R, Tinelli, C, Cancellieri, A, et al. Transbronchial needle aspiration in sarcoidosis: yield and predictors of a positive aspirate. J Thorac Cardiovasc Surg (2008). , 135, 837-842.

[36] Annema, J. T, Van Meerbeeck, J. P, Rintoul, R. C, et al. Mediastinoscopy vs endosonography for mediastinal nodal staging of lung cancer: a randomized trial. JAMA (2010). , 304, 2245-2252.

[37] Von Bartheld, M. B, Veselic-charvat, M, Rabe, K. F, et al. Endoscopic ultrasound-guided fine-needle aspiration for the diagnosis of sarcoidosis. Endoscopy (2010). , 42, 213-217.

[38] Iwashita, T, Yasuda, I, Doi, S, et al. The yield of endoscopic ultrasound-guided fine needle aspiration for histological diagnosis in patients suspected of stage I sarcoidosis. Endoscopy (2008). , 40, 400-405.

[39] Cetinkaya, E, Yildiz, P, Altin, S, et al. Diagnostic value of transbronchial needle aspiration by Wang 22-gauge cytology needle in intrathoracic lymphadenopathy. Chest (2004). , 125, 527-531.

[40] Trisolini, R, Agli, L. L, Cancellieri, A, et al. The value of flexible transbronchial needle aspiration in the diagnosis of stage I sarcoidosis. Chest (2003). , 124, 2126-2130.

[41] Feller-kopman, D, Yung, R. C, Burroughs, F, et al. Cytology of endobronchial ultrasound-guided transbronchial needle aspiration: a retrospective study with histology correlation. Cancer Cytopathol (2009). , 117, 482-490.

[42] Jacob-ampuero, M. P, Haas, A. R, Ciocca, V, et al. Cytologic accuracy of samples obtained by endobronchial ultrasound-guided transbronchial needle aspiration at Thomas Jefferson University Hospital. Acta Cytol (2008). , 52, 687-690.

[43] Brincker, H. Sarcoid reactions in malignant tumours. Cancer Treat Rev (1986). , 13, 147-156.

[44] Steinfort, D. P, & Irving, L. B. Sarcoidal reactions in regional lymph nodes of patients with non-small cell lung cancer: incidence and implications for minimally invasive staging with endobronchial ultrasound. Lung Cancer (2009). , 66, 305-308.

[45] Kennedy MP, Jimenez CA, Mhatre AD, et al. Clinical implications of granulomatous inflammation detected by endobronchial ultrasound transbronchial needle aspiration in patients with suspected cancer recurrence in the mediastinum. J Cardiothorac Surg 2008; 3:8

[46] Tomimaru, Y, Higashiyama, M, Okami, J, et al. Surgical results of lung cancer with sarcoid reaction in regional lymph nodes. Jpn J Clin Oncol (2007). , 37, 90-95.

[47] Kurata, A, Terado, Y, Schulz, A, et al. Inflammatory cells in the formation of tumor-related sarcoid reactions. Hum Pathol (2005). , 36, 546-554.

[48] Nakajima, T, Yasufuku, K, Nakagawara, A, et al. Multigene mutation analysis of metastatic lymph nodes in non-small cell lung cancer diagnosed by endobronchial ultrasound-guided transbronchial needle aspiration. Chest (2011). , 140, 1319-1324.

[49] Sakairi, Y, Nakajima, T, Yasufuku, K, et al. EML4-ALK fusion gene assessment using metastatic lymph node samples obtained by endobronchial ultrasound-guided transbronchial needle aspiration. Clin Cancer Res (2010). , 16, 4938-4945.

Treatment

Chapter 12

Treatment with Methotrexate in Patients with Sarcoidosis

Sonoko Nagai and Takateru Izumi

Additional information is available at the end of the chapter

1. Introduction

Sarcoidosis is a systemic inflammatory disease of unknown etiology. The hallmark histological feature of the disease is epithelioid cell granuloma derived from activated T cells and macrophages triggered by unknown immune stimuli such as bacterial protein or beryllium metal [1, 2]. Various inflammatory cytokines and growth factors can participate in the pathophysiological processes of sarcoidosis [1].

Sarcoidosis is fundamentally a chronic inflammatory disease. The pathological and clinical courses vary widely from spontaneous regression to fibrotic progression leading to various patterns of organ dysfunction [3].

Any of the following may be selected as therapeutic targets for sarcoidosis, depending on the pathophysiology and evolution of the disease: 1) delete the etiological agents, 2) attenuate the hyperimmune reactions directly underlying the epithelioid cell granuloma formation, 3) arrest any pathophysiological processes that tend to persist, 4) relieve functional disturbances caused by fibrotic lesions, 5) replace disabled organs by transplantation.

It is critical to grasp or predict the whole clinical course of sarcoidosis when considering therapies.

Corticosteroids, the established standard therapy for sarcoidosis, have drawbacks. While corticosteroids are reliably therapeutic, some patients manifest adverse effects during treatment or functional declines in spite of treatment [4]. Corticosteroids may also disturb the defensive function of granulomas surrounding etiological antigens or disturb healing processes by attenuating various inflammatory processes homogeneously.

In this article we review the widely variable clinical courses sarcoidosis is known to take. We also try to propose a therapeutic strategy for stably managing chronic sarcoidosis, especially for patients with involvement of vital organs such as the lung and heart.

2. Therapeutic problems and clinical courses

The clinical courses of sarcoidosis vary considerably. The disease spontaneously regresses in about 10-20 % of patients, persists in chronic form in another 30-50 %, relapses and recurs in another 20-30 %, and deteriorates in about 10 % [3].

The clinical phenotypes associated with the various clinical courses have been proposed based on a review of 400 sarcoidosis cases collected all over the world. The WASOG Task Force classified 9 phenotypes according to evaluations of clinical courses up to 5 years after detection (see Fig. 1) [5]. Among cases in Japan, sarcoidosis is presumed to reach the chronic stage when chest radiographic abnormalities persist for five years after detection [3]. According to the clinical phenotypes classified by WASOG, 17 % of cases spontaneously regress, 8 % deteriorate, 34 % manifest minimal remaining lesions with or without therapies, and 34 % progress to the chronic stage with or without treatment [5]. Among the patients who receive treatment, 40 % reportedly relapse after the corticosteroids are tapered or discontinued altogether [6]. The ACCESS study reported multiple lesion sites, lesion frequency by site, and various associations of clinical characteristics with the patient age, sex, number of lesions, and population differences [7]. Though the frequencies vary, functional deterioration has been reported in all affected organs. The clinical course of sarcoidosis is stable in 80 % of cases at 2 years after detection, though the prognosis tends to be worse in African Americans [8].

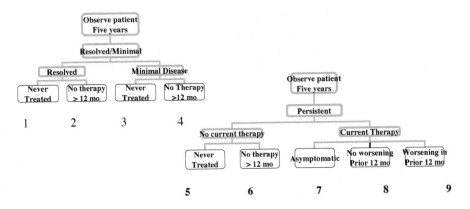

Figure 1. Clinical phenotypes of sarcoidosis patients proposed by WASOG 2005. Minimal disease is defined as less than 25 % of maximal lesions

3. Sarcoidosis therapy

Therapy is indicated for sarcoidosis patients with lesions of the heart, with pulmonary fibrosis in bronchovascular bundle areas, with neurosarcoidosis, and with systemic symptoms such as fever, malaise, and ocular lesions. The therapies administered tend to be prolonged in most patients with chronic lesions.

According to a meta-analysis by Reich, excessive corticosteroid therapy may unfavorably influence the long-term course of the disease in some individuals [9]. Among 948 sarcoidosis patients retrospectively reviewed by our group, 28 had advanced pulmonary sarcoidosis, 13 of those 28 advanced cases died, and 9 of those deceased cases had received corticosteroids [3]. Another retrospective study from Japan reported corticosteroid response in 70-80 % of 195 sarcoidosis patients, although the rate was lower, that is, only 48 %, in patients with cardiac sarcoidosis [4].

Methotrexate, one of the alternative drug treatments for sarcoidosis, is prescribed mainly for chronic sarcoidosis and can be expected to confer a steroid-sparing effect in addition to an immunomodulatory effect [10]. Methotrexate is reported to be therapeutically effective mainly in cases with skin lesions [11], ocular lesions [12], neuromuscular lesions [13],etc. In our clinical experience the agent is therapeutically effective, albeit incompletely, for sarcoidosis involving lesions of the lung, heart, and neuromuscular system. Long-term therapy is mandatory for chronic sarcoidosis, especially for the prevention of functional declines that can lead to congestive cardiac failure or sudden death in cases with cardiac lesions. Corticosteroid therapy may fail to prevent functional deteriorations longitudinally [12]. The Delphi study offered no precise guidance on how to treat sarcoidosis with corticosteroids or alternative agents [14,15].

In this chapter we try to introduce our own clinical experience with pulmonary and cardiac sarcoidosis.

3.1. Treatment for pulmonary sarcoidosis

Patients with sarcoidosis present with various types of pulmonary lesions, some of which spontaneously regress and some of which show fibrotic deterioration [16,17]. Fibrotic lesions situated along the bronchovascular bundle of the lung are likely to result in chronic airflow limitations [18] and bronchial distortions of a type often associated with infections such as nontuberculous mycobacterium, pseudomonas aeruginosa, and aspergillus fumigatus [16,19]. Some patients with pulmonary fibrosis also develop pulmonary hypertension [20]. Lung transplantation is considered when the disease progresses to a severe stage in patients under 60 years old [21,22].

Therapy itself might cause opportunistic infection under these circumstances. No medicines available at present are definitively effective at attenuating the fibrotic progression along the bronchovascular bundles. It usually takes 5-10 years before the fibrotic progression leads to chronic respiratory failure [3]. Longitudinal management and treatment must continue for long durations without adverse effects, as chronic respiratory failure persists for several years after it first manifests [3]. From this standpoint, methotrexate may be an available option for pulmonary sarcoidosis. Unlike methotrexate therapy for rheumatoid arthritis, methotrexate for sarcoidosis has seldom led to drug-related pneumonia in our clinical experience.

Presentation of two cases

Case 1: 59-year-old male, never-smoker, no occupational exposure

Patient 1 visited our institution, Central Clinic, with complaints of a severe cough and exertional dyspnea. His chest radiograph showed diffuse pulmonary lesions with fibrosis mainly distributed on the upper and middle lung fields (Figure 2). Transbronchial lung biopsy revealed epithelioid cell granuloma. Having found no obvious infection at the initial examination, we started the patient on prednisolone (10 mg /day) and methotrexate (6 mg/week). After therapy his symptoms gradually attenuated. The opacities decreased during treatment in radiological images, but not drastically on CT findings (Figure 3). Pulmonary function results showed improved diffusion capacity and the patient reported an abatement of his cough and exertional dyspnea. The airflow limitation, however, gradually worsened (Table 1).

	Initial exam.	3 years	5 years
%FVC (%)	55.6	58.2	55.0
FEV1 (l)	1.88 l	1.56 l	1.48 l
FEV1% (%)	89.9	79.6	76.2
%DLCO (%)	51.3	61.5	61.4
EF	67.6	53.9	57.4
Reg.	I	I	I
sPAP mmHg	32.9	31.8	42.4
ACE	14.1	14.3	15.3
1,25-(OH)2VD	75.3		

FVC: forced vital capacity, FEV1: forced expiratory vital capacity one second,

DLCO: diffusion lung capacity carbon monoxide

EF: ejection fraction, Reg. : regurgitation, sPAP : systolic pulmonary artery pressure

ACE: angiotensin converting enzyme, 1,25-(OH)2 VD: 1,25-OH)2 vitamine D

Table 1. Change in the functional or blood markers over time: 59 M Ns

No pulmonary hypertension appeared in a cardiac echogram. No blood markers suggestive of disease activity (serum ACE, 1,25-(OH)2 vitamin D) appeared in association with the treatment course (Table 1). The patient's symptoms almost wholly abated and his prednisolone and methotrexate were tapered to 3 mg/day and 2 mg/week, respectively. No adverse effects were found during treatment.

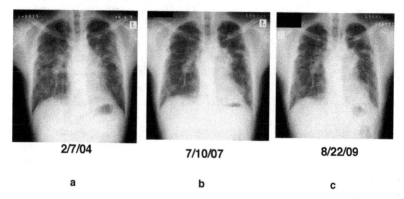

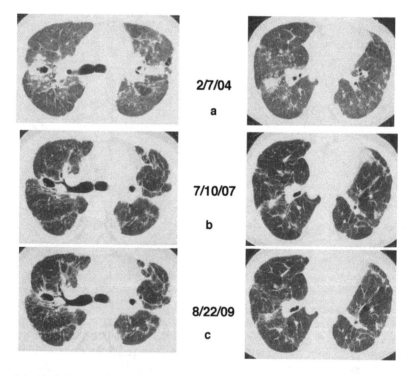

Figure 2. Longitudinal course of pulmonary fibrosis in patients with sarcoidosis: Plain chest radiograph 59-year-old male, nonsmoker, chief complaints of cough and exertional dyspnea a : when corticosteroids and methotrexate were introduced b: after 3 years of treatment c: after 5 years of treatment

Figure 3. Longitudinal course of pulmonary fibrosis in patients with sarcoidosis: High-resolution CT findings a : when corticosteroids and methotrexate were introduced b: after 3 years of treatment c: after 5 years of treatment

Case 2. 60-year-old male, ex-smoker, no occupational exposure

Ocular lesions and BHL were detected by a health survey 27 years earlier, in 1982. A transbronchial lung biopsy at the time revealed epithelioid cell granuloma, and few parenchymal lesions of the lung were evident on HRCT. After an initial examination at Kyoto University, the patient moved away from Kyoto for his work. In the intervening 27 years we had no opportunity to follow his condition. In 2008, the patient visited our clinic because of exertional dyspnea and a severe cough with sputum production. Bilateral fibrotic lung lesions had developed on his upper lungs (Figure 4). Having detected no obvious infection, we started the patient on prednisolone (5 mg/day) and methotrexate (6 mg/week). His symptoms improved considerably by the end of the third month after treatment and he remained stable thereafter. Pulmonary function results also demonstrated a mild increase in %DLCO 18 months after the treatment commenced (Table 2).

	27 yrs before	PSL+MTX	3 mos	12 mos	18 mos
%FVC (%)	68.2	61.3	66.1	70.4	69.1
FEV1 (l)	2.02	1.85	2.04	2.08	1.92
FEV1% (%)	86.3	86.0	ND	84.2	79.7
%DLCO (%)	ND	39.6	39.3	41.0	49.0
DOE	Grade 3	Grade 3	Grade 2	Grade 2	Grade 1
cough	severe	severe	moderate	mild	mild

FVC: forced vital capacity, FEV1: forced expiratory vital capacity one second,

DLCO: diffusion lung capacity carbon monoxide

DOE: dyspnea on exertion

Grade : Hugh Johns grade of exertional dyspnea

Table 2. Change in his symptoms and functions over time: 60, M, Ex, Eye, BHL, Lung 31 yrs,

While the therapeutic effects in these cases were by no means stellar, they did bring about symptomatic relief, relatively good functional stabilization, and improved radiographic findings. It remains unsolved whether antifibrotic drugs such as pirfenidone are effective for fibrotic lesions in patients with sarcoidosis.

3.2. Treatment for cardiac sarcoidosis

Cardiac lesions can be patchily distributed in the four chambers of the heart. The dysfunctions they cause range from arrhythmia to right bundle block, left bundle block, and complete atrioventricular block leading to cardiac failure or cardiac arrest [23].

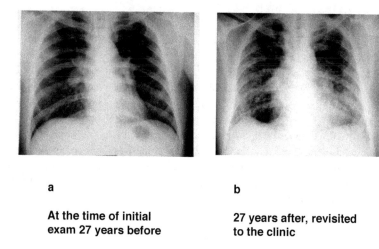

a   b

At the time of initial   **27 years after, revisited**
exam 27 years before   **to the clinic**

Figure 4. Longitudinal course of pulmonary fibrosis in patients with sarcoidosis: Plain chest radiograph 60-year-old male, ex-smoker, chief complaints of cough and exertional dyspnea Eye, BHL, and lung (30-year duration) a : at the initial exam in Kyoto University 27 years earlier b: at the revisit to the clinic 27 years later

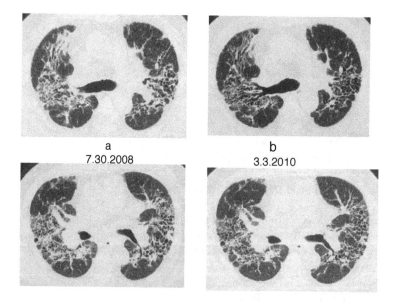

a   b
7.30.2008   3.3.2010

Figure 5. Longitudinal course of pulmonary fibrosis in patients with sarcoidosis: High-resolution CT findings 60-year-old male, ex-smoker, chief complaints of cough and exertional dyspnea Eye, BHL, and lung (30-year duration) a : when corticosteroids and methotrexate were introduced b: after 2 years of therapy

The Japanese Society of Sarcoidosis and Other Granulomatous Disorders published revised guidelines for the diagnosis of cardiac sarcoidosis [24]. These guidelines proposed criteria for definite diagnosis and clinical diagnosis: 1) Definite group, histological diagnosis by cardiac biopsy; 2) Clinical diagnosis group, negative biopsy with proven extracardiac sarcoidosis and satisfaction of 1 of 4 major criteria and 2 or more minor criteria. The major criteria were advanced AV block, basal thinning of the ventricular septum, positive cardiac gallium uptake, and left ventricular ejection fraction of less than 50 %. The minor criteria were abnormal ECG findings (ventricular tachycardia, multifocal frequent premature ventricular contractions, complete right bundle branch block pathologic Q waves, or abnormal axis deviation, UCG abnormality (regional wall motion abnormalities, ventricular aneurysm, or unexplained increase in wall thickness), perfusion defects detected by myocardial scintigraphy, delayed gadolinium enhancement of the myocardium on cardiac MRI scanning, and interstitial fibrosis or monocyte infiltration greater than moderate grade by endomyocardial biopsy. As the positive biopsy rate seems to be lower, the aforesaid guidelines are useful in a patients with proven noncardiac sarcoidosis and suspected cardiac involvement [23].

Regarding treatment, published data on several uncontrolled series of patients with cardiac sarcoidosis have suggested that steroids may be a valuable therapy for this condition. Yet no randomized control data are available to support this. In a retrospective series of 48 cases of cardiac sarcoidosis from Japan, high-dose steroid therapy seemed to be ineffective for patients with a pretreatment left ventricular ejection fraction of less than 30%, whereas improvement in ejection fraction and a decrease in left ventricular end-diastolic volume was seen in patients with a pretreatment ejection fraction of between 30% and 55% [4]. In a retrospective study from France, corticosteroid therapy improved abnormal echocardiographic parameters in 78% of cases and symptoms completely resolved in 9 of 17 patients presenting with congestive heart failure [25]. In a retrospective study of cardiac sarcoidosis in 30 Japanese patients who received 40 mg or more of prednisone daily and 45 patients who received less than 30 mg/d, there was no apparent survival benefit of high-dose prednisone over the lower dose [13].

No data are available to support the efficacy of additional immunosuppressive therapy for cardiac sarcoidosis with cyclophosphamide, methotrexate, or cyclosporine. Infliximab and etanercept, agents used against rheumatoid arthritis via their actions against tumor necrosis factor-α, have recently been proposed as treatments for some forms of chronic, refractory sarcoidosis [26].

3.3. Methotrexate for the treatment of cardiac sarcoidosis

This chapter presents the findings of a small open label comparative study by our group.

Long-term functional changes of ejection fraction on echocardiography were compared between patients who received combination therapy (low-dose prednisolone and methotrexate) and patients who received corticosteroids only.

As shown in table 3, there were no significant differences in sex distribution, duration of sarcoidosis, the number of lesions, or the frequency of pace maker implantation, though the age at the time of drug introduction tended to be higher in the patients treated with cortico-

	CS only	CS+MTX	p-value
No of the cases	7	13	
Age (years)	67±12.5*	56.5±13.7	0.07
M:W	2:05	5:08	0.66
duration (mos)	92.1±70.4	64.7±41.0	0.63
No of the extracardiac lesion	3.86±1.26	3.85±1.52	0.83
pace maker	6	11	0.95

CS:corticosteroid, MTX: methotrexate

M:man, W:woman, duration: from the detection to the introduction of the therapy,

* Figures express mean±standard deviation (SD)

p-value: less than 0.05 as statistically significant

Table 3. Clinical profiles in patients studied

steroids. There were no significant differences in the number of lesion sites, except for the number renal stones (higher in patients on corticosteroids). There were no significant differences in abnormal findings on electrocardiogram between the two groups (Table 4). Guided by these findings, we followed the ejection fraction (%) at one-year intervals after the introduction of the therapy. As shown in Table 5, ejection fraction stabilized in the combination therapy group 3 to 5 years after the first treatment.

	CS only	CS+MTX	p-value
Af	0	1	
PVC		1	0.463
CRBB	0	2	
LBBB	6	7	
CAVB			
basal thinning	7	9	0.101

Af:atrial fibrilation, PVC: premature ventricular contractions

CRBBB : complete right bundle branch block, LBBB: left bundle branchblock

CAVB: complete atrioventricular block

Basal thinning: basal thinning of the ventricular septum

p-value: less than 0.05 as statistically significant

Table 4. Comparison of the electrocardiographic abnormalities between the steroid treated and the combination therapy

EF %	CS only	CS+MTX	p-value
0*	56.1±13.1	58.4±15.3	0.812
12	48.0±16.7	55.5±15.3	0.383
36	41.2±9.8	58.6±11.6	0.007
60	41.0±13.1	56.2±12.3	0.069
96	48.7±9.2	55.0±25.2	

EF : ejection fraction (%) on echocardiography

CS: corticosteroid, MTX: methotrexate

* months from the intorduction of the treatment

Figures express mean±standard deviation (SD)

p-value: less than 0.05 as statistically significant

Table 5. Comparison of the ejection fraction on echocardiography between the steroid treated and the combination therapy

In the corticosteroid group, cardiac enlargement was found on plain chest radiographs at 3 to 5 years after the commencement of therapy in association with a decrease in ejection fraction (see, for example, **Figs. 6** and **7**). Meanwhile, combination therapy restored or stabilized the ejection fraction and cardiac enlargement on chest radiograph (see, for example, **Figs. 8** and **9**).

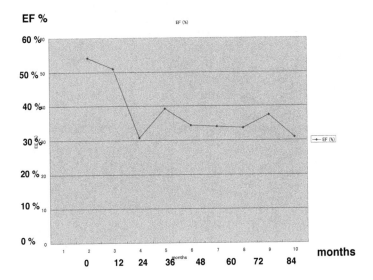

Figure 6. Longitudinal course of the ejection fraction on UCG 74-year-old female, nonsmoker, eye, renal stone, BHL, ACE 28.3, heart with complete AV block Ordinate: ejection fraction (%) on echocardiography Abscissa: months from the introduction of therapy

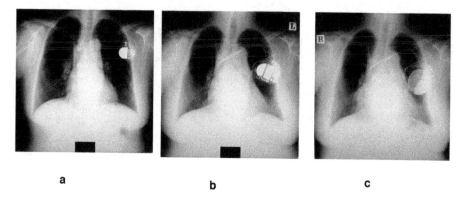

a   b   c

Figure 7. Longitudinal course of plain chest radiograph 74-year-old female, nonsmoker, eye, renal stone, BHL, ACE 28.3, heart with complete AV block a: when the corticosteroid therapy was introduced, b: after 5 years of treatment, c: after 7 years of treatment

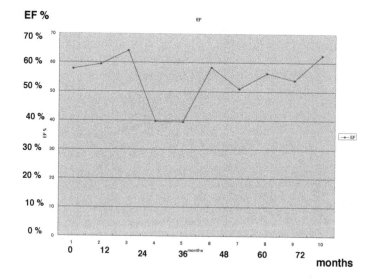

Figure 8. Longitudinal course of the ejection fraction on UCG 62-year-old female, nonsmoker, BHL, lung, ACE 29.0, heart with complete AV block Ordinate: ejection fraction (%) on echocardiography Abscissa: months from the introduction of therapy

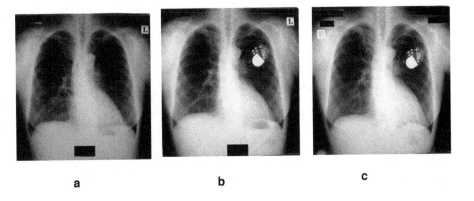

a   b   c

Figure 9. Longitudinal course of plain chest radiograph 62-year-old female, nonsmoker, BHL, lung, ACE 29.0, heart with complete AV block, a: when the introduction of corticosteroid and methotrexate therapy was introduced, b: after 2 years of treatment c: after 5 years of treatment

Eight patients received methotrexate in our clinic after treatment with corticosteroid therapy in another hospital. Some presented with decreased ejection fraction suggestive of congestive heart failure when they came to our clinic. Yet even for those patients, the add-on methotrexate improved the ejection fraction over a period years.

During long-term treatment with methotrexate and low-dose of prednisolone, there were no serious adverse effects such as bone marrow suppression, opportunistic infection, or drug-related pneumonia in our series.

At present we propose the following therapeutic strategy: in patients with cardiac sarcoidosis (especially those with pace makers because of complete AV block), a combination therapy of low-dose prednisolone and methotrexate as the initial treatment following long-term mainte-nance therapy will stabilize cardiac function with few adverse effects. A large-scale controlled prospective study to assess this approach will of course be warranted.

4. Conclusion

It is important to evaluate the whole clinical course in patients with sarcoidosis. Therapeutic decisions should be based on the clinical course, especially for chronic patients who need long-term treatment. As our studies on patients with cardiac lesions and patients with fibrotic pulmonary lesions demonstrate, weekly methotrexate therapy with or without small doses of corticosteroids may stabilize the deterioration without eliciting adverse effects during long-term treatment.

Nomenclature

WASOG: World Association of Sarcoidosis and Other Granulomatous Disorders

ACCESS: A Case Control Etiologic Study of Sarcoidosis

ACE: Angiotensin converting enzyme

1,25-(OH)2 vitamin D: 1,25-dihydroxy- vitamin D

HRCT: High Resolution Computed Tomography

DLCO: diffusion capacity for carbon monoxide

AV block: atrioventricular block

ECG: Electrocardiography

UCG: ultrasound cardiography

FVC: forced vital capacity, FEV1: forced expiratory volume one second,

EF: ejection fraction, Reg.: regurgitation, sPAP : systolic pulmonary artery pressure

DOE: dyspnea on exertion

Grade : Hugh Johns grade of exertional dyspnea

CS:corticosteroid, MTX: methotrexate

M:man, W:woman

Af:atrial fibrilation, PVC: premature ventricular contractions

CRBBB : complete right bundle branch block, LBBB: left bundle branchblock

CAVB: complete atrioventricular block

Acknowledgements

We thank all of our colleagues and staffs who support our clinical work longitudinally.

Author details

Sonoko Nagai and Takateru Izumi

Central Clinic, Clinical Research Center, Kyoto, Japan

References

[1] Hunninghake, G. W, Costabel, U, Ando, M, Baughman, R, & Cordier, J. F. du Bois R, Eklund A, Kitaichi M, Lynch J, Rizzato G, Rose C, Selroos O, Semenzato G, Sharma OP.ATS/ERS/WASOG statement on sarcoidosis. American Thoracic Society/European Respiratory Society/World Association of Sarcoidosis and other Granulomatous Disorders. Sarcoidosis Vasc Diffuse Lung Dis. (1999). , 16(2), 149-73.

[2] Ishige, I, Eishi, Y, Takemura, T, Kobayashi, I, Nakata, K, Tanaka, I, Nagaoka, S, Iwai, K, Watanabe, K, Takizawa, T, & Koike, M. Propionibacterium acnes is the most common bacterium commensal in peripheral lung tissue and mediastinal lymph nodes from subjects without sarcoidosis. Sarcoidosis Vasc Diffuse Lung Dis. (2005). , 22(1), 33-42.

[3] Nagai, S, Handa, T, Ito, Y, Ohta, K, Tamaya, M, & Izumi, T. Outcome of sarcoidosis. Clin Chest Med. (2008). , 29(3), 565-574.

[4] Sugisaki, K, Yamaguchi, T, Nagai, S, Ohmichi, M, Takenaka, S, Morimoto, S, Ishihara, M, Tachibana, T, & Tsuda, T. Clinical characteristics of 195 Japanese sarcoidosis patients with oral corticosteroids. Sar Vasculits Dissuse Lung Disease. (2003). , 20(3), 222-226.

[5] Baughman, R. P, Nagai, S, Balter, M, Costabel, U, & Drent, M. du Bois R, Grutters JC, Judson MA, Lambiri I, Lower EE, Muller-Quernheim J, Prasse A, Rizzato G, Rottoli P, Spagnolo P, Teirstein A. Defining the clinical outcome status (COS) in sarcoidosis: results of WASOG Task Force. Sarcoidosis Vasc Diffuse Lung Dis. (2011). , 28(1), 56-64.

[6] Gottlieb, J. E, Israel, H. L, Steiner, R. M, Triolo, J, & Patrick, H. Outcome in sarcoidosis. The relationship of relapse to corticosteroid therapy. Chest. (1997). , 111(3), 623-31.

[7] Baughman, R. P, Teirstein, A. S, Judson, M. A, & Rossman, M. D. Yeager H Jr, Bresnitz EA, DePalo L, Hunninghake G, Iannuzzi MC, Johns CJ, McLennan G, Moller DR, Newman LS, Rabin DL, Rose C, Rybicki B, Weinberger SE, Terrin ML, Knatterud GL, Cherniak R; Case Control Etiologic Study of Sarcoidosis (ACCESS) research group. Clinical characteristics of patients in a case control study of sarcoidosis. Am J Respir Crit Care Med. (2001). Pt 1):1885-9

[8] Judson, M. A, Baughman, R. P, Thompson, B. W, Teirstein, A. S, Terrin, M. L, & Rossman, M. D. Yeager H Jr, McLennan G, Bresnitz EA, DePalo L, Hunninghake G, Iannuzzi MC, Johns CJ, Moller DR, Newman LS, Rabin DL, Rose C, Rybicki BA, Weinberger SE, Knatterud GL, Cherniak R; ACCESS Research Group. Two year prognosis of sarcoidosis: the ACCESS experience. Sarcoidosis Vasc Diffuse Lung Dis. (2003). , 20(3), 204-11.

[9] Reich, J. M. Mortality of intrathoracic sarcoidosis in referral vs population-based settings: influence of stage, ethnicity, and corticosteroid therapy. Chest. (2002). , 121(1), 32-39.

[10] Baughman, R. P, & Lower, E. E. A clinical approach to the use of methotrexate for sarcoidosis. Thorax (1999). , 54, 742-746.

[11] Myers, T. D, Werthheim, M. S, Egan, R. A, Shults, W. T, & Rosenbaum, J. T. Use of corticosteroid spring systemic immunosuppression for treatement of corticosteroid dependent optic neuritis not associated with demyelinating disease. Br J Ophthalmol (2004). , 88, 673-680.

[12] Kaye, O, Palazzo, E, Grossin, M, Bourgeois, P, Kahn, M. F, & Malaise, M. G. Low dose methotrexate : an effective corticosteroid-sparing agent in the musculoskeletal manifestations of sarcoidosis. Br J Rheumatolo (1995). , 34, 642-644.

[13] Yazaki, Y, Isobe, M, Hiroe, M, Morimoto, S, Hiramitsu, S, Nakano, T, & Izumi, T. Sekiguchi M; Central Japan Heart Study Group. Prognostic determinants of long-term survival in Japanese patients with cardiac sarcoidosis treated with prednisone. Am J Cardiol. (2001). , 88(9), 1006-1010.

[14] Hamzeh, N. Y, Wamboldt, F. S, & Weinberger, H. D. Management of cardiac sarcoidosis in the United States: a delphi study. Chest. (2012). , 141(1), 154-62.

[15] Schutt, A. C, Bullington, W. M, & Judson, M. A. Pharmacotherapy for pulmonary sarcoidosis: a Delphi consensus study. Respir Med. (2010). , 104(5), 717-23.

[16] Akira, M, Kozuka, T, Inoue, Y, & Sakatani, M. Long-term follow-up CT scan evaluation in patients with pulmonary sarcoidosis. Chest. (2005). , 127(1), 185-91.

[17] Lynch, J. P. rd, Kazerooni EA, Gay SE. Pulmonary sarcoidosis. Clin Chest Med. (1997).

[18] Handa, T, Nagai, S, Fushimi, Y, Miki, S, Ohta, K, Niimi, A, Mishima, M, & Izumi, T. Clinical and radiographic indices associated with airflow limitation in patients with sarcoidosis. Chest (2006). , 130(6), 1851-6.

[19] Nardi, A, Brillet, P. Y, Letoumelin, P, Girard, F, Brauner, M, Uzunhan, Y, Naccache, J. M, Valeyre, D, & Nunes, H. Stage IV sarcoidosis: comparison of survival with the general population and causes of death. Eur Respir J. (2011). , 38(6), 1368-73.

[20] Handa, T, Nagai, S, Miki, S, Fushimi, Y, Ohta, K, Mishima, M, & Izumi, T. Incidence of pulmonary hypertension and its clinical relevance in patients with sarcoidosis. Chest. (2006). , 129(5), 1246-1252.

[21] The registry of the international society for heart and lung transplantation: 27 annual report 2010J Heart and Lung Transplantation (2010). , 29, 1083-1141.

[22] Shlobin, O. A, & Nathan, S. D. Management of end-stage sarcoidosis: pulmonary hypertension and lung transplantation. Eur Respir J. (2012). Epub ahead of print]

[23] Dubrey, S. W, & Falk, R. H. Diagnosis and management of cardiac sarcoidosis. Prog in Cardiovascular Dis. (2010). , 52, 336-346.

[24] Soejima, K. Yada H: The work-up and management of patients with apparent or sub-clinical cardiac sarcoidosis: with emphasis on the associated heart rhythm abnormalities. J Cardiovasc Electrophysiol (2009). , 20, 578-583.

[25] Chapelon-abric, C, De Zuttere, D, Duhaut, P, Veyssier, P, Wechsler, B, Huong, D. L, De Gennes, C, Papo, T, Blétry, O, Godeau, P, & Piette, J. C. Cardiac sarcoidosis : a retrospective study of 41 cases. Medicine (2004). , 83, 315-334.

[26] Baughman, R P, Drent, M, Kavuru, x, Judson, M, Costabel, M. A, Du, U, Bois, R. M, Albera, C, Brutsche, M, Davis, G, Donohue, J. F, Müller-quernheim, J, Schlenker-herceg, R, Flavin, S, Hung, K, & Oemar, L. B. Barnathan ES and on behalf of the Sarcoidosis Investigators Infliximab Therapy in Patients with Chronic Sarcoidosis and Pulmonary Involvement Am J Respir Crit care Med (2006). , 795-802.

Permissions

The contributors of this book come from diverse backgrounds, making this book a truly international effort. This book will bring forth new frontiers with its revolutionizing research information and detailed analysis of the nascent developments around the world.

We would like to thank Prof. Yoshinobu Eishi, for lending his expertise to make the book truly unique. He has played a crucial role in the development of this book. Without his invaluable contribution this book wouldn't have been possible. He has made vital efforts to compile up to date information on the varied aspects of this subject to make this book a valuable addition to the collection of many professionals and students.

This book was conceptualized with the vision of imparting up-to-date information and advanced data in this field. To ensure the same, a matchless editorial board was set up. Every individual on the board went through rigorous rounds of assessment to prove their worth. After which they invested a large part of their time researching and compiling the most relevant data for our readers. Conferences and sessions were held from time to time between the editorial board and the contributing authors to present the data in the most comprehensible form. The editorial team has worked tirelessly to provide valuable and valid information to help people across the globe.

Every chapter published in this book has been scrutinized by our experts. Their significance has been extensively debated. The topics covered herein carry significant findings which will fuel the growth of the discipline. They may even be implemented as practical applications or may be referred to as a beginning point for another development. Chapters in this book were first published by InTech; hereby published with permission under the Creative Commons Attribution License or equivalent.

The editorial board has been involved in producing this book since its inception. They have spent rigorous hours researching and exploring the diverse topics which have resulted in the successful publishing of this book. They have passed on their knowledge of decades through this book. To expedite this challenging task, the publisher supported the team at every step. A small team of assistant editors was also appointed to further simplify the editing procedure and attain best results for the readers.

Our editorial team has been hand-picked from every corner of the world. Their multi-ethnicity adds dynamic inputs to the discussions which result in innovative outcomes. These outcomes are then further discussed with the researchers and contributors who give their valuable feedback and opinion regarding the same. The feedback is then collaborated with the researches and they are edited in a comprehensive manner to aid the understanding of the subject.

Apart from the editorial board, the designing team has also invested a significant amount of their time in understanding the subject and creating the most relevant covers. They scrutinized every image to scout for the most suitable representation of the subject and create an appropriate cover for the book.

The publishing team has been involved in this book since its early stages. They were actively engaged in every process, be it collecting the data, connecting with the contributors or procuring relevant information. The team has been an ardent support to the editorial, designing and production team. Their endless efforts to recruit the best for this project, has resulted in the accomplishment of this book. They are a veteran in the field of academics and their pool of knowledge is as vast as their experience in printing. Their expertise and guidance has proved useful at every step. Their uncompromising quality standards have made this book an exceptional effort. Their encouragement from time to time has been an inspiration for everyone.

The publisher and the editorial board hope that this book will prove to be a valuable piece of knowledge for researchers, students, practitioners and scholars across the globe.

List of Contributors

Yoshinobu Eishi
Department of Human Pathology, Division of Surgical Pathology, Tokyo Medical and Dental University, Japan

Mitsuteru Akahoshi
Department of Medicine and Biosystemic Science, Kyushu University Graduate School of Medical Sciences, Fukuoka, Japan

Nabeel Y. Hamzeh and Lisa A. Maier
Division of Environmental and Occupational Health Sciences, National Jewish Health, Denver, CO, USA
Division of Pulmonary and Critical Care Sciences, Department of Medicine, School of Medicine, University of Colorado, Aurora, CO, USA

Birendra P. Sah and Michael C. Iannuzzi
SUNY, Upstate Medical University, Syracuse, New York, USA

Adam S. Morgenthau
The Mount Sinai School of Medicine, Department of Medicine, Division of Pulmonary, Critical Care and Sleep Medicine, New York, NY, USA

Luis Jara-Palomares, Candela Caballero-Eraso, Cesar Gutiérrez, Alvaro Donate and Jose Antonio Rodríguez-Portal
Pneumologist, Medical-Surgical Unit of Respiratory Diseases. University Hospital Virgen del Rocio, Seville, Spain

Kentaro Watanabe
Department of Respiratory Medicine, Fukuoka University School of Medicine, Fukuoka, Japan

Mohankumar Kurukumbi and Jayam-Trouth Annapurni
Department of Neurology, Howard University Hospital, Washington, DC, USA

Preema Mehta and Isha Misra
Howard University College of Medicine, Washington, DC, USA

Abiramy Jeyabalan and Andrew RL Medford
North Bristol Lung Centre, Southmead Hospital, Westbury-on-Trym, Bristol, UK

Paul S. Thomas
Inflammation and Infection Research Centre (IIRC), Faculty of Medicine, University of New South Wales, Sydney, NSW, Australia
Department of Respiratory Medicine, Prince of Wales Hospital, Randwick, NSW, Australia
Multidisciplinary Sarcoidosis Clinic, Prince of Wales Hospital, Randwick, NSW, Australia

Denis Wakefield
Inflammation and Infection Research Centre (IIRC), Faculty of Medicine, University of New South Wales, Sydney, NSW, Australia
Multidisciplinary Sarcoidosis Clinic, Prince of Wales Hospital, Randwick, NSW, Australia
Immunology of the Eye Clinic, St. Vincent's Clinic, Darlinghurst, NSW, Australia

Hasib Ahmadzai
Inflammation and Infection Research Centre (IIRC), Faculty of Medicine, University of New South Wales, Sydney, NSW, Australia
Department of Respiratory Medicine, Prince of Wales Hospital, Randwick, NSW, Australia

Atsushi Kitamura
Department of Medical Oncology, Graduate School of Medicine, Chiba University, Japan
Department of Respiratory Medicine, St. Luke's International Hospital, Japan

Yuichi Takiguchi
Department of Medical Oncology, Graduate School of Medicine, Chiba University, Japan

Sonoko Nagai and Takateru Izumi
Central Clinic, Clinical Research Center, Kyoto, Japan

Printed in the USA
CPSIA information can be obtained
at www.ICGtesting.com
JSHW011458221024
72173JS00005B/1128